Mike Reiners
Feb. 15, 2011

The Practice of Electroconvulsive Therapy

Recommendations for Treatment, Training, and Privileging

Second Edition

A TASK FORCE REPORT OF THE
AMERICAN PSYCHIATRIC ASSOCIATION

American Psychiatric Association
Committee on Electroconvulsive Therapy

Richard D. Weiner, M.D., Ph.D. (*Chairperson*)
C. Edward Coffey, M.D.
Laura J. Fochtmann, M.D.
Robert M. Greenberg, M.D.
Keith E. Isenberg, M.D.
Charles H. Kellner, M.D.
Harold A. Sackeim, Ph.D.
Louis Moench, M.D. (*Assembly Liaison*)

APA Staff

Harold Alan Pincus, M.D.
Laurie E. McQueen, M.S.S.W.

The Practice of Electroconvulsive Therapy

Recommendations for Treatment, Training, and Privileging

Second Edition

A Task Force Report of the
American Psychiatric Association

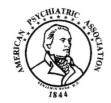

Published by the American Psychiatric Association
Washington, DC

Copyright © 2001 American Psychiatric Association
03 02 01 00   4 3 2 1
Second Edition

ALL RIGHTS RESERVED
Manufactured in the United States of America on acid-free paper

American Psychiatric Association
1400 K Street, N.W.
Washington, DC 20005
www.psych.org

Library of Congress Cataloging-in-Publication Data
[American Psychiatric Association. Committee on Electroconvulsive Therapy.
  The practice of electroconvulsive therapy : recommendations for treatment, training, and privileging : a task force report of the American Psychiatric Association / [American Psychiatric Association, Committee on Electroconvulsive Therapy, Richard D. Weiner, chairperson ... et al.].-- 2nd ed.
    p. ; cm.
  Includes bibliographical references and index.
  ISBN 0-89042-206-0 (alk. paper)
    1. Electroconvulsive therapy. I. Weiner, Richard D., 1945- II. Title.
    [DNLM: 1. Electroconvulsive Therapy--standards. WM 412 A512p 2000]
RC485 .A43 2000
616.89'122--dc21

00-032794

British Library Cataloguing in Publication Data
A CIP record is available from the British Library.

Contents

Contributors

C. Edward Coffey, M.D.
Dr. Coffey, a neuropsychiatrist, is Vice President of Behavioral Health, Chairman and Kathleen and Earl Ward Chair of Psychiatry, Henry Ford Health System, Detroit, Michigan; Professor of Psychiatry and of Neurology, Case Western Reserve University, Cleveland, Ohio; Clinical Professor of Psychiatry, Wayne State University, Detroit, Michigan; immediate President, Association for Convulsive Therapy; and current President, American Neuropsychiatric Association (1999–2000). He has authored over 150 scientific publications and chapters and has published several texts on ECT, neuropsychiatry, and related topics.

Laura J. Fochtmann, M.D.
Dr. Fochtmann, a psychiatrist, is Associate Professor of Psychiatry and Behavioral Sciences and Director of the ECT Service, State University of New York at Stony Brook, and a consultant for the Neurological Devices Advisory Panel of the Center for Devices and Radiological Health, U.S. Food and Drug Administration. She has published extensively on the neurobiology of ECT. Dr. Fochtmann has previously served as a consultant and has received research funding from Eli Lilly and Company.

Robert M. Greenberg, M.D.
Dr. Greenberg, a psychiatrist, is Director of Geropsychiatry and ECT Services, Bon Secours Health System of New Jersey, and President, Association for Convulsive Therapy (1998–2000). He has published on factors affecting the efficacy of ECT.

Keith E. Isenberg, M.D.
Dr. Isenberg, a psychiatrist, is Associate Professor of Psychiatry and Vice Chair for Clinical Affairs, Department of Psychiatry, Washington University; Director of ECT, Barnes-Jewish Hospital; and Medical Director, Behavioral Health Partners, a managed-care company that is a joint venture between Washington University and BJC Health Systems, St. Louis, Missouri. He has published on the use of ECT to prevent relapse and recurrence of illness and has also served as a consultant to Pfizer, Inc.

Charles H. Kellner, M.D.
Dr. Kellner, a psychiatrist and neurologist, is Professor of Psychiatry and Neurology and Director of the ECT Service, Medical University of South Carolina, Charleston, South Carolina. He has also been Editor-in-Chief since 1994 of the *Journal of ECT*. Dr. Kellner has published extensively on various topics dealing with the clinical use of ECT, and from 1993 to 1998 he organized an annual 2-day training course on ECT for practitioners that was sponsored in part by small educational grants from Somatics Inc. and MECTA Inc.

Louis A. Moench, M.D.
Dr. Moench, a psychiatrist, is Clinical Professor of Psychiatry, University of Utah School of Medicine, and a private practitioner of general and forensic psychiatry, Salt Lake Clinic, Salt Lake City, Utah. He is liaison to the Task Force on ECT from the American Psychiatric Association Assembly, where he also serves on the Assembly Executive Committee, the Steering Committee on Practice Guidelines, the Committee on Psychiatric Diagnosis and Assessment, and the Practice Research Network Steering Committee.

Harold A. Sackeim, Ph.D.
Dr. Sackeim, a neuropsychologist, is Chief, Department of Biological Psychiatry, New York State Psychiatric Institute, and Professor, Departments of Psychiatry and Radiology, College of Physicians and Surgeons, Columbia University, New York, New York. He has directed the ECT research program at Columbia University since 1979 and has published over 200 articles on this topic. He has received numerous national and international awards for his work on ECT, including a MERIT award from the National Institute of Mental Health, has served as a consultant to MECTA, Somatics, Pfizer, and Wyeth-Ayerst Corporations and Forest Laboratories. He has received research grant funding from Cyberonics Inc. and Magstim Company.

Richard D. Weiner, M.D., Ph.D.
Dr. Weiner, a psychiatrist and clinical neurophysiologist, is Professor of Psychiatry and Behavioral Sciences and Director, Duke ECT Program, Duke University Medical Center, and Chief, Mental Health Service Line, Durham Department of Veterans Affairs Medical Center, Durham, North Carolina. He has published over 140 clinical and scientific articles related to ECT. Dr. Weiner is also a coinventor on a patent licensed to MECTA Inc. and has provided consultation to MECTA Inc. and Somatics Inc.; he has received neither royalties nor personal payments for these activities.

CHAPTER 1

Introduction

The American Psychiatric Association (APA) first presented recommendations on the practice of electroconvulsive therapy (ECT) in 1978 with the publication of the landmark report *Electroconvulsive Therapy*, which offered a comprehensive overview of ECT (American Psychiatric Association Task Force on ECT 1978). Following a consensus conference on ECT sponsored by the National Institutes of Health (NIH) and the National Institute of Mental Health (NIMH) in 1985, the APA determined that development of new, up-to-date practice recommendations for ECT would be beneficial, as would recommendations regarding both education/training and the clinical privileging of ECT staff (Consensus Conference 1985). Accordingly, in the late 1980s, a new APA Task Force on ECT was given the mandate to develop these recommendations with partial financial support from the NIMH.

In 1990, the APA published the first edition of *The Practice of Electroconvulsive Therapy: Recommendations for Treatment, Training, and Privileging*, a comprehensive set of recommendations for the practice of ECT (American Psychiatric Association 1990). This work was well received and influenced clinical practice in a number of meaningful ways, including the encouragement of guideline development by other groups within the United States (Fink et al. 1996) and elsewhere (Gangadhar 1992; Royal Australian and New Zealand College of Psychiatrists 1992; Royal College of Psychiatrists 1995). In the ensuing decade, the field of ECT continued to advance, with a substantial amount of new scientific and clinical information forthcoming. Each year, hundreds of relevant publications have appeared as interest in this treatment modality continues to expand.

Because of this growing knowledge base, APA gave the Task Force on ECT (redesignated in mid-1999 as the Committee on ECT) a mandate to update the 1990 report. The revision process has been extensive. A review of the available clinical literature included a search of all clinical citations related to ECT published between 1989 and 1998 that had been entered into the MEDLINE database by December 1998. Supplementing this literature review were suggestions received at a Task Force workshop at the 1996 APA Annual Meeting and subsequent presentations at annual meetings of the Association for Convulsive Therapy (ACT) as well as informal input from experts in the field and other interested parties. These efforts were also made known to the APA membership on an ongoing basis through published summaries of component activities and notification of the APA Assembly.

To ensure that these recommendations would be clinically useful as well as scientifically, ethically, and legally sound, input was sought from a large number of professional organizations (covering the fields of psychiatry, neurology, anesthesiology, nursing, nurse anesthesia, and psychology), individual experts in related areas (including child, adult, and geriatric psychiatry, neurology, neuropsychiatry, psychology, anesthesiology, cardiology, obstetrics, medical ethics, and law), regulatory bodies (Joint Commission on Accreditation of Healthcare Organizations and the U.S. Food and Drug Administration [FDA]), and major lay mental health organizations (see Appendix A). As the initial draft of the revised document neared completion, an article was published in the APA newspaper *Psychiatric News* soliciting input from additional members with an interest in reviewing the draft. This request ensured that rank and file practitioners would also have the opportunity to participate. Finally, the APA's own internal review process ensured that drafts were examined from a wide variety of perspectives. Input from these diverse sources was taken into consideration in writing the final document.

This revised volume offers a set of recommendations to assist practitioners and facilities in the safe and effective use of ECT. We have once again made the scope of these recommendations as comprehensive as possible, including coverage of the important issues of education, training, and privileging. In each section, recommendations are preceded by applicable background information, including pertinent literature citations (with a particular focus on recent work). This format differs from that of the original 1990 report, in which background information was placed in a separate Rationale section that followed an overall Recommendations section. The goal of this change in format was an improved integration of the recommendations with their justification. As before, the bibliography and appendices provide additional source material of use to practitioners. Consistent with the literature review noted above, the bibliography in this revised report has been greatly expanded to four times the original number of citations, with particular representation of those published within the past decade. In addition to citations focused on specific topics, a number of general texts on ECT geared toward practitioners are available (Abrams 1997a; Beyer et al. 1998; Coffey 1993; Endler and Persad 1988; Goodwin 1994; Kellner 1991; Kellner et al. 1997). Other books are oriented to the layperson (Endler 1990; Fink 1999; Manning 1994). Finally, one journal, *The Journal of ECT*, is dedicated to articles on ECT.

Since the development of pharmacoconvulsive therapy in 1934 (Fink 1984) and of ECT itself in 1938 (Endler 1988), the practice of ECT has evolved into a complex procedure about which much has been learned, but many questions remain. To provide a comprehensive set of recommendations, it was necessary to include material based on empirical findings as well as clinical consensus for those situations in which well-controlled clinical trials are either unavailable or not applicable. It was also apparent that, in some cases, courses of action existed that were reasonable alternatives to those presented in these recommendations. Where applicable, attempts have been made to describe a number of such alternatives. For such reasons, these recommendations should be viewed as suggestions rather than requirements.

In writing recommendations for a complex procedure such as ECT, it is impossible to cover all situations or deal with all possible exceptions. Accordingly, there will be times when overriding factors lead a reasonable and prudent practitioner to alter practice from that recommended here. In addition, new, clinically relevant information is continually appearing and should be readily incorporated into clinical practice whenever it is shown to either maximize efficacy or minimize adverse effects.

To aid the practitioner in weighing the importance of individual recommendations, we have distinguished between recommendations that we believe are critical to the delivery of safe and effective treatment and those we believe advisable but not essential. The categorical term "should" is used to designate crucial recommendations, whereas other recommendations are described in more permissive terms such as "encouraged," "suggested," "recommended," or "considered."

As a final caveat, the practitioner should be aware that legal regulations exist regarding ECT, particularly concerning informed consent procedures (see Chapter 8). Because applicable regulations vary considerably among jurisdictions and over time, the recommendations contained here may not always be compatible with all requirements of present or future statutes. Accordingly, practitioners should seek out information on relevant regulations before beginning practice of ECT and should be aware of substantive statutory changes as they unfold.

We encourage practitioners and trainees in psychiatry as well as those in related disciplines to read this document and to integrate its recommendations into their clinical practice. This report is designed to offer a comprehensive yet practical overview of the safe and effective use of ECT, with recommendations that should be applicable across a wide spectrum of clinical settings.

CHAPTER 2

Indications for Use of Electroconvulsive Therapy

2.1. General Issues

The clinical literature establishing the efficacy of ECT in specific disorders is among the most substantial for any medical treatment (Abrams 1997a; Krueger and Sackeim 1995; Mukherjee et al. 1994; Sackeim et al. 1995; Weiner and Coffey 1988). As in other medical treatments, various sources of evidence support the efficacy of ECT in specific conditions. The indications for ECT have been defined by randomized, controlled trials comparing ECT with sham interventions or treatment alternatives and similar trials comparing modifications of ECT technique. The indications for ECT have also been supported by reports of uncontrolled clinical series, case studies, and surveys of expert opinion.

The decision to recommend the use of ECT derives from a risk/benefit analysis for the specific patient. This analysis considers the diagnosis of the patient and the severity of the presenting illness, the patient's treatment history, the anticipated speed of action and efficacy of ECT, the medical risks and anticipated adverse effects, and the likely speed of action, efficacy, and safety of alternative treatments.

2.2. Primary and Secondary Use of ECT

2.2.1. Primary Use of ECT

There is considerable variability among practitioners and geographic regions in the extent to which ECT is used as a first-line or primary treatment or is considered only secondarily after patients have not responded to other interventions. As a major treatment in psychiatry with well-defined indications, ECT should not be reserved for use only as a "last resort." Such practice may deprive patients of an effective treatment, may delay response and prolong suffering, and may possibly contribute to treatment resistance. In major depression, the chronicity of the index episode is one of the few consistent predictors of clinical outcome with ECT or pharmacotherapy (Black et al. 1989c, 1993; Dunn and Quinlan 1978; Hamilton and White 1960; Hobson 1953; Kindler et al. 1991; Kukopulos et al. 1977; Magni et al. 1988; Prudic et al. 1996). Patients with a longer duration of current illness have a reduced probability of responding to antidepressant treatments. The possibility has been raised that exposure to longer episode durations or ineffective treatment actively contributes to treatment resistance (Fava and Davidson 1996; Flint and Rifat 1996).

The likely speed and efficacy of ECT are factors that influence its use as a primary intervention. Particularly in major depression and acute mania, substantial clinical improvement often occurs soon after the start of ECT. It is common for patients to manifest appreciable improvement after a few treatments (Nobler et al. 1997; Segman et al. 1995). In addition, the time to achieve maximal response is often more rapid than that with psychotropic medications (Quitkin et al. 1996; Sackeim et al. 1995). Besides speed of action, the likelihood of obtaining significant clinical improvement is often more certain with ECT than with other treatment alternatives. Therefore, primary use of ECT should be considered when a rapid or a higher probability of response is needed, such as when patients are severely medically ill or at risk to harm themselves or others.

Additional considerations for the first-line use of ECT relate to the patient's medical status, treatment history, and treatment preference. Depending on the patient's medical status, ECT may be safer than alternative treatments (Sackeim 1993, 1998; Weiner et al. 2000). This circumstance most commonly arises among the physically debilitated, the elderly, and during pregnancy (see Sections 4.2 and 4.3). Positive response to ECT in the past, particularly in the context of medication resistance or intolerance, also should lead to early consideration of ECT. At times, patients will prefer ECT over alternative treatments, but commonly the opposite will be the case. Patient preferences should be discussed and considered before making treatment recommendations.

Some practitioners also base a decision for primary use of ECT on other factors, including the nature and severity of symptoms. Severe major depression with psychotic features, mania with psychotic features, and catatonia are conditions for which there is a clear consensus favoring early reliance on ECT (American Psychiatric Association 1993, 1994a; Weiner and Coffey 1988).

2.2.2. Secondary Use of ECT

ECT is most often used in patients who have not responded to other treatments. During the course of pharmacotherapy, reasons to consider using ECT include lack of clinical response, intolerance of side effects, deterioration in psychiatric condition, appearance of suicidality, or inanition.

The definition of psychotropic medication resistance and its implications with respect to a referral for ECT have been the subject of considerable discussion (Kroessler 1985; Keller et al. 1986; Prudic et al. 1990, 1996; Quitkin et al. 1984; Sackeim et al. 1990a, 1990b; Thase and Rush 1995). At present, there are no accepted standards by which to define medication resistance. In practice, when assessing the adequacy of pharmacologic treatment, psychiatrists rely on factors such as the type and dosage of medication used, blood levels, duration of treatment, compliance with the medication regimen, adverse effects, degree of therapeutic response, and type and severity of clinical symptoms (Prudic et al. 1996). For example, patients with psychotic depression should not be viewed as pharmacologic nonresponders unless a trial of an antipsychotic medication has been attempted in combination with an antidepressant (Chan et al. 1987; Nelson et al. 1986; Spiker et al. 1985). Regardless of diagnosis, patients who have not responded to psychotherapy alone should not be considered treatment resistant in the context of referral for ECT.

In general, a diagnosis of major depression with failure to respond to one or more antidepressant medication trials does not preclude a favorable response to ECT (Avery and Lubrano 1979; Magni et al. 1988; Paul et al. 1981; Prudic et al. 1996). Indeed, compared with other treatment alternatives, the probability of response to ECT may be favorable among patients with medication-resistant depression. On the other hand, medication resistance may also predict a poorer clinical outcome of ECT. Patients who have not responded to one or more adequate antidepressant medication trials have a lower probability of responding to ECT compared with patients treated with ECT without having received an adequate medication trial during the index episode (Prudic et al. 1990, 1996; Shapira et al. 1996). In addition, patients with medication resistance may require particularly intensive ECT treatment to achieve symptomatic improvement. Consequently, most patients who fail to benefit from ECT are also likely to be patients who have not responded to adequate pharmacotherapy. The relationship between medication resistance and poorer ECT outcome may be stronger with tricyclic antidepressants (TCAs) than with selective serotonin reuptake inhibitors (SSRIs) (Prudic et al. 1996). Little information is available about the predictive significance of resistance to other pharmacologic agents (e.g., mirtazepine, nefazodone, venlafaxine).

2.3. Principal Diagnostic Indications

2.3.1. Major Depression

2.3.1.1. Efficacy

The efficacy of ECT in depressive disorders is documented by an impressive body of research, including the open trials of the 1940s (Kalinowsky and Hoch 1946, 1961; Sargant and Slater 1954), the comparative ECT/pharmacotherapy trials of the 1960s (Greenblatt et al. 1964; Medical Research Council 1965), the comparisons of ECT and sham ECT in both the 1950s and the more recent British studies (Brandon et al. 1984; Freeman et al. 1978; Gregory et al. 1985; Johnstone et al. 1980; Lambourn and Gill 1978; Sackeim 1989 [review]; West 1981), and the recent studies contrasting variations in ECT technique (Letemendia et al. 1993; Sackeim et al. 1987a, 1993, 2000; Scott et al. 1992; Weiner et al. 1986a, 1986b).

Although ECT was first introduced as a treatment for schizophrenia, it was quickly found to be especially effective in patients with mood disorders, including both depressive and manic states. In the 1940s and 1950s, ECT was a mainstay of mood disorder treatment, with response rates between 80% and 90% commonly reported (Kalinowsky and Hoch 1946; Sargant and Slater 1954). The results of these early, largely impressionistic studies have been summarized by Abrams (1997a), the American Psychiatric Association Task Force on ECT (1978), Fink (1979), Kiloh et al. (1988), and Mukherjee et al. (1994).

Post (1972) suggested that, prior to the introduction of ECT, elderly patients with depression often manifested a chronic course or died of intercurrent medical illnesses in psychiatric institutions. Several studies have contrasted the clinical outcome of depressed patients who received inadequate or no biologic treatment with that of patients who received ECT. Although none of this work used prospective, random assignment designs, most studies indicated that ECT resulted in decreased chronicity and morbidity and decreased rates of mortality (Avery and Winokur 1976; Babigian and Guttmacher 1984; Black et al. 1989b; Philibert et al. 1995; Wesner and Winokur 1989). In much of this work, the advantages of ECT were particularly pronouced in elderly patients. For example, in a recent retrospective comparison of elderly depressed patients treated with ECT or pharmacotherapy, Philibert et al. (1995) found higher rates of mortality and significant depressive symptoms in the pharmacotherapy group at long-term follow-up.

With the introduction of the TCAs and monoamine oxidase inhibitors (MAOIs), random assignment trials were conducted in patients with depression in which ECT was used as the "gold standard" for measuring efficacy of these medications. Three such studies involved random assignment and blind ratings, and each found a significant therapeutic advantage for ECT over TCAs and placebo (Gangadhar et al. 1982; Greenblatt et al. 1964; Medical Research Council 1965). Other studies also reported ECT to be equal to or more effective than TCAs (Bruce et al. 1960; Davidson et al. 1978; Fahy et al. 1963; Hutchinson and Smedberg 1963; Kristiansen 1961; McDonald et al. 1966; Norris and Clancy 1961; Robin and Harris 1962; Stanley and Fleming 1962; Wilson et al. 1963) or MAOIs (Davidson et al. 1978; Hutchinson and Smedberg 1963; Kiloh et al. 1960; King 1959; Stanley and Fleming 1962). In a meta-analysis of this work, Janicak et al. (1985) reported an average response rate to ECT that was 20% higher than that of TCAs and 45% higher than that of MAOIs.

It should be noted that standards for adequate pharmacologic treatment have changed over the decades (Quitkin 1985; Sackeim et al. 1990a) and that, by current criteria, few of these early comparative trials used aggressive pharmacotherapy in terms of dosage or duration (Rifkin 1988). In addition, these studies usually focused on depressed patients who were receiving their first biologic treatment during the index episode. More recently, in a small study, Dinan and Barry (1989) randomized patients who did not respond to monotherapy with a TCA to treatment with either ECT or a combination of a TCA and lithium carbonate. The groups had equivalent efficacy, but the pharmacotherapy group may have had an advantage in terms of speed and response.

Only one study has compared the efficacy of ECT with that of an SSRI. Folkerts et al. (1997) found ECT to be markedly superior in short-term benefit compared with paroxetine in patients with medication-resistant depression. No studies have compared the efficacy of ECT with that of other, newer antidepressant medications such as bupropion, mirtazepine, nefazodone, or venlafaxine. However, no trial has ever found an antidepressant medication regimen to be more effective than ECT. Among patients who are receiving ECT as a first-line treatment or who have received inadequate pharmacotherapy during the index episode because of medication intolerance, response rates continue to be reported in the range of 80%–90% (Prudic et al. 1990, 1996). Among patients who have not responded to one or more adequate antidepressant trials the response rate remains substantial, falling in the range of 50%–60% (Prudic et al. 1996; Sackeim et al. 1990b, 2000).

The time to achieve full symptomatic improvement with antidepressant medications is typically estimated as 4–6 weeks (Quitkin et al. 1984, 1996). This delay until response may be longer in older patients (Salzman et al. 1995). In contrast, the average ECT course for major depression consists of eight or nine treatments (Prudic et al. 1996; Sackeim et al. 1993). Thus, when ECT is administered at a schedule of three treatments per week, full symptomatic improvement usually occurs more rapidly than with pharmacologic treatment (Nobler et al. 1997; Sackeim et al. 1995).

ECT is a highly structured treatment involving a complex, repeatedly administered procedure accompanied by high expectations of therapeutic success. Such conditions may augment placebo effects. Given this concern, a set of double-blind, random assignment trials were conducted in England during the late 1970s and 1980s that contrasted "real" ECT with "sham" ECT—the repeated administration of anesthesia alone. With one exception (Lambourn and Gill 1978), real ECT was found to be consistently more efficacious than sham treatment (Brandon et al. 1984; Freeman et al. 1978; Gregory et al. 1985; Johnstone et al. 1980; Sackeim 1989 [review]; West 1981). In the single exception, Lambourn and Gill (1978) used a form of real ECT involving low stimulus intensity and right unilateral electrode placement that is now known to be ineffective (Sackeim et al. 1987a, 1993). Overall, the real-versus-sham ECT studies demonstrated that passage of an effective electrical stimulus capable of eliciting a generalized seizure is necessary for the antidepressant effects of ECT. After the randomized acute treatment period, patients who participated in these studies were free to receive other forms of acute or continuation treatment, including ECT. Consequently, information about the duration of symptomatic improvement with real versus sham treatment could not be obtained in this research.

Finally, several studies in the treatment of major depression have contrasted variations in ECT technique by manipulating factors such as stimulus waveform, electrode placement, and stimulus dosage. An important practical observation that emerged was that the efficacy of ECT is equivalent regardless of whether sine wave or brief pulse stimulation is used, but sine wave stimulation results in more severe cognitive impairments (Carney et al. 1976; Scott et al. 1992; Weiner et al. 1986a). More critical in establishing the efficacy of ECT was the demonstration that clinical outcome with ECT depends on electrode placement and stimulus dosage (McCall et al. 2000; Sackeim et al. 1987a, 1993, 2000). These factors can dramatically affect the efficacy of the treatment. This work went beyond sham-controlled studies, because the forms of ECT that differed markedly in outcome all involved electrical stimulation and production of a generalized seizure. Thus, technical factors in ECT administration can strongly influence efficacy (see Chapter 11).

2.3.1.2. Prediction of Response

ECT is an effective antidepressant in major depressive episodes, whether they occur in the context of unipolar or bipolar disorder. Nonetheless, many attempts have been made to determine whether particular subtypes or clinical features of depressive illness have prognostic value with respect to the efficacy of ECT.

In the 1950s and 1960s, a series of studies in patients with depression showed impressive power to predict clinical outcome on the basis of pre-ECT symptomatology and history (Abrams 1997a [review]; Black et al. 1987a; Carney et al. 1965; Hamilton and White 1960; Hobson 1953; Mendels 1967; Nobler and Sackeim 1996 [review]; Rose 1963). This work is now largely of historical interest (Hamilton 1986). Whereas early research emphasized the importance of vegetative or melancholic features as prognostic of positive ECT outcome, recent studies restricted to patients with major depression suggest that subtyping as endogenous or melancholic has little predictive value (Abrams et al. 1973; Black et al. 1993; Coryell and Zimmerman 1984; Prudic et al. 1989; Sackeim and Rush 1995; Zimmerman et al. 1985, 1986b). It is likely that the early positive associations were due to the inclusion in the sample of patients who had "neurotic depression," or dysthymia, which does not respond to ECT. Similarly, the distinction between unipolar and bipolar depressive illness generally has been found to be unrelated to therapeutic outcome (Abrams and Taylor 1974; Aronson et al. 1988; Black et al. 1986, 1993; Perris and d'Elia 1966; Zorumski et al. 1986). However, some evidence indicates that psychomotor retardation may predict a favorable response (Hickie et al. 1990, 1996; Sobin et al. 1996).

In recent research, a few clinical features have been related to ECT therapeutic outcome. In the majority of studies that have examined the distinction between psychotic and nonpsychotic depression, superior response rates were found among patients within the psychotic subtype (Avery and Lubrano 1979; Buchan et al. 1992; Clinical Research Centre 1984; Hamilton and White 1960; Hobson 1953; Kroessler 1985; Lykouras et al. 1986; Mandel et al. 1977; Mendels 1965a, 1965b; Pande et al. 1990; Parker et al. 1992; Sobin et al. 1996). This finding is of particular note given the established inferior response rate of psychotic or delusional depression to monotherapy with an antidepressant or antipsychotic medication (Chan et al. 1987; Parker et al. 1992; Spiker et al. 1985). To be effective, a pharmacologic trial in psychotic depression should involve combination treatment with an antidepressant and an antipsychotic medication (Nelson et al. 1986; Parker et al. 1992; Rothschild et al. 1993; Wolfersdorf et al. 1995). However, relatively few patients with psychotic depression who are referred for ECT have been administered such combination treatment in sufficient dosage and duration to be considered adequate (Mulsant et al. 1997). Multiple factors may be contributory. Many such patients cannot tolerate the dosage of traditional antipsychotic medications generally viewed as necessary for an adequate medication trial (Nelson et al. 1986; Spiker et al. 1985). Patients with psychotic depression commonly have severe symptoms and are at increased risk for suicide (Roose et al. 1983). The rapid onset and high probability of improvement with ECT makes this treatment of particular value for these patients.

Several studies have also noted that, as with pharmacologic treatment, patients with long duration of current episode are less likely to respond to ECT (Black et al. 1989c, 1993; Dunn and Quinlan 1978; Hamilton and White 1960; Hobson 1953; Kindler et al. 1991; Kukopulos et al. 1977; Magni et al. 1988; Prudic et al. 1996). As already discussed, the treatment history of patients may provide a useful predictor of ECT outcome, with patients who have failed one or more adequate medication trials showing a diminished but still substantial rate of ECT response (Prudic et al. 1990, 1996). In most relevant studies, patient age has also been associated with ECT outcome (Black et al. 1993; Coryell and Zimmerman 1984; Folstein et al. 1973; Gold and Chiarello 1944; Greenblatt et al. 1962; Roberts 1959a, 1959b; Mendels 1965a, 1965b; Nystrom 1964; Strömgren 1973; Tew et al. 1999). Older patients are more likely than younger patients to show marked benefit (see Sackeim 1993, 1998 for reviews). Gender, race, and socioeconomic status do not predict ECT outcome.

Catatonia or catatonic symptoms may be a particularly favorable prognostic sign. Catatonia occurs in patients with severe affective disorders (Abrams and Taylor 1976; Taylor and Abrams 1977) and is now recognized in the DSM-IV (American Psychiatric Association 1994a) as a specifier of a major depressive or manic episode. Catatonia may also occur as a consequence of some severe medical illnesses (Breakey and Kala 1977; Hafeiz 1987; O'Toole and Dyck 1977) as well as in patients with schizophrenia. The clinical literature suggests that ECT is effective in treating catatonic symptoms regardless of diagnosis, including the more malignant form of "lethal catatonia" (Bush et al. 1996; Geretsegger and Rochowanski 1987; Mann et al. 1986, 1990; Philbrick and Rummans 1994; Rohland et al. 1993).

Major depression occurring in individuals with preexisting psychiatric or medical disorders is termed *secondary depression*. Uncontrolled studies suggest that patients with secondary depression respond less well to somatic treatments, including ECT, than do patients with primary depressions (Bibb and Guze 1972; Black et al. 1988, 1993; Coryell et al. 1985; Zorumski et al. 1986). Patients with major depression and a comorbid personality disorder also may have a reduced probability of ECT response (Black et al. 1988, Zimmerman et al. 1986a). However, there is sufficient variability in outcome with ECT that each case of secondary depression must be considered on its own merits. For example, patients with poststroke depression are believed to have a relatively good prognosis with ECT (Allman and Hawton 1987; DeQuardo and Tandon 1988; Gustafson et al. 1995; House 1987; Krystal and Coffey 1997; Murray et al. 1986). Patients with major depression superimposed on a personality disorder (e.g., borderline personality disorder) should not be denied ECT out of hand.

Dysthymia as the sole clinical diagnosis has been rarely treated with ECT. However, a history of dysthymia preceding a major depressive episode is common and does not appear to have predictive value with regard to ECT outcome. Indeed, recent evidence suggests that the degree of residual symptoms after ECT is equivalent in patients with major depression superimposed on a dysthymic baseline, that is, "double depression," and in patients with major depression without a history of dysthymia (Prudic et al. 1993).

Patient features such as psychosis, medication resistance, and episode duration have only statistical associations with ECT outcome. This information may be considered in the overall risk/benefit analysis of ECT; for example, a patient with a nonpsychotic, chronic major depression who has failed to respond to multiple robust medication trials may be less likely than other patients to respond to ECT. Nonetheless, the probability of response with alternative treatments may be still lower, and the use of ECT may be justified.

2.3.2. Mania

Mania is a syndrome that, when fully expressed, is potentially life threatening because of its attendant exhaustion, excitement, and violence. Early case literature first suggested that ECT is rapidly effective in mania (Impastato and Almansi 1943; Kino and Thorpe 1946; Smith et al. 1943). A series of retrospective studies included either naturalistic case series or comparisons of outcome using ECT with outcome using lithium carbonate or chlorpromazine (Alexander et al. 1988; Black et al. 1986, 1987c; McCabe 1976; McCabe and Norris 1977; Mukherjee and Debsikdar 1992; Strömgren 1988; Thomas and Reddy 1982). This literature supported the efficacy of ECT in acute mania and suggested equivalent or superior antimanic properties relative to lithium and chlorpromazine (see Mukherjee et al. 1994 for a review). Three prospective comparative studies of the clinical outcome of ECT in acute mania have been published. One study primarily compared ECT with lithium treatment (Small et al. 1988); another compared ECT with combined treatment with lithium and haloperidol (Mukherjee et al. 1988, 1994); and the third study compared real and sham ECT in patients receiving neuroleptic treatment (Sikdar et al. 1994). Although each of the prospective studies had small samples, the findings supported the conclusion that ECT was efficacious in acute mania and likely resulted in better short-term outcome than did the comparison pharmacologic conditions. In a review of the English-language literature on ECT, Mukherjee et al. (1994) reported that ECT was associated with remission or marked clinical improvement in 80% of 589 patients with acute mania. However, no comparisons of ECT and newer antimanic medication regimens have been made.

With the availability of lithium and anticonvulsant and antipsychotic medications, ECT generally has been reserved for patients with acute mania who do not respond to adequate pharmacologic treatment. Evidence from retrospective and prospective studies has indicated that a substantial number of medication-resistant patients with mania benefit from ECT (Black et al. 1986; McCabe 1976; Mukherjee et al. 1988). For example, one such study required patients to have failed an adequate trial of lithium and/or an antipsychotic medication before randomization to ECT or intensive pharmacotherapy. Clinical outcome with ECT was superior to that with a combination treatment of lithium and haloperidol (Mukherjee 1989). Nonetheless, evidence suggests that, as with major depression, medication resistance predicts poorer response to ECT in acute mania (Mukherjee et al. 1994). Although most patients with medication-resistant acute mania respond to ECT, the response rate is lower than that among patients in whom ECT is used as a first-line treatment.

The rare syndrome of manic delirium represents a primary indication for the use of ECT because it is rapidly effective with a high margin of safety (Constant 1972; Heshe and Röder 1975; Kramp and Bolwig 1981; Strömgren 1997). In addition, patients with mania who cycle rapidly may be particularly unresponsive to medications, and ECT may represent an effective alternative treatment (Berman and Wolpert 1987; Mosolov and Moshchevitin 1990; Vanelle et al. 1994).

Other than medication resistance, few attempts have been made to examine the clinical features predictive of ECT response in acute mania. One study suggested that symptoms of anger, irritability, and suspiciousness were associated with poorer ECT outcome (Schnur et al. 1992). In this respect, some overlap may exist between the clinical features predictive of ECT response and of lithium response in acute mania (Goodwin and Jamison 1990).

2.3.3. Schizophrenia

Convulsive therapy was first used as a treatment for schizophrenia (as reviewed by Fink 1979). Early in its use, it became evident that the efficacy of ECT was greater in mood disorders than in schizophrenia. The introduction of effective antipsychotic medications markedly reduced the use of ECT in patients with schizophrenia. However, ECT remains an important treatment modality, particularly for patients with schizophrenia who do not respond to pharmacologic treatment (Fink and

Sackeim 1996). In the United States, schizophrenia and related conditions (schizophreniform and schizoaffective disorders) constitute the second most common diagnostic indications for ECT (Thompson and Blaine 1987; Thompson et al. 1994).

2.3.3.1. Efficacy

The earliest reports on the efficacy of ECT in patients with schizophrenia largely comprised uncontrolled case series (Danziger and Kendwall 1946; Guttmann et al. 1939; Kalinowsky 1943; Kalinowsky and Worthing 1943; Kennedy and Anchel 1948; Kino and Thorpe 1946; Miller et al. 1953; Ross and Malzberg 1939; Zeifert 1941), historical comparisons (Bond 1954; Currier et al. 1952; Ellison and Hamilton 1949; Gottlieb and Huston 1951), and comparisons of ECT with milieu therapy or psychotherapy (Goldfarb and Kieve 1945; McKinnon 1948; Palmer et al. 1951; Rachlin et al. 1956; Wolff 1955). These early reports lacked operational criteria for diagnosis, and patient samples and outcome criteria were often poorly characterized. It is likely that the samples included patients with mood disorder, given the overinclusiveness of the diagnosis of schizophrenia in that era (Kendell 1975; Pope and Lipinski 1978). Nonetheless, these reports were enthusiastic about the efficacy of ECT, noting that a large proportion of patients with schizophrenia, typically on the order of 75%, showed remission or marked improvement (see Krueger and Sackeim 1995, Salzman 1980, and Small 1985 for reviews). In this early work, it was also noted that ECT was considerably less effective in schizophrenic patients with insidious onset and long duration of illness (Chafetz 1943; Cheney and Drewry 1938; Danziger and Kendwall 1946; Herzberg 1954; Kalinowsky 1943; Lowinger and Huddleson 1945; Ross and Malzberg 1939; Shoor and Adams 1950; Zeifert 1941). It was also suggested that schizophrenic patients commonly required particularly long courses of ECT to achieve full benefit (Baker et al. 1960b; Kalinowsky 1943).

Several trials have used a real-versus-sham-ECT design to examine efficacy in patients with schizophrenia (Abraham and Kulhara 1987; Brandon et al. 1985; Brill et al. 1957, 1959a, 1959b, 1959c; Heath et al. 1964; Krueger and Sackeim 1995 [review]; Miller et al. 1953; Taylor and Fleminger 1980; Ulett et al. 1954, 1956). Studies prior to 1980 failed to demonstrate a therapeutic advantage of real ECT relative to sham treatment (Brill et al. 1959a, 1959b, 1959c; Heath et al. 1964; Miller et al. 1953). In contrast, three later studies all found a substantial advantage for real

ECT in short-term therapeutic outcome (Abraham and Kulhara 1987; Brandon et al. 1985; Taylor and Fleminger 1980). The factors that likely account for this discrepancy are the chronicity of the patients studied and the use of concomitant antipsychotic medication (Krueger and Sackeim 1995). The early studies focused mainly on patients with a chronic, unremitting course, whereas patients with acute exacerbations were more common in the more recent studies. All of the recent studies involved the use of antipsychotic medications in both the real ECT and the sham groups. As discussed below, there is evidence that the combination of ECT and antipsychotic medication is more effective in schizophrenia than either treatment alone.

The utility of monotherapy with ECT or antipsychotic medication was compared in a variety of retrospective (Ayres 1960; Borowitz 1959; DeWet 1957; Rohde and Sargant 1961) and prospective (Bagadia et al. 1970, 1983; Baker et al. 1958, 1960a; Childers 1964; Exner and Murrillo 1973, 1977; King 1960; Langsley et al. 1959; May 1968; May and Tuma 1965; May et al. 1976, 1981; Murrillo and Exner 1973a, 1973b; Ray 1962) studies of patients with schizophrenia. In general, short-term clinical outcome in schizophrenia with antipsychotic medication was found to be equivalent or superior to that of ECT, although there were exceptions (Murrillo and Exner 1973a). However, a consistent theme in this literature was the suggestion that patients with schizophrenia who had received ECT had better long-term outcome compared with those who received medication (Ayres 1960; Baker et al. 1958; Exner and Murrillo 1977; May et al. 1976, 1981). This research was conducted in an era when the importance of continuation and maintenance treatment was not appreciated and none of the studies controlled the treatment received after resolution of the schizophrenic episode. Nonetheless, the possibility that ECT may have long-term beneficial effects in schizophrenia merits attention.

Various prospective studies have compared the efficacy of combination treatment using ECT and antipsychotic medication with that of monotherapy using ECT or antipsychotic medication (Abraham and Kulhara 1987; Childers 1964; Das et al. 1991; Janakiramaiah et al. 1982; Ray 1962; Small et al. 1982; Smith et al. 1967; Ungvári and Pethö 1982). Relatively few of these studies involved random assignment and blind outcome assessment. Nonetheless, in each of the three studies in which ECT alone was compared with an ECT/antipsychotic combination, evidence indicated that the combination was more effective (Childers 1964; Ray 1962; Small et al. 1982). With the exception of Janakiramaiah et al. (1982), all of the studies that compared the combination treatment with antipsychotic medication alone found the combination treatment to be more effective (Abraham and Kulhara 1987; Childers 1964; Das et al. 1991; Ray 1962; Small et al. 1982; Smith et al. 1967; Ungvári and Pethö 1982). This pattern held even though the dosage of the antipsychotic medication was often lower when combined with ECT. The few findings on the persistence of benefit suggested that the rate of relapse was reduced in patients who had received the ECT/antipsychotic combination as acute-phase treatment. A new study has also found that the combination of ECT and antipsychotic medication is more effective as a continuation therapy than either treatment used alone in patients with medication-resistant schizophrenia who respond to the combination treatment in the acute phase (Chanpattana et al. 1999a, 1999b). These results support the recommendation that, in the treatment of patients with schizophrenia and possibly other psychotic conditions, the combination of ECT and antipsychotic medication may be preferable to the use of ECT alone.

In current practice, ECT is rarely used as a first-line treatment for patients with schizophrenia. ECT is most commonly considered in patients with schizophrenia only after unsuccessful treatment with antipsychotic medication. Thus, the key clinical issue concerns the efficacy of ECT in patients with medication-resistant schizophrenia.

With one exception (Agarwal and Winny 1985), prospective, blinded studies in which patients with medication-resistant schizophrenia are randomized to continued treatment with antipsychotic medication or to ECT (alone or in combination with antipsychotic medication) have yet to be performed. Most information on this issue comes from naturalistic case series (Chanpattana et al. 1999b; Childers and Therrien 1961; Friedel 1986; Gujavarty et al. 1987; König and Glatter-Götz 1990; Lewis 1982; Milstein et al. 1990; Rahman 1968; Sajatovic and Meltzer 1993). This body of work suggests that a substantial number of patients with medication-resistant schizophrenia benefit when treated with combination ECT and antipsychotic medication. ECT has been reported to be safe and effective when administered in combination with traditional antipsychotic medications (Friedel 1986; Gujavarty et al. 1987; Sajatovic and Meltzer 1993) or those with atypical properties, particularly clozapine (Benatov et al. 1996; Cardwell and Nakai 1995; Farah et al. 1995; Frankenburg et al. 1993; Klapheke 1991, 1993; Landy 1991; Masiar and Johns 1991; Safferman and Munne 1992). Although some practitioners have been concerned that clozapine may increase the likelihood of prolonged or spontaneous (tardive) seizures when combined with ECT (Bloch et al. 1996), such adverse events appear to be rare.

2.3.3.2. Prediction of Response

Since the earliest research was published, the clinical feature most strongly associated with the therapeutic outcome of ECT in patients with schizophrenia has been the duration of the episode of illness. Patients with acute onset of symptoms (i.e., psychotic exacerbations) and shorter episode duration are more likely to benefit from ECT than are patients with persistent, unremitting symptoms (Cheney and Drewry 1938; Danziger and Kendwall 1946; Dodwell and Goldberg 1989; Herzberg 1954; Kalinowsky 1943; Landmark et al. 1987; Lowinger and Huddelson 1945; Ross and Malzberg 1939; Zeifert 1941). Less consistently, preoccupation with delusions and hallucinations (Landmark et al. 1987), fewer schizoid and paranoid premorbid personality traits (Dodwell and Goldberg 1989; Wittman 1941), and the presence of catatonic symptoms (Ellison and Hamilton 1949; Hamilton and Wall 1948; Kalinowsky and Worthing 1943; Pataki et al. 1992; Wells 1973) have been linked to positive therapeutic effects. In general, the features associated with the clinical outcome of ECT in patients with schizophrenia overlap substantially with the features that predict outcome with pharmacotherapy (Leff and Wing 1971; Watt et al. 1983; World Health Organization 1979). Although patients with unremitting, chronic schizophrenia are the least likely to respond, it has also been argued that such patients should not be denied a trial of ECT (Fink and Sackeim 1996). The probability of significant improvement with ECT may be low in such patients, but alternative therapeutic options may be even more limited, and a small minority of patients with chronic schizophrenia may show dramatic improvement after ECT.

ECT may also be considered in the treatment of patients with schizoaffective or schizophreniform disorder (Black et al. 1987b, 1987c; Pope et al. 1980; Ries et al. 1981; Tsuang et al. 1979). The presence of perplexity or confusion in patients with schizoaffective disorder may be predictive of positive clinical outcome (Dempsey et al. 1975, Dodwell and Goldberg 1989; Perris 1974). Many practitioners believe that the manifestation of affective symptoms in patients with schizophrenia is predictive of positive clinical outcome. However, the evidence supporting this view is inconsistent (Dodwell and Goldberg 1989; Folstein et al. 1973; Wells 1973).

2.4. Other Diagnostic Indications

ECT has been used successfully in some other conditions, although this use has been rare in recent years (American Psychiatric Association 1990; American Psychiatric Association Task Force on ECT 1978; Thompson et al. 1994). Much of this usage has been reported as case material and typically reflects the administration of ECT only after other treatment options have been exhausted or when the patient presents with life-threatening symptoms. Because of the absence of controlled studies, which in any event would be difficult to carry out given the low utilization rates, any such referrals for ECT should be well substantiated in the clinical record. Psychiatric or medical consultation from individuals experienced in the management of the specific condition may be a useful component of the evaluation process.

2.4.1. Psychiatric Disorders

Besides the major diagnostic indications discussed above, there is limited evidence for the efficacy of ECT in the treatment of other psychiatric disorders. As noted earlier, major diagnostic indications for ECT may coexist with other conditions, and the presence of secondary diagnoses should not dissuade practitioners from recommending ECT when it is otherwise indicated, for example, a major depressive episode in a patient with a preexisting anxiety disorder. However, no evidence of beneficial effects has been found for patients with Axis II disorders or most other Axis I disorders who do not also have one of the major diagnostic indications for ECT. Although case reports of favorable outcome in some selected conditions do exist, evidence for efficacy is limited. For example, some patients with medication-resistant obsessive-compulsive disorder may show improvement with ECT (Dubois 1984; Gruber 1971; Janike et al. 1987; Khanna et al. 1988; Maletzky et al. 1994; Mellman and Gorman 1984). However, no controlled studies in this disorder have been performed, and the longevity of the beneficial effect is uncertain.

2.4.2. Mental Disorders due to Medical Conditions

Severe affective and psychotic conditions secondary to medical and neurologic disorders, as well as certain types of deliria, may be responsive to ECT. The use of ECT in such conditions is rare and should be reserved for patients who are resistant to or intolerant of more standard medical treatments or who require an urgent response. Prior to ECT, attention should be given to determining the underlying etiology of the medical disorder, and treatment should be targeted at the specific causes. It is largely of historical interest that ECT has been reported to be of benefit in conditions such as alcoholic delirium (Dudley and Williams 1972; Kramp and Bolwig 1981), toxic delirium secondary to phencyclidine (PCP) (Dinwiddie et al. 1988; Rosen et al. 1984), and in mental syndromes caused by enteric fevers (Breakey and Kala 1977; Hafeiz 1987; O'Toole and Dyck 1977), head injury (Kant et al. 1995), and other causes (Strömgren 1997). ECT has been effective in mental syndromes secondary to lupus erythematosus (Allen and Pitts 1978; Douglas and Schwartz 1982; Guze 1967; Mac and Pardo 1983). Catatonia may be secondary to a variety of medical conditions and is usually responsive to ECT (Bush et al. 1996; Fricchione et al. 1990; Rummans and Bassingthwaighte 1991). Additionally, ECT may be effective in the treatment of some chronic pain syndromes associated with mood disorders (Bloomstein et al. 1996).

When evaluating potential secondary mental syndromes, it is important to recognize that cognitive impairment may be a manifestation of major depressive disorder. Indeed, many patients with major depression have cognitive deficits (Sackeim and Steif 1988; Zakzanis et al. 1998). There is a subgroup of patients with severe cognitive impairment that resolves with treatment of the major depression. This condition has been termed *pseudodementia* (Caine 1981; Kiloh 1961). Occasionally, the cognitive impairment may be sufficiently severe to mask the presence of affective symptoms. When such patients have been treated with ECT, recovery has often been dramatic (Allen 1982; Bulbena and Berrios 1986; Burke et al. 1985; Fink 1989; Grunhaus et al. 1983; McAllister and Price 1982; O'Shea et al. 1987). It should be noted, however, that the presence of preexisting neurologic impairment or disorder (including dementia) may increase the risks for ECT-induced delirium and for more severe and persistent amnestic effects (Figiel et al. 1990; Krystal and Coffey 1997). Furthermore, among patients with major depression without known neurologic disease, the extent of pre-ECT cognitive impairment also appears to predict the severity of amnesia at follow-up. Thus, patients with baseline impairment thought to be secondary to the depressive episode may show improved global cognitive function at follow-up; however, they may also be subject to greater retrograde amnesia (Sobin et al. 1995).

2.4.3. Medical Disorders

The physiologic effects associated with ECT may result in therapeutic benefit in certain medical disorders, independent of antidepressant, antimanic, and antipsychotic actions. Because effective alternative treatments are usually available for these medical disorders, ECT should be reserved for use when patients are resistant to standard treatments.

There is now considerable experience in the use of ECT in patients with Parkinson's disease (see Faber and Trimble 1991; Kellner et al. 1994a; Rasmussen and Abrams 1991 for reviews). Independent of effects on psychiatric symptoms, ECT commonly results in general improvement in motor function (Ananth et al. 1979; Atre-Vaidya and Jampala 1988; Dysken et al. 1976; Jeanneau 1993; Lebensohn and Jenkins 1975; Pridmore and Pollard 1996; Roth et al. 1988; Stern 1991). Patients with the "on–off" phenomenon, in particular, may show considerable improvement (Andersen et al. 1987; Balldin et al. 1980, 1981). However, the beneficial effects of ECT on the motor symptoms of Parkinson's disease are highly variable in duration. Preliminary evidence indicates that continuing or maintaining ECT may be helpful in prolonging the therapeutic effects, particularly in patients who are resistant or intolerant to standard pharmacotherapy (Pridmore and Pollard 1996).

Neuroleptic malignant syndrome (NMS) is a medical condition that repeatedly has been shown to improve after ECT (Addonizio and Susman 1987; Casey 1987; Davis et al. 1991; Hermesh et al. 1987; Hermle and Oepen 1986; Kellam 1987; Nisijima and Ishiguro 1999; Pearlman 1986b; Pope et al. 1986; Troller and Sachdev 1999; Weiner and Coffey 1987). ECT is usually considered in such patients after autonomic stability has been achieved and should not be used without discontinuing neuroleptic medications. Because the presence of NMS restricts pharmacologic treatment options for the psychiatric condition, ECT may have the advantage of being effective in treating the manifestations of both the NMS and the psychiatric disorder.

ECT has marked anticonvulsant properties (Coffey et al. 1995b; Post et al. 1986; Sackeim 1999; Sackeim et al. 1983) and its use as an anticonvulsant has been reported in patients with seizure disorders since the 1940s (Caplan 1945, 1946; Kalinowsky and Kennedy 1943; Sackeim et al. 1983; Schnur et al. 1989). ECT may be of value in patients with intractable epilepsy or status epilepticus that is unresponsive to pharmacologic treatment (Carrasco Gonzalez et al. 1997; Dubovsky 1986; Fink et al. 1999; Griesemer et al. 1997; Hsiao et al. 1987; Krystal and Coffey 1997).

RECOMMENDATIONS

2.1. General Issues

a. Referrals for ECT are based on a combination of factors, including the patient's diagnosis, type and severity of symptoms, treatment history, consideration of the anticipated risks and benefits of ECT and alternative treatment options, and patient preference.
b. There are no diagnoses that should automatically lead to treatment with ECT.
c. In most cases ECT is used after treatment failure with psychotropic medications (see Section 2.2.2), although specific criteria exist for the use of ECT as a first-line treatment (see Section 2.2.1).

2.2. Primary and Secondary Use of ECT

2.2.1. Primary Use of ECT

Situations in which ECT may be used prior to a trial of psychotropic medication include, but are not limited to, any of the following:

- A need for rapid, definitive response because of the severity of a psychiatric or medical condition
- When the risks of other treatments outweigh the risks of ECT
- A history of poor medication response or good ECT response in one or more previous episodes of illness
- The patient's preference

2.2.2. Secondary Use of ECT

In other situations, one or more antidepressant medication trials should be considered prior to referral for ECT. Subsequent referral for ECT should be based on at least one of the following:

- Treatment resistance (taking into account issues such as choice of medication, dosage and duration of trial, and compliance)
- Intolerance to or adverse effects with pharmacotherapy that are

deemed less likely or less severe with ECT

- Deterioration of the patient's psychiatric or medical condition creating a need for a rapid, definitive response

2.3. Principal Diagnostic Indications

For major diagnostic indications, there is either compelling data supporting the efficacy of ECT or a strong consensus in the field supporting the use of ECT.

2.3.1. Major Depression

a. ECT is an efficacious treatment for unipolar major depression, including major depression, single episode (296.2x) and major depression, recurrent (296.3x) (DSM-IV; American Psychiatric Association 1994a).
b. ECT is an efficacious treatment for bipolar major depression, including bipolar disorder, depressed (296.5x) and bipolar disorder, mixed (296.6x).

2.3.2. Mania

ECT is an efficacious treatment for mania, including bipolar disorder, mania (296.4x) and bipolar disorder, mixed (296.6x).

2.3.3. Schizophrenia

a. ECT is an efficacious treatment for psychotic exacerbations in patients with schizophrenia in any of the following situations:

- When psychotic symptoms in the present episode have an abrupt or recent onset
- When schizophrenia is of the catatonic type (295.20)
- When there is a history of a favorable response to ECT

b. ECT is an efficacious treatment for related psychotic disorders, notably schizophreniform disorder (295.40) and schizoaffective disorder (295.70).
c. ECT may also be useful in patients with psychotic disorders not otherwise specified (298.9) when the clinical features are similar to those of other major diagnostic indications.

2.4. Other Diagnostic Indications

For other diagnoses, the efficacy data for ECT are only suggestive, or only a partial consensus exists in the field supporting its use. In such cases, ECT should be recommended only after standard treatment alternatives have been considered as a primary intervention. The presence of such disorders, however, should not deter the use of ECT for treatment of patients who also have a concurrent major diagnostic indication.

2.4.1. Psychiatric Disorders

Although ECT has sometimes been useful in the treatment of psychiatric disorders other than the principal diagnostic indications described above (see Section 2.3), such usage is not adequately substantiated and should be carefully justified in the clinical record on a case-by-case basis.

2.4.2. Mental Disorders due to Medical Conditions

ECT may be effective in the management of severe secondary affective and psychotic conditions displaying symptoms similar to those of primary psychiatric diagnoses, including catatonic states. There is some evidence that ECT may be effective in treating deliria of various etiologies, including toxic and metabolic.

2.4.3. Medical Disorders

The neurobiologic effects of ECT may be of benefit in a small number of medical disorders. Such conditions include Parkinson's disease (including those with the "on–off" phenomenon), neuroleptic malignant syndrome, and intractable seizure disorder

CHAPTER 3

Medical Conditions Associated with Substantial Risk

Electroconvulsive therapy is often administered to patients with severe medical illness (see Section 4.1). In fact, it may be the treatment of choice in some medically ill patients because of its speed of action and safety profile. No absolute medical contraindications to ECT exist; instead, an assessment of the relative risks and benefits of ECT should be undertaken in each individual case. This risk/benefit analysis, performed by the attending physician and the ECT psychiatrist, should include 1) consideration of the severity and duration of the psychiatric illness and its threat to life; 2) the likelihood of therapeutic success with ECT; 3) the medical risks of ECT and the degree to which these risks can be diminished; and 4) the benefits and risks of alternative treatments and of no treatment. After such an analysis, a choice can be made regarding the optimal intervention for an individual patient.

Some medical conditions substantially increase the risk of ECT treatment. In treating such high-risk patients with ECT, attempts should be made to improve and stabilize the medical conditions as well as to decrease the level of risk at the time of ECT (usually through pharmacologic intervention) (see Section 4.1 and Chapter 7). Careful medical evaluation is an essential component of this process and may include consultations with internists, cardiologists, neurologists, and other specialists (see Chapter 6). Management of medical conditions in patients referred for ECT is discussed in Sections 4.1 and 11.4.4 as well as in Chapter 7.

The organ systems of most importance when considering the medical risks of ECT are the cardiovascular, central nervous, and pulmonary systems. The majority of the medical complications and mortality associated with ECT are referable to the heart. The type and severity of preexisting cardiac disease impacts the likelihood, type, and severity of cardiac complications during ECT (Zielinski et al. 1993). Recent myocardial infarction is believed to represent a risk for reinfarction during ECT (Applegate 1997). In the absence of relevant supporting data, this concept of "recency" is difficult to define. For example, the risks at 6 weeks after a mild myocardial infarction without adverse sequelae may be less than those present at 6 months after a severe, complicated infarction.

Perianesthetic risk in general is believed to be greatly elevated in the presence of uncompensated congestive heart failure, severe valvular heart disease, or unstable angina (Dolinsky and Zvara 1997; Rayburn 1997). Again, pharmacologic strategies may be used to diminish such risk during ECT (see Section 4.1.3). A similar situation exists with respect to vascular aneurysms. Here, lesions of particular concern are those that have an increased risk of rupture with transient elevations in blood pressure.

Regarding the central nervous system, conditions associated with increased intracranial pressure, such as some brain tumors, are theoretically of great concern (Krystal and Coffey 1997). In the presence of these conditions, the rise in intracranial pressure that occurs with ECT could lead to brain herniation (see also Section 4.1.2). Such events are rare in practice, however (Kellner 1996b). Most reports of dire outcomes are from the distant past, when ECT technique was far less sophisticated (Maltbie et al. 1980). The type and size of a brain tumor also correlate with the degree of danger; smaller and slow-growing neoplasms pose less risk. For example, there are now several case reports of successful ECT in the presence of meningiomas (Fried and Mann 1988; Greenberg et al. 1988; Hsiao and Evans 1984; Kellner and Rames 1990; Malek-Ahmadi and Sedler 1989; McKinney et al. 1998; Zwil et al. 1990). Clearly, clinical judgment must be exercised in determining the risk/benefit ratio in each case. Only rarely would one treat a patient with a large brain tumor; likewise, only rarely would one need to avoid ECT in a patient with a small, stable meningioma.

ECT may pose additional risks in a patient with a recent cerebral infarction. Reports of stroke (either hemorrhagic or ischemic) during or shortly after ECT are surprisingly rare, given the magnitude of hemodynamic changes that occur during the treatment and the number of patients with cerebrovascular disease who receive ECT (Miller and Isenberg 1998; Zwil et al. 1992).

Severe pulmonary conditions may lead to difficulties in airway management during and after the ECT procedure (Smetana 1999). Consultation with anesthesiology or other staff regarding management (e.g., pre-ECT use of bronchodilators, attention to pretreatment oxygenation) is often indicated.

Another potentially high-risk situation with ECT occurs when patients are rated a level 4 or 5 on the American Society of Anesthesiologists (ASA; 1963) physical status classification, typically because of severe cardiopulmonary or other organ system disease. Medical consultation before ECT may be indicated to optimize the patient's medical status (see Chapters 4.1 and 6).

In addition to medical conditions that increase the risks of ECT, certain medication regimens may also contribute to risk (see Chapter 7).

RECOMMENDATIONS

a. There are no "absolute" medical contraindications to ECT.
b. In situations in which ECT is associated with an increased likelihood of serious morbidity or mortality, the decision to administer ECT should be based on the premise that the patient's psychiatric condition is grave and that ECT is the safest treatment available.
c. Careful medical evaluation of risk factors should be carried out prior to ECT with specific attention to modifications in patient management or ECT technique that may diminish the level of risk (see Section 4.1).
d. Specific conditions that may be associated with substantially increased risk include the following:

  • Unstable or severe cardiovascular conditions such as recent myocardial infarction, unstable angina, poorly compensated congestive heart failure, and severe valvular cardiac disease
  • Aneurysm or vascular malformation that might be susceptible to rupture with increased blood pressure
  • Increased intracranial pressure, as may occur with some brain tumors or other space-occupying cerebral lesions
  • Recent cerebral infarction
  • Pulmonary conditions such as severe chronic obstructive pulmonary disease, asthma, or pneumonia
  • Patient status rated as ASA level 4 or 5

CHAPTER 4

Use of Electroconvulsive Therapy in Special Populations

4.1. Concurrent Medical Illness

4.1.1. General Considerations

Coexisting medical illnesses and their treatments may have an impact on both the likelihood of response and the risks of ECT. Use of ECT to treat certain medical disorders such as Parkinson's disease is discussed in Chapter 2 and represents a different situation from the use of ECT to treat mental disorders in people with coexisting medical conditions. Indeed, effective management of medical conditions is often more difficult in patients with mental disorders because of factors such as diminished compliance with medical treatment (Koenig and Kuchibhatla 1998). Furthermore, effective psychiatric treatment often improves the medical outcome (Thompson et al. 1998). Relative to these considerations, there is evidence that ECT reduces long-term mortality from medical conditions in patients with major depression (Avery and Winokur 1976; Philibert et al. 1995).

In patients referred for ECT, it is especially important to understand the interactions among coexisting medical conditions, physiologic events associated with anesthetic induction, electrical stimulation of the brain, and induced seizure activity. The pre-ECT evaluation (see Chapter 6) is designed to identify coexisting medical illnesses, elucidate their impact on risks and benefits of ECT, and suggest potential means of minimizing adverse effects. Additional laboratory evaluation and specialist consultations are often a necessary part of this information-gathering process. This material facilitates the treatment team's ability to arrive at a medically sound decision about whether ECT should be recommended and, if so, whether any procedural modifications are indicated.

Potential modifications of ECT technique include use of medications before, during, and after the ECT procedure; changes in technical aspects of the electrical stimulation (e.g., electrode placement or electrical dosage); and use of additional types of physiologic monitoring. In certain high-risk situations, the presence of specialty medical or anesthesiologic consultants at one or more of the treatments may be indicated. If a higher level of potential acute medical intervention is required, ECT may need to be administered in a more intensive setting, either locally or in a different facility.

A large number of specific medical conditions may have an impact on the risks or benefits of ECT. There are several recent reviews in this area (Abrams 1991, 1997a; Welch 1993; Weiner et al. 2000; Zwil and Pelchat 1994) as well as reviews focusing on patients with neurologic (Folkerts 1995; Kellner and Bernstein 1993; Krystal and Coffey 1997) and cardiovascular (Applegate 1997; Dolinski and Zvara 1997; Rayburn 1997) disease.

4.1.2. Neurologic Disorders

Traditionally, a major concern has been intracerebral masses such as brain tumors and hematomas (see Chapter 3). Present evidence suggests that small or chronic space-occupying cerebral lesions pose minimal increased risk unless associated with increased intracranial pressure or other signs of a mass effect (Malek-Ahmadi and Sedler 1989; Malek-Ahmadi et al. 1990; McKinney et al. 1998; Starkstein and Migliorelli 1993; Wijeratne and Shome 1999; Zwil et al. 1990). However, patients with increased intracranial pressure or focal cerebrovascular fragility are at substantial risk of acute neurologic decompensation (Krystal and Coffey 1997). Although there are strategies to diminish this risk with ECT (e.g., use of potent antihypertensive agents, steroids, diuretics, and hyperventilation), the risk remains high and must be weighed against the risk of not giving ECT.

Patients with preexisting cerebrovascular disease are commonly referred for ECT (Zwil et al. 1992). Although the risk of an intracerebral infarct or bleed is believed to be small in patients with stable lesions (Farah et al. 1996; Weisberg et al. 1991), concern is greater for individuals with very recent strokes or cerebral aneurysms. The acute ECT-related hypertensive surge should be pharmacologically blunted when ECT is given to patients at risk for a bleed (Bader et al. 1995; Kolano et al. 1997; Krystal and Coffey 1997; Najjar and Guttmacher 1998; Viguera et al. 1998) (see also Section 11.4.4). However, patients with ischemic cerebrovascular disease generally should not receive aggressive antihypertensive medication because of the risk of hypotensive morbidity. Patients with clinically silent cerebrovascular disease, as evidenced by subcortical hyperintensities on magnetic resonance imaging (MRI) scans, do not appear to be at increased risk with ECT (Coffey 1996; Coffey et al. 1987a). The likelihood of ECT-induced delirium may be increased in some patients who have had strokes (Martin et al. 1992) or hyperintensities on MRI scans in the basal ganglia (Figiel et al. 1991).

Patients with a coexisting diagnosis of dementia (Beale et al. 1997a; Goetz and Price 1993; Mulsant et al. 1991; Krystal and Coffey 1997; Price and McAllister 1989) may have an increased risk of transient cognitive worsening with ECT. However, ECT is often of value in the pseudodementia syndrome of depression (Nelson and Rosenberg 1991; Price and McAllister 1989).

Because of its anticonvulsant effects, ECT may be associated with an improvement in seizure control in patients with epilepsy (Griesemer et al. 1997; Kalinowsky and Kennedy 1943; Krystal and Coffey 1997; Sackeim et al. 1983; Schnur et al. 1989). However, such patients may be at slightly increased risk for prolonged or spontaneous seizures during ECT (Devinsky and Duchowny 1983). Anticonvulsant medications may complicate ECT by raising seizure threshold or by adversely affecting seizure expression and, possibly, clinical efficacy. Thus, the indication for anticonvulsant treatment should be confirmed and dosage should be kept as low as clinically feasible during ECT. In the presence of an anticonvulsant medication, the use of a stimulus dose-titration procedure at the time of the first treatment is particularly desirable because it allows the most accurate assessment of the patient's actual seizure threshold (see Section 11.7). For general suggestions on management of anticonvulsant agents during ECT, see Chapter 7.

Patients with a history of brain trauma may be at risk for increased cognitive changes with ECT, although the available literature is not definitive (Kant et al. 1999). It is clear, however, that stimulation over a skull defect should be avoided (Crow et al. 1996; Everman et al. 1999; Hartman and Saldivia 1990; Wijeratne and Shome 1999). Such situations should be detected during the pre-ECT evaluation (see Chapter 6) and modified stimulus electrode placement should be used (Everman et al. 1999; Kant et al. 1999) (see also Section 11.6). Patients with intracerebral shunts should have shunt patency assessed, and the presence of any skull defects should also be noted (Cardno and Simpson 1991; Coffey et al. 1987b).

Patients with multiple sclerosis generally tolerate ECT without experiencing major adverse effects (Coffey et al. 1987d; Krystal and Coffey 1997), although those with active cerebral demyelination may experience deterioration in neurologic function (Mattingly et al. 1992). Gadolinium-enhanced brain MRI has been suggested as a possible means of detecting high-risk patients.

Because myasthenia gravis is associated with an increased resistance to and slow recovery from depolarizing muscle relaxants, a decrease in dosage should be considered (Pande and Grunhaus 1990; Wainwright and Broderick 1987). A switch to a nondepolarizing agent may be problematic because of increased sensitivity to such medications in patients with myasthenia gravis (Eisenkraft et al. 1988). Increased sensitivity to succinylcholine may also be seen in patients with upper motor neuron disease such as quadriplegia and amyotrophic lateral sclerosis (Janis et al. 1995) (see Section 11.4).

As noted in Chapter 2, ECT often has beneficial, although transient, effects on symptoms of idiopathic Parkinson's disease (Andersen et al. 1987; Balldin et al. 1981; Douyon et al. 1989; Faber and Trimble 1991; Kellner et al. 1994a; Krystal and Coffey 1997; Rasmussen and Abrams 1991; Zwil et al. 1990; Zwil and Pelchat 1994). These effects may be extended by continuation or maintenance ECT treatment (Aarsland et al. 1997; Friedman and Gordon 1992; Kramer 1999; Pridmore and Pollard 1996; Wengel et al. 1998). There is also evidence that parkinsonism and extrapyramidal symptoms due to other etiologies (e.g., neuroleptic-induced) may improve with ECT (Faber and Trimble 1991; Goswami et al. 1989; Hermesh et al. 1992; Moellintime et al. 1998; Mukherjee and Debsikdar 1994), although contrary data have been reported (Hanin et al. 1995; Yassa et al. 1990). Some reports have indicated that patients with Parkinson's disease may have greater cognitive dysfunction after ECT, particularly with respect to an increased incidence of delirium (Figiel et al. 1991; Kellner et al. 1994a). This potential complication may be minimized by the use of unilateral ECT and a less frequent schedule of treatments. The increased dopaminergic tone produced by ECT may also result in psychosis or dyskinesia. These effects may be limited by careful reduction in any concomitant dopaminergic medications (McGarvey et al. 1993; Nymeyer and Grossberg 1997; Zervas and Fink 1992).

Use of ECT in the acute management of neuroleptic malignant syndrome (NMS) is also discussed in Section 2.4.3. More commonly, ECT is used to treat mental disorders in patients with current or past NMS. In such patients, dopamine blocking agents such as neuroleptics, metoclopramide, prochlorperazine, and promethazine should be avoided. Patients with a history of NMS generally do not require specific changes in the ECT or anesthetic protocol (Addonizio and Susman 1987; Davis et al. 1991; Scheftner and Shulman 1992). However, switching to a nondepolarizing relaxant agent should be considered in those with NMS symptoms, particularly in the presence of extensive muscular rigidity, because of the risk of hyperkalemia after succinylcholine administration (see Section 11.4.3). It is important for patients with active NMS symptoms to be observed for metabolic or cardiovascular instability throughout the ECT course (Lazarus 1986; Scheftner and Shulman 1992). It has been suggested that two seizure inductions in a single ECT session (see Section 11.11) may hasten the time to recovery in severe NMS (McKinney and Kellner 1997).

4.1.3. Cardiovascular Disorders

With the trend toward increased use of ECT in the elderly (Olfson et al. 1998; Thompson et al. 1994) as well as the availability of more effective means to diminish the cardiovascular risks of ECT (see Chapter 3 and Sections 5.2, 11.4, and 11.8.3), it is not surprising that the prevalence of cardiovascular disease in patients referred for ECT may be increasing.

The cardiovascular risks of ECT derive primarily from the marked changes in heart rate and blood pressure that typically occur during and immediately after the electrical stimulus and induced seizure (Dolinski and Zvara 1997; Fuenmayor et al. 1997; Messina et al. 1992; Webb et al. 1990; Zielinski et al. 1993) (see Sections 5.2 and 11.4). In general, patients with cardiovascular disease can be safely managed during ECT (Abrams 1991, 1997a; Applegate 1997; Dolinski and Zvara 1997; Rayburn 1997; Weiner et al. 2000; Welch 1993; Zwil and Pelchat 1994).

As noted in Chapter 3, however, individuals with certain cardiovascular conditions (i.e., recent myocardial infarction, unstable angina, uncompensated congestive heart failure, severe valvular heart disease, clinically significant cardiac arrhythmias, and fragile vascular aneurysms) are believed to be at increased risk with ECT. In addition to these conditions, some increased risk is also believed to be present for patients with unstable angina or other evidence of active cardiac ischemia, uncontrolled hypertension, high-grade atrioventricular block, symptomatic ventricular arrhythmias, and supraventricular arrhythmias with uncontrolled ventricular rate (Applegate 1997). In this regard, the type of condition appears to predict the type of cardiac complication (Zielinski et al. 1993).

If a high cardiovascular risk of ECT is believed to be present, a physician with expertise in the assessment and treatment of such conditions should be consulted (Applegate 1997). As with any pre-ECT medical consultation, the consultant should be asked to comment on both the degree of risk and the means of diminishing it but should not be asked to "clear" the patient for ECT (McCall 1997). High-risk situations should also be discussed with the consentor as part of the informed consent procedure (see Chapter 8). At the same time, it is important to recognize that patients with untreated mood disorders are exposed to a higher level of cardiovascular risk (Avery and Winokur 1976; Frasure-Smith et al. 1993; Glassman and Shapiro 1998). There is evidence that such individuals also have increased morbidity or mortality with alternatives to ECT such as psychopharmacologic agents (McElroy et al. 1995; Thorogood et al. 1992).

Assessment of the presence, type, and severity of cardiovascular risk of ECT as well as the potential means of ameliorating adverse effects depends on a careful medical evaluation of patients with cardiovascular disease (see Chapter 6). In addition to cardiopulmonary history and examination, patients with cardiovascular disease should have an electrocardiogram (ECG) prior to ECT. A chest radiograph and measurement of serum electrolyte levels are considered optional (Abramczuk and Rose 1979). In patients for whom the evaluation raises the possibility of ischemic disease, functional cardiac testing (i.e., stress test with or without imaging) may be helpful in the assessment of risk (Eagle et al. 1996).

Regardless of the type and degree of cardiovascular disease, optimization prior to ECT should be attempted, keeping in mind any risks that may be associated with delaying the start of ECT. Unless there is clear evidence to the contrary, current medications likely to diminish cardiovascular risk with ECT should be continued, including administration prior to ECT, when such medication would have been provided in any case (see Chapter 7). If the pre-ECT evaluation (see Chapter 6) or the patient's response to previous ECT treatments suggests that additional cardiovascular medications will decrease risk (see Section 11.4.4), these should be considered at the time of ECT. Such agents include, but are not limited to, sympatholytic medications, short-acting nitrates, other antihypertensive drugs, and anticholinergics (Figiel et al. 1993; Fu et al. 1998; Maneksha 1991; McCall 1996; McCall et al. 1991; Petrides et al. 1996; Rice et al. 1994; Weinger et al. 1991; Welch and Drop 1989; Zielinski et al. 1993). At the same time, iatrogenic hypotension should be avoided during and after the ECT treatment. In this regard, the half-life of the medication should be taken into account and precautions against orthostatic hypotension and falls during the post-ECT recovery period should be considered when applicable. Because of its pronounced anticonvulsant effects, lidocaine should be avoided prior to and during the induced seizure, unless a potentially life-threatening complication is present (Devanand and Sackeim 1988; Hood and Mecca 1983; Ottosson 1960; Weinger et al. 1991).

Because implanted cardiac pacemakers improve control of cardiac rate and rhythm, they generally have a protective effect during ECT (Alexopoulous 1980; Grossman 1986; Morgan 1987; Pearlman 1986a). To prevent unnecessary pacemaker triggering at the time of ECT, some practitioners choose to convert a demand pacemaker to a fixed mode (using a magnet). Implanted cardiac defibrillators are not generally problematic with ECT (Goldberg and Badger 1993; Pornnoppadol and Isenberg 1998), although a cardiac electrophysiologist should be consulted to determine whether the unit's defibrillator function should be inhibited at the time of each treatment. (In such cases, the pacemaker function should be left operative.) Because ECT may convert atrial fibrillation to a sinus rhythm, some practitioners recommend routine anticoagulation of patients with this condition to diminish risk of embolism from mural thrombi (Harsch 1991; Petrides and Fink 1996a). If cardiac function is normal, patients who have undergone cardiac transplant do not present a specific cardiac risk during ECT (Bloch et al. 1992; Kellner et al. 1991a; Pargger et al. 1995).

4.1.4. Other Disorders

ECT may necessitate changes in management of diabetes (Finestone and Weiner 1984; Reddy and Nobler 1996; Weiner and Sibert 1996; Williams et al. 1992). Dosing of antidiabetic agents should account for the fasting period prior to each ECT treatment as well as the typical hyperglycemic effect of electrically induced seizures. Blood glucose should be monitored closely during the ECT course, including assessment within the hour before each treatment to allow hypoglycemic states to be detected and treated. Infusion of intravenous glucose solutions is indicated in such situations and also may be helpful before ECT in some patients with brittle, insulin-dependent diabetes. Endocrinologic or medical consultation should be considered for individuals whose diabetes is unstable or insulin dependent.

Clinically significant hyperthyroidism substantially increases risk of thyroid storm at the time of ECT (Farah and McCall 1995). Treatment of hyperthyroid states should be optimized with the assistance of specialty consultation, and β-blocking agents should be used at the time of ECT unless otherwise contraindicated. However, mild subclinical elevations in thyroid function on test results, which may occur in conjunction with episodes of mood disorder, are not a risk factor and may resolve with ECT (Diaz-Cabal et al. 1986). Hypothyroidism (Garrett 1985), hypoparathyroidism (Cunningham and Anderson 1995), and pseudohypoparathyroidism (McCall et al. 1989) have not been reported to be problems with ECT, although case reports primarily have described relatively stable cases. Although pheochromocytoma does represent a significant risk with ECT, this can be minimized with β-blockers, α-blockers, and blockers of tyrosine hydroxylase (Carr and Woods 1985; Weiner et al. 2000). Because ECT treatments are associated with transient adrenocortical stimulation, patients with Addison's disease and other patients with steroid dependence may require an increased does of steroid before each treatment (Cumming and Kort 1956). With Cushing's disease, no specific risks or special precautions appear to be necessary with ECT (Ries and Bokan 1979).

Various metabolic disorders may increase ECT risk or require alterations in ECT technique. Patients with hyperkalemia are at increased risk of cardiotoxic effects because of the transient rise in serum potassium with succinylcholine (Bali 1975) (see also Section 11.4.3). If serum potassium cannot be normalized prior to treatment, a switch to a nondepolarizing muscle relaxant should be made (see Section 11.4.3). Such a switch should also be considered for patients with either genetic or acquired pseudocholinesterase deficiencies (Hicks 1987; Messer et al. 1992) as well as in those with diffuse muscle membrane dysfunction, for example, extensive severe muscular rigidity or widespread acute third-degree burns (Dwersteg and Avery 1987; Mashimo et al. 1997). Hypokalemia may be associated with prolonged paralysis and apnea after ECT and should also be corrected before starting treatment.

Hyponatremia can lead to spontaneous seizures and should be corrected prior to ECT treatment, particularly if it is severe or acute (Finlayson et al. 1989; Greer and Stewart 1993). Dehydration, on the other hand, is more common in patients referred for ECT (Mashimo et al. 1996) and may be associated with other types of electrolyte imbalance, particularly hypernatremia and hyperkalemia. Dehydration may raise seizure threshold, although this has not been proven. Electrolyte imbalance is common in patients undergoing renal dialysis (Pearlman et al. 1988). In addition to ongoing monitoring of electrolyte levels, ECT treatments should be scheduled on the day after dialysis when possible. Patients with porphyria are intolerant to barbiturates and must be switched to an alternative anesthetic agent (Shaw and McKeith 1998) (see Section 11.4.2).

Patients with chronic obstructive pulmonary disease should receive pretreatment with any prescribed bronchodilators as well as preoxygenation at each ECT treatment (Wingate and Hansen-Flaschen 1997) (see Section 11.3). At the same time, theophylline should be discontinued or levels should be kept as low as clinically feasible to minimize the risk of prolonged seizures (Devanand et al. 1988a; Fink and Sackeim 1998; Peters et al. 1984; Rasmussen and Zorumski 1993) (see Chapter 7). Patients with asthma should have bronchodilators available for use both before and after each ECT treatment (Fawver and Milstein 1985).

Esophageal reflux with or without hiatal hernia is a common clinical problem associated with an increased risk of aspiration during procedures involving general anesthesia (Weiner et al. 2000). Reflux is particularly common in patients with gastroparesis, morbid obesity, and pregnancy, most notably in the third trimester (see Section 4.3). Histamine-2 antagonists such as ranitidine (150 mg) given orally the night before and the morning of a treatment will diminish gastric acidity. Other agents that may be used include metoclopramide (which promotes gastric emptying but has neuroleptic side effects), cisapride, or sodium citrate (which neutralizes gastric contents). Metoclopramide is particularly useful in patients with gastroparesis. With patients at moderate to high risk of reflux, some anesthetists use cricoid pressure during the period of anesthesia, although the effectiveness of this technique is unclear (Brimacomb and Berry 1997). Because of the morbidity associated with multiple intubations over an ECT course, endotracheal intubation should be reserved for situations in which the risk of aspiration is high (see Section 11.3).

Urinary retention should be avoided during ECT because of the remote possibility of bladder rupture (O'Brien and Morgan 1991). In severe cases, placement of a foley catheter or straight catheterization should be considered before treatment when the bladder has not been adequately emptied (Irving and Drayson 1984).

Patients with joint or bone disease, including moderate to severe osteoporosis, often need an increased dosage of muscle relaxant (Coffey et al. 1986; Dighe-Deo and Shah 1998; Hanretta and Malek-Ahmadi 1995; Kellner et al. 1991b; Mashimo et al. 1995; Milstein et al. 1992; Weller and Kornhuber 1992) (see Section 11.4.3). When suggested by medical history or examination, radiologic evaluation prior to ECT can help establish the extent and severity of such conditions (see Chapter 6). Postsurgical patients whose wounds are still healing also may fall into this category. At the time of ECT, a peripheral nerve stimulator can supplement usual means of ascertaining maximal muscle relaxation and, although not always the case, may make this determination more precise (Beale et al. 1994a) (see Section 11.4.3). The existence of skull defects from injury, surgery, or disease should be established prior to ECT (see Chapter 6) and stimulus electrodes should not be placed over or adjacent to a skull defect (Crow et al. 1996; Hartmann and Saldivia 1990; Krahn et al. 1993) (see Section 11.6).

The pre-ECT evaluation should include an assessment of the patient's teeth (see Chapter 6 and Section 5.2) (McCall et al. 1992a; Minneman 1995; Weiner and McCall 1992). When teeth are unstable or unlikely to withstand pressure associated with the contraction of jaw muscles during the ECT stimulus (see Section 11.3), the applicable teeth may need to be removed or the usual mouth protection may need to be modified during ECT. Examples of such modifications range from the use of rolled-up gauze to custom-made prostheses specifically designed to protect teeth at the time of ECT. Dental consultation may be useful when the assessment of risk is unclear or management requires specific expertise. Removable dental appliances, such as dentures, should be taken out before each ECT treatment unless dental consultation indicates that the appliances will protect oral structures from injury.

Patients with dermatologic disease may have problems with stimulus or recording electrode contact (see Sections 11.6.3 and 11.8.1.3).

At the present time, either warfarin or heparin is often used in the management of patients with thrombophlebitis and other hypercoagulable states during ECT (Weiner et al. 2000). In the former case, a target

International Normalized Ratio (INR) of 1.5–2.5, generally viewed as being compatible with surgical procedures, appears to be reasonable for ECT (Petrides and Fink 1996a). Recently, there has been growing interest in the use of low molecular weight heparin preparations, such as enoxaparin, as a substitute for warfarin, particularly because INR does not need to be monitored (Nurmohamed et al. 1992). With thrombophlebitis, some practitioners also increase muscle relaxant dosage or use acute antihypertensive treatment to minimize the hypertensive surge during the seizure. Sickle cell disease represents a contraindication to use of the cuff technique (La Grone 1990). No special precautions appear indicated in patients with thrombocytopenic (Kardener 1968) or thrombocythemic states (Hamilton and Walter-Ryan 1986).

Despite a transient increase in blood-brain barrier permeability during and shortly after electrically induced seizures, no evidence exists of spread of infection to the brain with ECT. A growing number of patients with HIV, including those with AIDS, are being safely treated with ECT (Kessing et al. 1994; Schaerf et al. 1989). In patients with neoplastic disease, ECT technique requires modification only if a mass effect occurs in the brain (see above), if affected organ systems raise the risk associated with transient ECT-induced autonomic changes (see Chapter 5), or if the patient's antineoplastic agents adversely interact with medications used at the time of ECT (Beale et al. 1997b; Magen and D'Mello 1995) (see Chapter 7 and Section 11.4).

Administration of ECT is associated with a brief increase in intraocular pressure, presumably by multiple mechanisms (Edwards et al. 1990). Although this effect is theoretically a concern in patients with open-angle glaucoma, such complications have not been reported (Van den Berg and Honjol 1998). Still, most practitioners administer antiglaucoma medications before each treatment for patients who take them on a routine basis. Long-acting anticholinesterase ophthalmic solutions, such as demecarium and echothiophate, could greatly prolong succinylcholine-induced apnea and therefore should be replaced by alternative agents for an appropriate time period prior to ECT (Messer et al. 1992; Packman et al. 1978). Closed- or narrow-angle glaucoma is a medical emergency and represents a greater risk with ECT, although no reports have been made of such patients being referred for ECT. In the past, acute or evolving retinal detachment has been considered a substantial risk with ECT. However, no reports of such problems have been made (Karliner 1958). Still, ophthalmologic consultation should be considered and attempts should be made to avoid unnecessary movement of the head during ECT. Some practitioners also pharmacologically blunt the acute hypertensive surge associated with ECT in such patients.

4.2. Elderly

ECT has a special role in the treatment of late-life depression and other psychiatric conditions in the elderly (Coffey and Kellner 2000; Sackeim 1993, 1998), who as a group constitute a particularly high proportion of the patients who receive ECT. For example, a survey of practice in California between 1977 and 1983 indicated that the probability of receiving ECT increased with patient age. Although 1.12 persons per 10,000 in the general adult population were treated with ECT, the rate was 3.86 persons per 10,000 among people aged 65 years and older (Kramer 1985). Similarly, a national survey of inpatient psychiatric facilities conducted by the National Institute of Mental Health (NIMH) indicated that patients aged 61 and older composed the largest age group to receive ECT (Thompson and Blaine 1987). In this survey, overall use of ECT had declined substantially in comparisons between the years 1975 and 1980. However, the rate of use for patients aged 61 years and older was not changed. In a follow-up NIMH national survey, Thompson et al. (1994) observed that the use of ECT increased somewhat between 1980 and 1986. Hospital type and patient age were particularly strong predictors of the use of this modality: ECT was far more commonly administered in private general and psychiatric hospitals than in the public sector, and individuals aged 65 and older received ECT at a higher rate than any other age group. Indeed, the overall increase in the use of ECT between 1980 and 1986 was fully attributable to its greater use in elderly patients. In 1986, the national estimate was that 15.6% of inpatients with mood disorders received ECT if they were 65 years of age or older, whereas the rate was 3.4% among younger inpatients with mood disorders. Further evidence for increased use of ECT in the elderly comes from a survey of Medicare part B claims data between the years 1987 and 1992 (Rosenbach et al. 1997).

Despite frequent use of ECT among the elderly, age per se does not constitute a particular indication for ECT in major depression or other diagnostic groups. Rather, elderly patients are particularly likely to be characterized by the diagnostic indications and other factors that impact on a referral for ECT (see Chapter 2). Intolerance to antidepressant medications and the presence of medical conditions are known to be age related. This relationship is particularly true for some forms of cardiovascular disease that may preclude or limit pharmacologic options, although such limitations may be less likely with the newer antidepressant agents (Roose et al. 1998a, 1998b). At least in terms of the morbidity and mortality associated with traditional heterocyclic antidepressants, ECT is believed to present less medical risk, making its use particularly likely in elderly and medically compromised patients (Abrams 1997a; Benbow 1989; Rice et al. 1994; Sackeim 1998; Weiner et al. 2000; Zielinski et al. 1993). It is also suspected, but not well documented, that resistance to the therapeutic effects of antidepressant medication is age related, with depression in late life more likely to be medication resistant (Gerson et al. 1988; Himmelhoch et al. 1980; Prudic et al. 1990). Some evidence has indicated that this medication resistance may be the case particularly in late-onset major depression (Alexopoulos et al. 1996). Because the likelihood and speed of a full clinical response is greater with ECT than with antidepressant medications (Janicak et al. 1985; Rifkin 1988; Sackeim 1989; Segman et al. 1995), ECT is also considered when patients present with medical and psychiatric conditions of heightened urgency. Severe inanition, refusal to eat, psychosis, and suicidality are features of depression that may be more common in the elderly.

The impact of aging on the short-term efficacy of ECT has been examined repeatedly (Sackeim 1993, 1998). Although the findings in this area have been somewhat inconsistent, approximately half of the studies reported superior therapeutic effects of ECT in older, relative to younger, depressed patients. Indeed, an impressive number of both early and recent investigations found positive associations between patient age and the degree of clinical improvement after ECT (Black et al. 1993; Coryell and Zimmerman 1984; Folstein et al. 1973; Gold and Chiarello 1944; Greenblatt et al. 1962; Herzberg 1954; Mendels 1965a, 1965b; Nystrom 1964; Roberts 1959a, 1959b; Strömgren 1973; Tew et al. 1999). In contrast, a variety of studies have not found aging effects and some data suggest that older individuals may have a diminished response to unilateral ECT but not to bilateral ECT (Heshe et al. 1978; Pettinati et al. 1986) or that older patients may require longer courses of treatment to achieve the same level of remission as younger patients (Ottosson 1960; Rich et al. 1984).

In general, the findings in this area suggest that older patients with depression have a better outcome with ECT than do younger patients.

This pattern is unusual in the somatic treatment of major depression. It is also of particular note because most of the work in this area preceded the discovery that the extent to which the intensity of the electrical stimulus in ECT exceeds the patient's seizure threshold greatly influences the efficacy of right unilateral ECT and the speed of response, regardless of electrode placement (Sackeim et al. 1987a, 1991, 1993, 2000). This discovery is of special relevance because age is a reliable but modest predictor of seizure threshold (Beale et al. 1994b; Boylan et al. 2000; Coffey et al. 1995a; Colenda and McCall 1996; Enns and Karvelas 1995; Krueger et al. 1993; Rasmussen et al. 1994; Sackeim et al. 1987b, 1987c; Shapira et al. 1996; Watterson 1945; Weiner 1980), with the oldest patients generally having the highest thresholds. Because in most early ECT studies all patients in a given study received the same fixed electrical dosage, therapeutic response could have been delayed or diminished in elderly patients relative to younger patients. This consideration makes the findings of positive association between patient's age and short-term clinical outcome all the more impressive.

This positive association between patient age and ECT outcome may reflect some of the clinical factors that influence ECT referral and outcome (see Chapter 2). Because of the overrepresentation of medication intolerance, medical complications, and psychotic depression in elderly compared with younger patients, elderly patients treated with ECT often have a shorter duration of current episode and a lower rate of medication resistance. As indicated in Chapter 2, short duration of index episode (Black et al. 1989c; Coryell and Zimmerman 1984; Fraser and Glass 1980; Hobson 1953; Kindler et al. 1991) and absence of medication resistance (Flint and Rifat 1996; Prudic et al. 1990, 1996; Shapira et al. 1996) are consistent predictors of positive ECT outcome. Unlike pharmacotherapy, there is also evidence that patients with delusional or psychotic depression may respond preferentially to ECT (Buchan et al. 1992; Mulsant et al. 1991; Nobler and Sackeim 1996). However, elderly patients with psychotic depression are less likely to be given an adequate medication trial (combined neuroleptic and antidepressant) before receiving ECT (Mulsant et al. 1997). Although this has not been substantiated, the elderly may also have a lower rate of comorbid Axis II pathology, and this factor may also contribute to a superior ECT response rate (Black et al. 1993).

Administration of ECT in the elderly presents certain age-related issues. As indicated, seizure threshold may rise with increasing age, and effective seizures may be difficult to induce (Boylan et al. 2000; Coffey et al. 1995a; Sackeim et al. 1987b). Especially when treated with bilateral ECT, some elderly patients may have seizure thresholds that exceed the maximum output of current-generation ECT devices in the United States (Krystal et al. 2000; Lisanby et al. 1996; Sackeim 1991). In the context of an elevated seizure threshold, the clinician should consider reducing or withdrawing sedative/hypnotic or other anticonvulsant agents (including benzodiazepines), replacing prophylactic lidocaine with another antiarrhythmic medication (Devanand and Sackeim 1988; Hood and Mecca 1983), minimizing doses of barbiturate anesthesia, and ensuring adequate ventilation. In addition, because of altered metabolism in the elderly, dosages of all medications used with ECT may need to be reduced.

In the recent past, preadministration of intravenous caffeine was used to augment ECT in the context of short seizures (Calev et al. 1993; Coffey et al. 1987d, 1990; Hinkle et al. 1987; Shapira et al. 1985, 1987). However, although pretreatment with caffeine lengthens the duration of evoked seizures, it does not appear to reduce seizure threshold (Fochtmann 1994; McCall et al 1993). Because seizure duration per se is not related to the efficacy of ECT (Nobler et al. 1993; Sackeim et al. 1991), the rationale for using caffeine or related agents (Swartz and Lewis 1991) as an augmentation strategy is questionable. In addition, caffeine augmentation of ECT has been associated in rare cases with cardiovascular (Acevedo and Smith 1988; Beale et al. 1994c; Jaffe et al. 1990b) and perhaps other (Enns et al. 1996) adverse effects.

Elderly patients may be at greater risk for more persistent confusion and greater memory deficits during and after ECT treatment. Various retrospective studies have indicated that patient age and medical status are predictors of the development of persistent confusion during the ECT course (Alexopoulos et al. 1984; Burke et al. 1985, 1987; Fraser and Glass 1978, 1980; Gaspar and Samarasinghe 1982; Kramer 1987a; Miller et al. 1986; Tomac et al. 1997). Older patients and those with compromised medical status are at highest risk for prolonged confusion. Relative to younger patients, Zervas et al. (1993) found that older patients with depression had more severe anterograde and retrograde amnesia immediately following the end of the ECT course, with some of these differences persisting at 1-month follow-up. Unfortunately, in this work, a cutoff of 65 years was used for the oldest patients in the sample. Sobin et al. (1995) examined the relationship between preexisting cognitive impairment and the magnitude of retrograde amnesia for autobiographic information immediately and 2 months after the end of an ECT course. In a sample of patients with major depression without known neurologic disease or insult, pre-ECT baseline scores on the modified Mini-Mental State Examination (MMSE) predicted the magnitude of retrograde amnesia at both time points. Patients with global cognitive impairments at pre-ECT baseline manifested the greatest retrograde amnesia following ECT. In this work, both the duration of postictal disorientation and the baseline MMSE score uniquely predicted long-term retrograde amnesia. At 2-month follow-up, patients who had had global cognitive impairment at baseline showed the greatest improvement in MMSE scores, indicating a dissociation between the severity of amnesia and improvement in global cognitive status after ECT.

Elderly patients, particularly those with preexisting cognitive impairment, should be carefully assessed on an ongoing basis for such changes in cognitive status (see Chapter 12). Electrode placement, stimulus intensity, and treatment frequency (e.g., twice instead of three times weekly) should be modified as needed to minimize adverse cognitive effects (see Table 1, Chapter 5).

4.3. Pregnancy and the Puerperium

4.3.1. Pregnancy

Recent case material supports the use of ECT as a treatment with low risk and high efficacy in the management of specific disorders in all three trimesters of pregnancy (Altshuler et al. 1996; Ferrill et al. 1992; Miller 1994; Nurnberg 1989; Oates 1986; Walker and Swartz 1994; Wise et al. 1984; Wisner et al. 1988). In addition, the APA practice guidelines for major depressive disorder and bipolar disorder endorse the safety and efficacy of ECT and suggest ECT as a primary treatment for these disorders during pregnancy (American Psychiatric Association 1993, 1994b). Severe postpartum depressive or manic states, with or without psychosis, are also responsive to ECT (Herzog et al. 1976; Katona 1982; Nonacs et al. 1998; Protheroe 1969; Robinson and Stewart 1986).

During the first trimester of pregnancy, the risk of teratogenicity must be considered when patients require pharmacologic treatment. Teratogenic risks have been identified for benzodiazepines, antipsychotics, lithium, and other mood stabilizers (Altshuler et al. 1996; Delgado-Escueta and Janz 1992; Edlund and Craig 1984; Ferrill et al. 1992; Kuller et al. 1996; McElhatton 1992, 1994; Miller 1998; Nurnberg 1989; Oates 1986; Wisner and Perel 1988). Specific teratogenic risks have not been identified with tricyclic antidepressants and selective serotonin reuptake inhibitors (Chambers et al. 1996; Cohen and Rosenbaum 1998; Cohen et al. 1994; Goldstein et al. 1997; Kulin et al. 1998; Malone and D'Alton 1997; Miller 1998; Pastuszak et al. 1993).

During later stages of pregnancy and particularly near term, neonatal toxicity has been reported with chronic administration of all major classes of psychotropic agents (Cohen and Rosenbaum 1998; Miller 1998). For example, neuroleptics have been associated with tremor, motor restlessness, abnormal movements, and hypertonicity in neonates (Ananth 1976; Auerbach et al. 1992; McElhatton 1992), whereas benzodiazepines have been reported to cause hypotonicity, apnea, and impaired temperature regulation (Altshuler et al. 1996; Ananth 1976; Kanto 1982; McElhatton 1994). Chronic treatment with antidepressants has been associated with anticholinergic symptoms in the neonate as well as withdrawal syndromes consisting of jitteriness, irritability, and convulsions (Altshuler et al. 1996; Ananth 1976; Chambers et al. 1996; Schimmell et al. 1991; Spencer 1993). Use of lithium in the third trimester has been associated with premature labor, polyhydramnios, and neonatal hypothyroidism or lithium toxicity (Altshuler et al. 1996; Ananth 1976; Ang et al. 1990).

From the standpoints of teratogenicity and neonatal toxicity, ECT is considered relatively safe. In treating pregnant patients with ECT, the risks to the fetus from anesthetic agents are likely to be less than those of psychopharmacologic alternatives. Succinylcholine has a relatively low ratio of placental transfer and is not expected to have a major impact on the fetus (Guay et al. 1998; Moya et al. 1961; Wingard and Cook 1977). In the Collaborative Perinatal Project, no fetal abnormalities were noted in the 26 women who received succinylcholine in the first trimester (Heinonen et al. 1977). For methohexital and thiopental, the teratogenic risks are not fully studied (Ferrill et al. 1992; Middaugh 1986), although data from the Collaborative Perinatal Project do not suggest any increase in teratogenesis (Friedman 1988; Heinonen et al. 1977). Also, brief exposures to such agents during ECT are not likely to be problematic, because at ordinary therapeutic doses teratogenesis is largely a function of exposure duration (Shnider et al. 1993). Placental transfer of barbiturates does occur, but the infrequent doses of methohexital used in ECT do not appear to produce neonatal toxicity when used in the third trimester of pregnancy (Elliot et al. 1982; Ferrill et al. 1992). Nonetheless, the informed consent process should include discussions of potential neonatal toxicity and teratogenic effects (see Chapter 8). It should also be kept in mind that lack of effective treatment could adversely affect the health and welfare of both the patient and the fetus (Cohen and Rosenbaum 1998; Coverdale et al. 1996; Miller et al. 1992; Spielvogel and Wile 1992; Wrede et al. 1980).

An obstetrician should be consulted prior to ECT to clarify the risks to the patient and fetus and to suggest any indicated treatment modifications (Oates 1986; Walker and Swartz 1994). Special emphasis should be placed on assessing risk factors for spontaneous abortion, preterm labor, abruption, and uteroplacental insufficiency (Echevarria Moreno et al. 1998; Polster and Wisner 1999; Sherer et al. 1991). To maximize delivery of oxygen to the fetus, patients should be well oxygenated during the ECT (Aldrich et al. 1994). However, hyperventilation should be avoided because this can diminish fetal oxygenation by decreasing placental blood flow and by reducing the dissociation of oxygen from hemoglobin (Cousins 1999; Motoyama et al. 1967). After 20 weeks of gestation, a wedge should be placed under the patient's right hip to displace the uterus from the aorta and vena cava (Aldrich et al. 1995). Before each treatment, intravenous hydration with a non–glucose-containing solution is also suggested.

Because of the increased risks of gastric reflux and possible aspiration, it is suggested that pregnant women be premedicated with a nonparticulate antacid such as sodium citrate. Aspiration risk can also be reduced by administering agents that enhance gastric motility or histamine-2 blockers (Rowe 1997). Of the available agents, cimetidine, ranitidine, and metoclopromide have been used most widely during pregnancy without apparent teratogenicity or fetal toxicity (Katz and Castell 1998; Koren and Zemlickis 1991; Koren et al. 1998; Magee et al. 1996). Beyond 24 weeks of gestation and particularly near term, some practitioners consider intubation with each ECT treatment (Livingston et al. 1994; Walker and Swartz 1994; Wise et al. 1984). However, the risks of aspiration should be weighed against the risks of repeated intubations, both of which are greater in the pregnant patient. Anticholinergic agents decrease the tone of the lower esophageal sphincter and may augment aspiration risk in patients who are not intubated (Shnider and Levinson 1993). When an anticholinergic agent is indicated in the pregnant patient, glycopyrrolate is usually preferable because its placental transfer rate is more limited than that of atropine (Abboud et al. 1983; Ali-Melkkila et al. 1990; Proakis and Harris 1978).

For post-ECT headache and muscle soreness during pregnancy, acetaminophen is the treatment of choice (Koren et al. 1998). Particularly in the third trimester of pregnancy, aspirin and nonsteroidal anti-inflammatory agents should not be administered because they may contribute to altered maternal and fetal hemostasis and to early constriction or closure of the fetal ductus arteriosus (Adverse Drug Reactions Advisory Committee 1998; Ostensen 1998; Pfaffenrath and Rehm 1998; Schoenfeld et al. 1992). Metoclopramide, prochlorperazine, or meclizine can be used for symptomatic treatment of nausea (Broussard and Richter 1998).

When gestational age is more than 14–16 weeks, fetal heart rate should be measured before and after each treatment (Miller 1994; Remick et al. 1987; Walker and Swartz 1994). With near-term and high-risk patients, additional monitoring may be needed so that signs of fetal distress can be detected (Livingston et al. 1994; Sherer et al. 1991; Walker and Swartz 1994; Wise et al. 1984). After 24 weeks and particularly in the context of fetal heart rate abnormalities, some specialists recommend a non-stress test with a tocometer (a 30- to 60-minute fetal heart rate strip) before and after each treatment (Miller 1994; Remick and Maurice 1978; Walker and Swartz 1994). Facilities intending to use ECT in pregnant women should have resources available to deal with obstetric and neonatal emergencies (Bhatia et al. 1999; Miller 1994).

4.3.2. Puerperium

Breastfeeding has clear benefits for the infant as well as for the mother and is an increasingly common form of infant nutrition (American Academy of Pediatrics Work Group on Breastfeeding 1997; Llewellyn and Stowe 1998). In general, breastfeeding need not be interrupted during a course of index or continuation/maintenance ECT. However, the informed consent process should discuss the potential impact of ECT as well as psychopharmacologic treatment alternatives on the breastfed infant (See Chapter 8).

Virtually all known psychotropic agents enter breast milk to some degree (American Academy of Pediatrics Committee on Drugs 1994; Pons et al. 1994). Little systematic data are available on the safety to breastfed infants of psychotropic medications given to the mother

(Llewellyn and Stowe 1998; Yoshida et al. 1999). However, at therapeutic maternal dosages, serum levels of tricyclic antidepressants are generally low or undetectable in the nursing infant (Llewellyn and Stowe 1998; Miller 1998; Pons et al. 1994). Less is known about other antidepressants, antipsychotics, and benzodiazepines, but the American Academy of Pediatrics has categorized these agents as being "of special concern when given to nursing mothers for long periods" (American Academy of Pediatrics Committee on Drugs 1994). In terms of mood-stabilizing agents, valproic acid is compatible with breastfeeding, whereas lithium should be avoided (American Academy of Pediatrics Committee on Drugs 1994; Dillon et al. 1997).

In contrast, anesthetic agents administered with ECT pose little risk to the nursing infant. Infant exposure to succinylcholine is minimal and absorption of succinylcholine from the gastrointestinal tract is poor (Lee and Rubin 1993). For methohexital, the relative infant exposure from breast milk has been estimated to be less than 1% of the maternal dose (Borgatta et al. 1997). The small concentrations of atropine that appear in breast milk are generally safe for the suckling infant (American Academy of Pediatrics Committee on Drugs 1994), but some infants have exhibited sensitivity to the toxic effects of anticholinergic medications (Dillon et al. 1997).

Other medications administered during ECT may also be excreted into breast milk. Consequently, the indications for such medications and their potential effects on the nursing infant should be evaluated prior to administration. Of the histamine-2 receptor antagonists, cimetidine is recommended during breastfeeding (American Academy of Pediatrics Committee on Drugs 1994), although newer agents may have less secretion into breast milk (Hagemann 1998). Antihypertensive agents compatible with breastfeeding include β-adrenergic receptor antagonists (propranolol, labetalol, metoprolol, and atenolol), angiotensin-converting enzyme inhibitors (captopril and enalapril), and the peripheral vasodilator hydralazine (American Academy of Pediatrics Committee on Drugs 1994). Acetaminophen, codeine, or nonsteroidal anti-inflammatory drugs may be used to treat headache or muscle soreness after ECT (Dillon et al. 1997; Lee and Rubin 1993). Aspirin is contraindicated because of its association with Reye's syndrome in children (Unsworth et al. 1987).

In general, exposure of breastfeeding infants to medications may be lessened if the mother delays the feeding for a period of several hours after an ECT treatment. Another strategy is to collect and store the breast milk prior to ECT for administration by bottle during the 24-hour period after an ECT treatment.

4.4. Children and Adolescents

Few studies address the use of ECT in children and adolescents (Fink and Coffey 1998; Kellner et al. 1998; Rey and Walter 1997; Walter et al. 1999b). ECT is only rarely used in such patients because affective syndromes in children and adolescents often go unrecognized, because child and adolescent psychiatrists tend to lack knowledge about the use of ECT in this population (Walter et al. 1997), and because of concerns that induced seizures may have greater sequelae in a developing nervous system. First-line use of ECT in children and adolescents is particularly rare. Despite this low utilization, evidence indicates that when an affective disorder is well defined, the response to ECT is likely to be favorable (Bertagnoli and Borchardt 1990; Cohen et al. 1997; Ghaziuddin et al. 1996; Guttmacher and Cretella 1988; Hill et al. 1997; Moise and Petrides 1996; Rey and Walter 1997; Walter and Rey 1997; Walter et al. 1999a, 1999b; Willoughby et al. 1997).

Each institution should have policies for the use of ECT in minors, including those pertaining to informed consent. These policies should be compatible with applicable state and federal regulations, particularly with regard to the circumstances under which such individuals should be considered adults for the purposes of consent for medical procedures (see Chapter 8). ECT treatment should be provided with the concurrence of two consultants experienced in treating psychiatric disorders of children. These consultants should deliver their opinion only after interviewing the patient and family or other collateral sources, reviewing the clinical record, and discussing the case with the patient's attending physician. The consent process, including discussion of the risks and benefits of ECT, should involve the parents or guardians of the child. Given a more substantial literature documenting the safety and efficacy of ECT in adolescents (Cohen et al. 1997, 2000; Moise and Petrides 1996; Schneekloth et al. 1993; Strober et al. 1998), one consultant should suffice for this age group.

Stimulus dosing must take into account the fact that seizure thresholds in children and adolescents are likely to be considerably lower than those in adults (Cohen et al. 1997; Fink 1993; Fink and Coffey 1998; Kellner et al. 1998). Use of empirical dose titration with low initial dosage settings is particularly encouraged in this age group (see Section 11.7). In addition, because of the possibly increased likelihood of prolonged seizures in children and adolescents (Bertagnoli and Borchardt 1990; Ghaziuddin et al. 1996; Walter and Rey 1997), the treatment team should be prepared to intervene with appropriate medication to terminate the seizure (see Section 11.9.3).

Comprehensive guidelines for the use of ECT in adolescents are presently under development by the American Academy of Child and Adolescent Psychiatry.

RECOMMENDATIONS

4.1. Concurrent Medical Illness

4.1.1. General Considerations

a. The decision to administer ECT should include consideration of the anticipated impact of the patient's medical status, including present medical treatments, on the risks and benefits of ECT (see Chapter 3).

b. Pre-ECT evaluation of medical conditions should include pertinent laboratory tests and specialist consultation when indicated to clarify the presence and optimize the treatment of coexisting medical illnesses, elucidate their impact on the risks and benefits of ECT, and suggest potential means of minimizing adverse effects (see Chapter 6).

c. The presence and implications of conditions associated with significantly increased risk should be included in the informed consent process (see Chapter 5).

d. To lower morbidity or augment efficacy, the ECT procedure should be modified when indicated. Such modifications may include changing ECT technique, altering pharmacologic regimens, administering ECT in a different hospital or clinic location, and using additional medical specialists or monitoring procedures.

4.1.2. Neurologic Disorders

a. Patients with increased intracranial pressure have substantially elevated risk with ECT; its use must be justified in terms of risk/benefit considerations. To diminish risk for such patients, treatment modifications should be considered, such as the use of potent antihypertensive agents, steroids, diuretics, and hyperventilation.

b. Short-acting antihypertensive agents should be considered at the time of ECT in patients at risk for hemorrhagic cerebrovascular events (e.g., aneurysms, arteriovenous malformations).

c. Care should be taken to avoid hypotension in patients with ischemic cerebrovascular disease who are receiving ECT.

d. Although certain neurologic conditions may be associated with an increased severity of cognitive dysfunction during and immediately after ECT (e.g., dementia, brain trauma, Parkinson's disease, multiple sclerosis), ECT is not contraindicated in these conditions.

e. In patients with epilepsy, dosage of anticonvulsant agents should be optimized to maintain effective seizure control yet still permit adequate seizure induction with ECT.

f. In patients with Parkinson's disease, dosage of dopaminergic agents should be optimized to maintain control of motor symptoms while also adjusting for increased dopaminergic effects with ECT.

g. Patients who have a history of NMS but no or mild active symptoms do not generally require modification of the ECT procedure other than avoiding neuroleptic medications. If more substantial symptoms of NMS are present, nondepolarizing muscle relaxants should be considered at the time of ECT, particularly if extensive or severe muscular rigidity is present. Such patients should also be observed for metabolic and cardiovascular instability.

4.1.3. Cardiovascular Disorders

a. Consultation with a physician who has expertise in the assessment and treatment of cardiovascular diseases should be considered if the pre-ECT evaluation suggests significantly increased cardiovascular risk. Conditions associated with increased risk include (but are not limited to) coronary artery disease, active angina, congestive heart failure, valvular heart disease, vascular aneurysms, uncontrolled hypertension, high-grade atrioventricular block, symptomatic ventricular arrhythmias, and supraventricular arrhythmias with uncontrolled ventricular rate. For such patients, the treatment team should request both an evaluation of the risk of the specific conditions and suggestions, if any, for clinical management as well as risk reduction. The team should not request "clearance" for ECT (see Chapter 6). Consultation should also be considered for patients with demand pacemakers or implanted defibrillators during ECT .

b. All patients referred for ECT who have clinically significant cardiovascular disease should have an ECG, a chest radiograph, and measurement of serum electrolytes as part of the pre-ECT evaluation. Functional cardiac imaging study should be considered if specifically indicated by history or physical examination (see Chapter 6).

c. Unstable cardiovascular disease should be stabilized as much as possible prior to ECT.

d. When standing and PRN cardiovascular medications are likely to decrease the risks of ECT, they should be continued prior to and during the ECT course, including administration of scheduled doses before ECT on treatment days (see Chapter 7).

e. Additional short-acting cardiovascular medications, including anticholinergics, sympatholytics, nitrates, and other antihypertensive agents, should be considered at the time of ECT if there are specific reasons to believe they will decrease risks (see Section 11.4.4). Care should be taken to avoid iatrogenic hypotensive effects. Whenever possible, systemic lidocaine should be avoided until after the induced seizure.

4.1.4. Other Disorders

a. Patients with unstable or insulin-dependent diabetes mellitus should be considered for medical consultation before ECT to help ensure appropriate adjustments in diabetic management, particularly with respect to the period of pre-ECT fasting. Diabetic conditions should be stabilized as much as possible before treatment. To help prevent hypoglycemia, fingerstick glucose monitoring should be done within an hour before each treatment.

b. Patients with clinically significant hyperthyroidism should receive specialty consultation prior to ECT and should receive β-blocking agents before each treatment unless otherwise contraindicated.

c. Specialty consultation should be used to help assess risk/benefit considerations for patients with pheochromocytoma who are referred for ECT. If ECT is to be administered, pharmacologic means should be used to diminish risk.

d. Patients with steroid dependence may need an increased dose of steroid prior to each treatment.

e. Clinically significant hyperkalemia, hypokalemia, and hyponatremia should be corrected prior to ECT if possible. Patients at risk for hyperkalemia during ECT should receive a nondepolarizing muscle relaxant instead of succinylcholine.

f. Patients with porphyria should receive a nonbarbiturate anesthetic during ECT.

g. Patients with chronic obstructive pulmonary disorder or asthma should get adequate doses of bronchodilator medication before ECT and, if clinically indicated, during the post-ECT recovery period. However, theophylline should be discontinued or its level should be kept as low as clinically feasible.

h. Patients at risk for esophageal reflux should receive medication before each ECT treatment to diminish the risk of aspiration.

i. Urinary retention should be avoided during ECT.

j. An increased dosage of muscle relaxant should be considered in patients with clinically significant bone or joint disease.

k. Unstable or loose teeth should be either removed or specially protected during each ECT treatment (see Section 11.3).

l. Patients with glaucoma should receive any prescribed ophthalmic medication before each ECT treatment, with the exception of long-acting anticholinesterase agents.

m. Patients with recent or evolving retinal detachment should undergo ophthalmologic consultation prior to ECT to establish risk and to determine means to diminish morbidity.

4.2. Elderly

a. ECT may be used with the elderly, regardless of age.

b. The efficacy of ECT does not diminish with advancing age and may be enhanced.

c. All somatic treatments, including ECT, are associated with increased risk in the elderly, particularly those with concurrent physical illness. However, clinical experience suggests that ECT may have a lower risk of complications than some forms of pharmacotherapy among the elderly.

d. Doses of anticholinergic, anesthetic, and relaxant agents may need to be modified based on the physiologic changes associated with aging.

e. ECT stimulus intensity should be selected with an awareness that seizure threshold generally increases with age.

f. Decisions about ECT technique should be guided by the possibility that ECT-induced cognitive dysfunction may be greater in elderly patients, particularly those with preexisting cognitive or neurologic impairment.

4.3. Pregnancy and the Puerperium

4.3.1. Pregnancy

a. ECT may be used in all three trimesters of pregnancy and during the puerperium.
b. In pregnant patients, obstetric consultation should be obtained prior to ECT.
c. The risks of ECT anesthetic agents to the fetus are likely to be less than the risks of alternative pharmacologic treatments for psychiatric disorders and also less than the risks of untreated mental illness. Nonetheless, potential teratogenic effects and neonatal toxicities should be discussed in the informed consent process.
d. Pregnant patients should be well oxygenated but not hyperventilated during ECT.
e. The risk of aspiration is increased in pregnant patients and should be assessed on an individual basis. Modifications in ECT procedure should be considered in order to diminish this risk and may include withholding anticholinergic agents; administering nonparticulate antacids, gastrointestinal motility enhancing agents, or histamine-2 blockers; or endotracheal intubation.
f. Medications used to minimize the risk of aspiration or for symptomatic treatment of nausea, headache, or muscle soreness should be appropriate for use during pregnancy.
g. Intravenous hydration with a non–glucose-containing solution is suggested before each ECT treatment.
h. When gestational age is more than 14–16 weeks, noninvasive monitoring of fetal heart rate should be done before and after each ECT treatment.
i. After 20 weeks of gestation, uterine blood flow should be optimized by placing a wedge under the patient's right hip to displace the uterus from the aorta and vena cava.
j. If the pregnancy is high risk or close to term, additional monitoring may be indicated at the time of ECT.
k. At facilities administering ECT to pregnant women, resources for managing obstetric and neonatal emergencies should be readily accessible.

4.3.2. Puerperium

a. Breastfeeding does not usually need to be interrupted during an index or continuation/maintenance course of ECT. However, the informed consent process should include a discussion of the potential risks to the infant of breastfeeding during the ECT course.
b. Anesthetic agents administered with ECT generally pose little risk to the nursing infant.
c. Because other medications given during ECT may be excreted into breast milk, the indications for such medications and their potential effects on the nursing infant should be evaluated before they are administered.
d. Infant medication exposure from breastfeeding immediately after an ECT treatment may be lessened by delaying feeding for several hours or by collecting and storing breast milk for administration by bottle.

4.4. Children and Adolescents

a. In children and adolescents, ECT should be reserved for instances in which other viable treatments have not been effective or cannot be safely administered.
b. Use of ECT in children and adolescents should be limited to the diagnostic indications described in Chapter 2.
c. For children under the age of 13, concurrence with the recommendation for ECT should be provided by two consultants who are experienced in the treatment of children. For adolescents, concurrence needs to be provided by only a single consultant.
d. Stimulus dosing should take into account the likelihood of lower seizure thresholds in children and adolescents.
e. Each facility offering ECT for children or adolescents should have policies covering the use of ECT, including informed consent, in this patient population.

CHAPTER 5

Adverse Effects

5.1. General Issues

Precise rates of mortality attributable to ECT are difficult to determine because of methodologic issues intrinsic to studies of medical mortality, such as uncertainty about cause of death, the time frame for linking death to ECT, and variability in reporting requirements. The rate of mortality attributed to ECT is estimated to be approximately the same as that associated with minor surgery (Badrinath et al. 1995; Brand et al. 1994; Hall et al. 1997; McCabe 1985; Warner et al. 1993) or childbirth (Salanave et al. 1999). Published estimates from large and diverse patient series over several decades report up to 4 deaths per 100,000 treatments (Abrams 1997b; Babigian and Guttmacher 1984; Crowe 1984; Fink 1979; Heshe and Röder 1976; Kramer 1985; Reid et al. 1998; Weiner 1979). Despite the frequent use of ECT in elderly patients or those with significant medical complications (Sackeim 1993, 1998; Weiner et al. 2000), the mortality rate appears to have decreased in recent years. A reasonable current estimate is that the rate of ECT-related mortality is 1 per 10,000 patients or 1 per 80,000 treatments. This rate may be higher in patients with severe medical conditions. The rate of significant morbidity and mortality is believed to be lower with ECT than with some types of antidepressant medication (e.g., tricyclics) (Sackeim 1998). Some evidence from longitudinal follow-up studies has shown that mortality rates following hospitalization are lower among depressed patients who received ECT than among patients who received other treatment modalities or no treatment (Avery and Winokur 1976; Philibert et al. 1995), although there is also a report that found no advantage for ECT (Black et al. 1989b).

To some extent, medical adverse events can be anticipated. Patients with preexisting cardiac illness, compromised pulmonary status, a history of brain insult, or medical complications after earlier courses of anesthesia or ECT are especially likely to be at increased risk (Weiner and Coffey 1988; Zieliniski et al. 1993). Whenever possible, the risks of medical adverse events should be minimized by optimizing the patient's medical condition prior to ECT or by modifying ECT procedures. ECT psychiatrists should review the medical work-up and history of prospective ECT patients (see Chapter 6). Specialist consultations, additional laboratory studies, or changes in medication regimens may be indicated. In spite of careful pre-ECT evaluation, medical complications may arise that have not been anticipated. ECT facilities should be appropriately equipped and staffed with personnel to manage potential clinical emergencies (see Chapters 9 and 10). Because cardiovascular complications are the most likely source of significant medical adverse events and occur most frequently in the immediate postictal period, the treatment team should be capable of managing the major classes of cardiovascular complications, including cardiac arrest, arrhythmias, ischemia, hypertension, and hypotension. It is also helpful to have a predetermined set of procedures for dealing with instances of prolonged apnea, prolonged or spontaneous (tardive) seizures, and status epilepticus.

Major adverse events that occur during or soon after the ECT course should be documented in the patient's medical record. Documentation should delineate the steps taken to manage the event, including consultation with a specialist, use of additional procedures, and administration of medications.

5.2. Cardiovascular Complications

When mortality occurs with ECT, it typically happens immediately after the seizure or during the postictal recovery period. Cardiovascular and pulmonary complications are the leading cause of death and of significant morbidity (Burke et al. 1987; Pitts 1982; Rice et al. 1994; Welch and Drop 1989; Zielinski et al. 1993). Despite the short-lived increases in cerebral blood flow and intracranial pressure, cerebrovascular complications are notably rare (Hsiao et al. 1987). Given the high rate of cardiac arrhythmias in the immediate postictal period, most of which are benign and resolve spontaneously, electrocardiograms (ECGs) should be monitored during and immediately after the procedure (see Section 11.8.3). Vital signs (pulse and systolic and diastolic pressure) should be stable before the patient leaves the recovery area (Section 11.10). Patients with preexisting cardiac illness are at greater risk for post-ECT cardiac complications (Prudic et al. 1987; Rice et al. 1994; Zielinski et al. 1993). Indeed, evidence has indicated that the type of preexisting cardiac disease predicts the type of complication that may be encountered after ECT (Zielinski et al. 1993). Management of cardiac complications is discussed in Chapter 11.

5.3. Prolonged Seizures

Two other possible sources of morbidity are prolonged seizures (seizures lasting longer than 3 minutes) and status epilepticus (continuous seizure activity lasting longer than 30 minutes or two or more seizures occurring without return of consciousness between seizure activity) (Engel 1989; Working Group on Status Epilepticus 1993). Management of prolonged seizures is described in Section 11.9.3. Failure to terminate seizures within a period of 3–5 minutes may increase postictal confusion and amnesia. Inadequate oxygenation during prolonged seizures increases the risk of hypoxia and cerebral dysfunction as well as cardiovascular complications. In animal studies, seizure activity sustained for periods exceeding 30–60 minutes is associated with an increased risk of structural brain damage and cardiovascular and cardiopulmonary complications, regardless of steps taken to maintain appropriate levels of blood gases (Devanand et al. 1994; Ingvar 1986; Meldrum 1986; Meldrum et al. 1974; O'Connell et al. 1988; Siesjö et al. 1986).

Prolonged seizures and status epilepticus may be more likely in patients receiving medications or having medical conditions that lower seizure threshold or interfere with seizure termination. These situations include use of theophylline, even at therapeutic levels (Abrams 1997a; Devanand et al. 1988a; Fink and Sackeim 1998; Peters et al. 1984); preexisting electrolyte imbalance (Finlayson et al. 1989); repeated induction of seizures within the same treatment session (e.g., multiple monitored ECT) (Maletzky 1981; Strain and Bidder 1971); and possibly concomitant lithium therapy (Weiner et al. 1980b).

Nonconvulsive status epilepticus may also occur in the interictal period, with an abrupt onset of delirium, unresponsiveness, or agitation as distinguishing clinical features (Grogan et al. 1995; Solomons et al. 1998). Cessation of abnormalities on electroencephalogram (EEG) and improved cognitive function after short-acting anticonvulsant treatment (e.g., intravenous lorazepam or diazepam) may prove diagnostic (Weiner and Krystal 1993).

Whether the rate of seizure disorder is increased after the course of ECT has raised some concern (Assael et al. 1967; Devinsky and Duchowny 1983). Evidence indicates, however, that the rate of occurrence of such events is extremely low and probably not different from population base rates (Blackwood et al. 1980; Small et al. 1981).

Rarely, patients may have a spontaneous seizure that occurs within hours of an ECT treatment. These events have been referred to as tardive seizures. No data are available about rates of tardive seizures. As noted in Section 11.9.3, prolonged or tardive seizures occurring during the immediate postictal period are often not accompanied by motor manifestations, underscoring the need for EEG seizure monitoring (Parker et al. 2000; Rao et al. 1993). As with status epilepticus, when a tardive seizure occurs, the practitioner should investigate its etiology.

5.4. Prolonged Apnea

Prolonged postictal apnea is a rare event that occurs primarily in patients who have slow metabolism of succinylcholine (Packman et al. 1978) (see Section 11.4.3). Maintaining adequate oxygenation is critical in instances of prolonged apnea, which will usually resolve spontaneously within 30–60 minutes. When prolonged apnea is encountered, it is helpful to determine etiology by obtaining a dibucaine number assay or a pseudocholinesterase level to establish etiology before the next treatment. At subsequent treatments, either a very low dose of succinylcholine may be used or a nondepolarizing muscle relaxant, such as atracurium, may be substituted (Hickey et al. 1987; Hicks 1987; Kramer and Afrasiabi 1991; Lui et al. 1993; Stack et al. 1988).

Rarely, patients may be partially conscious while paralyzed. This experience can be frightening and results from an insufficient dose of the anesthetic agent or an insufficient interval between administration of the anesthetic and muscle relaxant. For this reason, it is preferable to establish onset of the anesthetic effect before administering the muscle relaxant (see Section 11.4.3).

5.5. Headache, Muscle Soreness, and Nausea

Headache is a common side effect of ECT and is observed in as many as 45% of patients during and shortly after the postictal recovery period

(Devanand et al. 1995; Freeman and Kendell 1980; Gomez 1975; Sackeim et al. 1987d; Tubi et al. 1993; Weiner et al. 1994). However, the precise incidence of post-ECT headache is difficult to determine because of methodologic issues, including the high baseline (pre-ECT) occurrence of headache in patients with depression, the potential effects of concurrent medication or medication withdrawal, and differences in headache assessment across studies. Post-ECT headache appears to be particularly common in younger patients (Devanand et al. 1995), especially children and adolescents (Rey and Walter 1997; Walter and Rey 1997). It is not known whether preexisting headache syndromes (e.g., migraine) increase the risk of post-ECT headache, but ECT may exacerbate a previous headache condition (Weiner et al. 1994). Occurrence of post-ECT headache does not appear to be related to stimulus electrode placement (at least bifrontotemporal vs. right unilateral) (Devanand et al. 1995; Fleminger et al. 1970; Sackeim et al. 1987d; Tubi et al. 1993), stimulus dosage (Devanand et al. 1995), or therapeutic response to ECT (Devanand et al. 1995; Sackeim et al. 1987d).

In most patients, post-ECT headache is mild (Freeman and Kendell 1980; Sackeim et al. 1987d), although a sizable minority report severe pain associated with nausea and vomiting. Typically the headache is frontal in location with a throbbing character.

The etiology of post-ECT headache is not known. Its throbbing character suggests a similarity to vascular headache, and ECT may be associated with a temporary change in headache quality from muscle contraction type to vascular type (Weiner et al. 1994; Weinstein 1993). Indeed, ECT upregulates $5\text{-}HT_2$ receptors, and $5\text{-}HT_2$ receptor sensitization has been associated with development of vascular headache (Weiner et al. 1994). Other suggested mechanisms include electrically induced temporalis muscle spasm or an acute increase in blood pressure and cerebral blood flow (Abrams 1997a; Weiner et al. 1994). It is also possible that nitrates used to control blood pressure during ECT contribute to post-ECT headache (Cleophas et al. 1996; Lewis et al. 1999; Tassorelli et al. 1999).

Treatment of post-ECT headache is symptomatic. Aspirin, acetaminophen, and the nonsteroidal anti-inflammatory drugs (NSAIDs) typically are highly effective, particularly if given promptly after the onset of pain. Sumatriptan, a serotonin $5HT_{1D}$ receptor agonist, has also been effective at doses of 6 mg subcutaneously (DeBattista and Mueller 1995) or 25–100 mg orally (Fantz et al. 1998). Some patients require more potent analgesics (e.g., codeine), although narcotics may produce nausea, reduce respiratory effort, and delay recovery. Most patients also benefit from bed rest in a quiet, darkened environment.

Post-ECT headache may occur after any ECT treatment in a course, regardless of its occurrence at any prior treatment. Patients who experience frequent post-ECT headaches may benefit from prophylactic treatment such as aspirin, acetaminophen, or NSAIDs (e.g., intravenous ketorolac) given as soon as possible after ECT or even immediately before the ECT treatment. In a patient with severe refractory post-ECT headache, 6 mg subcutaneous sumatriptan given several minutes before ECT was also found to provide effective prophylaxis (DeBattista and Mueller 1995).

Some patients report general muscle soreness following ECT. These complaints are most common after the first treatment, and may not be reported subsequently. Muscle soreness due to intense fasciculations following administration of a depolarizing muscle relaxant (succinylcholine) can be alleviated at subsequent treatments by blocking the fasciculations with a nondepolarizing agent, as described in Section 11.4.3. Alternatively, muscle soreness due to excessively vigorous convulsive movements should be managed with an increase in the dose of muscle relaxant. In either case, muscle soreness can be treated symptomatically with analgesic agents such as aspirin, acetaminophen, or NSAIDs.

The ECT stimulus results in direct stimulation of the pterygoid, masseter, and temporalis muscles. Nerves in these muscles are depolarized, producing a clamping action of the jaw not attenuated by the muscle relaxant (Minneman 1995). Firm pressure, ensuring closure of the teeth around the bite-block, may minimize jaw pain. Such pain can be treated with aspirin, acetaminophen, or NSAIDs.

Estimates of the prevalence of nausea after ECT vary from 1% to 23% of patients (Gomez 1975; Sackeim et al. 1987d), but as with headache, methodologic issues make the incidence difficult to quantify. Nausea may occur secondary to headache or its treatment with narcotics, particularly in patients with vascular-type headache. Nausea may also occur independently as a side effect of anesthesia, because of the withdrawal or institution of psychotropic medications, or by other unknown mechanisms. When nausea accompanies the headache, the primary treatment should focus on the relief of the headache as outlined above. Otherwise, post-ECT nausea is typically well controlled with dopamine-blocking agents such as phenothiazine derivatives (e.g., prochlorperazine and others), butyrophenones (haloperidol, droperidol), trimethabenzamide, or metoclopramide. If nausea is severe or accompanied by vomiting, these agents should be administered parenterally or by suppository. All of these agents have the potential to cause hypotension and motoric side effects and lower seizure threshold. If nausea does not respond to these treatments or if side effects are problematic, the serotonin 5-HT$_3$ receptor antagonists ondansetron and dolasetron may be useful alternatives. These medications may be given in a single intravenous dose of 4 mg or 12.5 mg, respectively, several minutes before or after ECT. Routine use of 5-HT$_3$ receptor antagonists may be limited by their greater expense and lack of proven superiority over traditional antiemetics in the setting of ECT. If problematic nausea routinely follows the use of a particular anesthetic, an alternative anesthetic agent may be considered.

5.6. Treatment-Emergent Mania

As with pharmacologic antidepressant treatments, a small minority of patients with depression or those in mixed affective states switch into hypomania or mania during the ECT course (Andrade et al. 1988b, 1990; Angst et al. 1992; Devanand et al. 1988b, 1992). Although this reaction is rare, patients with bipolar disorder may be the most likely to exhibit it. In some patients, the severity of manic symptoms may worsen with further ECT treatments. In such cases, it is important to distinguish treatment-emergent manic symptoms from delirium with euphoria (Devanand et al. 1988b). These two conditions have a number of phenomenologic similarities. However, in delirium with euphoria, patients are typically confused and have pronounced memory disturbance. Confusion or disorientation should be continuously present and evident from the period immediately following the treatment. In contrast, hypomanic or manic symptoms may occur in the context of a clear sensorium. Therefore, evaluating cognitive status may be particularly helpful in distinguishing between these states. In addition, states of delirium with euphoria are often characterized by a giddiness in mood or a carefree disposition, whereas the classical features of hypomania such as racing thoughts, hypersexuality, irritability, and others may be absent. In delirium with euphoria, resolution of the condition may be facilitated by increasing the time between treatments, decreasing the stimulus intensity, or changing from bilateral to unilateral electrode placement.

No established strategy exists for managing manic symptoms that emerge during the ECT course. Some practitioners continue ECT in order to treat both the mania and any residual depressive symptoms. Other practitioners postpone further ECT and observe the patient's course. At times, manic symptoms remit spontaneously without further intervention. If the mania persists or the patient relapses into depression, reinstitution of ECT may be considered. However, other practitioners terminate the ECT course and treat manic symptoms by starting pharmacotherapy, often with lithium carbonate or other mood stabilizer or antipsychotic medication.

5.7. Postictal Delirium

At one or more treatments, a minority of patients develop postictal delirium or excitement (Devanand et al. 1989) characterized by motor agitation, disorientation, and poor response to commands. For some patients, postictal delirium may occur at one or two treatments and never recur, or it may be manifested at all treatments. Recovery may take from 5 to 45 minutes, and patients are usually amnestic for the episode. Postictal delirium may result in physical injury either to a patient who thrashes against hard objects or to staff members who attempt to protect the patient. In addition, patients may dislodge the intravenous line, complicating management. Depending on severity, postictal delirium may be managed supportively or pharmacologically. Pharmacologic prophylaxis should be considered for patients who repeatedly manifest postictal delirium. Methods to manage postictal delirium are described in Section 11.10.3.

5.8. Cognitive Side Effects

5.8.1. Objective Effects

Cognitive side effects produced by ECT have been the subject of intense investigation (McElhiney et al. 1995; Sackeim 1992; Squire 1986) and are the major complications limiting its use. ECT psychiatrists should be familiar with the nature and variability of cognitive side effects, and this information should be conveyed during the consent process (see Chapter 8).

The cognitive side effects of ECT have four essential features. First, the type and severity of cognitive alterations change rapidly with time following each treatment. The most severe cognitive side effects are observed in the postictal period. Immediately after seizure induction, patients experience a variable but usually brief period of disorientation with impairments in attention, praxis, and memory (Sackeim 1986). These deficits recede at variable rates over time. Consequently, the magnitude of deficits observed during the course of ECT is a function, in part, of the time of assessment relative to the last treatment as well as the number of treatments received (Daniel and Crovitz 1983a; Squire et al. 1985).

Second, the methods used in ECT administration have a profound impact on the nature and magnitude of cognitive deficits. For example, ECT treatment technique is a major determinant of the percentage of patients who develop delirium characterized by continuous disorientation (Daniel and Crovitz 1986; Miller et al. 1986; Sackeim et al. 1986, 1993). In general, as summarized in Table 5–1, bilateral electrode placement, sine wave stimulation, high electrical dosage relative to seizure threshold, closely spaced treatments, larger numbers of treatments, and high dosage of barbiturate anesthetic agents are each independently associated with more intense cognitive side effects compared with right unilateral electrode placement, brief pulse waveform, lower electrical intensity, more widely spaced treatments, fewer treatments, and lower dosage of barbiturate anesthesia (Lerer et al. 1995; Lisanby et al. 2000; McElhiney et al. 1995; Miller et al. 1985; Sackeim et al. 1986, 1993, 2000; Weiner et al. 1986b). Optimization of these parameters can minimize short-term cognitive side effects and likely reduce the magnitude of long-term changes (Sackeim et al. 2000; Sobin et al. 1995). In patients who develop severe cognitive side effects such as delirium (Miller et al. 1986; Mulsant et al. 1991; Summers et al. 1979), the attending physician and ECT psychiatrist should review and adjust the treatment technique being used. Such modification may include switching to unilateral ECT, lowering the electrical dose administered, increasing the time interval between treatments and decreasing the dose, or discontinuing any medications that may exacerbate cognitive side effects.

Third, patients vary considerably in the extent and severity of their cognitive side effects following ECT. Available information about the factors that contribute to these individual differences is limited. Among depressed patients without known neurologic disease or insult, evidence has indicated that the extent of pre-ECT global cognitive impairment (as measured by Mini-Mental State Exam [MMSE] scores) predicts the magnitude of retrograde amnesia for autobiographic information at

Table 5–1. *Treatment factors that may increase or decrease the severity of adverse cognitive side effects*

Treatment factor	Associated with increased cognitive side effects	Steps to be taken to reduce cognitive side effects
Stimulus waveform	Sine wave	Change to brief pulse
Electrode placement	Bilateral	Change to right unilateral
Stimulus intensity	Grossly suprathreshold	Decrease electrical dose
Spacing of treatments	ECT administered 3–5 times per week	Decrease frequency or stop ECT
Number of seizures per session	Multiple (two or more) seizures per session	Change to a single seizure per session
Concomitant psychotropic medications	Lithium or agents with independent adverse cognitive effects	Reduce dose or stop psychotropics
Anesthetic medications	High dose may contribute to amnesia	Reduce dose as appropriate for light level of anesthesia

long-term follow-up. In these patients, ECT typically results in improved global cognitive status as a function of symptomatic response. Nonetheless, these same patients may have greater persistent amnesia for personal memories (Sobin et al. 1995). Similarly, evidence has shown that the duration of disorientation immediately after ECT treatment is an independent predictor of the magnitude of retrograde amnesia for autobiographic information. Patients who require prolonged periods in order to recover their orientation may be at greater risk for more profound and persistent retrograde amnesia (Sobin et al. 1995). Patients who have preexisting neurologic disease or insult (e.g., Alzheimer's disease, Parkinson's disease, stroke) may also have an increased risk of ECT-induced delirium and memory deficits (Figiel et al. 1991; Mulsant et al. 1991). Magnetic resonance imaging findings of basal ganglia lesions and severe white matter hyperintensities have also been linked to the development of an ECT-induced delirium (Figiel et al. 1990). Some medications may exacerbate ECT-induced cognitive side effects, including lithium carbonate (Small et al. 1980; Weiner et al. 1980b) and medications with marked anticholinergic properties, particularly in elderly patients.

Fourth, ECT results in highly characteristic cognitive changes. Across diagnostic groups and prior to receiving ECT, many patients have deficits in attention and concentration that limit their capacity to learn new information (Byrne 1977; Pogue-Geile and Oltmanns 1980; Sackeim and Steif 1988; Zakzanis et al. 1998). For example, patients with severe psychopathology often have deficient recall of information just presented to them (immediate memory). In patients with depression, these deficits are most marked for unstructured material that requires effortful processing in order to impose organization (Burt et al. 1995; Roy-Byrne et al. 1986; Weingartner and Silberman 1984). However, such patients are less likely to have deficits in retaining new information that they do learn (delayed memory) (Cronholm and Ottosson 1961; Steif et al. 1986; Sternberg and Jarvik 1976). During the ECT course, deficits in attention and concentration may be accentuated (Calev et al. 1995; Sackeim et al. 1992b). In contrast, with symptomatic improvement following ECT these deficits usually resolve. Consequently, measures of immediate memory are either unchanged or improved within a few days of ECT termination (Cronholm and Ottosson 1961; Rossi et al. 1990; Sackeim et al. 1993, 2000; Steif et al. 1986; Weiner et al. 1986b).

Because attention and concentration are essential to many aspects of cognitive function, it is not surprising that shortly after completion of the ECT course improvement may be observed in a wide variety of neuropsychologic domains, including global cognitive status (Sackeim et al. 1993; Sobin et al. 1995) and measures of general intelligence (IQ) (Huston and Strother 1948; Malloy et al. 1982; Sackeim et al. 1992a; Squire et al. 1975; Stieper et al. 1951). There is no evidence that ECT results in lasting impairments of executive functions (e.g., the capacity to shift mental sets), abstract reasoning, creativity, semantic memory, implicit memory, or skill acquisition or retention (Frith et al. 1983; Jones et al. 1988; Squire et al. 1984; Taylor and Abrams 1985; Weeks et al. 1980).

Against this background of unchanged or improved neuropsychologic performance, ECT selectively results in anterograde and retrograde amnesia. The anterograde amnesia is characterized by rapid forgetting of newly learned information (Cronholm and Ottosson 1961; Frith et al. 1987; Sackeim et al. 1993; Squire 1986; Steif et al. 1986; Weiner et al. 1986b). As noted, compared with pre-ECT baseline, patients tested a few days after ECT may recall more items from a list that was just presented. However, recall after a delay is often impaired (Calev et al. 1989; Cronholm and Molander 1964; Cronholm and Ottosson 1961; d'Elia 1976; Korin et al. 1956; Robertson and Inglis 1978; Sackeim et al. 1993; Squire and Chace 1975; Squire and Miller 1974; Steif et al. 1986; Weiner et al. 1986b). The extent and persistence of this rapid forgetting of newly learned information varies among patients and should be considered when making recommendations for the post-ECT convalescence period. Until the patient's anterograde amnesia substantially resolves, returning to work, making important financial or personal decisions, or driving may need to be restricted. Following termination of ECT, the anterograde amnesia rapidly resolves. Indeed, no study has documented anterograde amnestic effects of ECT more than a few weeks after the ECT course (Bidder et al. 1970; Fraser and Glass 1980; Frith et al. 1983; Gangadhar et al. 1982; Heshe et al. 1978; Jackson 1978; Sackeim et al. 1993; Strain et al. 1968; Weeks et al. 1980; Weiner et al. 1986b). It is unlikely that ECT has any long-term effect on the capacity to learn and retain new information.

Following ECT, patients also display retrograde amnesia. Deficits in recalling both personal (autobiographic) and public information are usually evident and are typically greatest for events that occurred temporally closest to the treatment (Cronholm and Molander 1961; Janis 1950; McElhiney et al. 1995; Sackeim et al. 1986, 1993, 2000; Squire 1975; Squire et al. 1975, 1976, 1981; Strain et al. 1968; Weeks et al. 1980, Weiner et al. 1986b). The magnitude of the retrograde amnesia is greatest immediately after treatment. A few days after the ECT course, memory for events in the remote past is usually intact, but there may be difficulty in recalling events that transpired several months to years prior to ECT. The retrograde amnesia over this time span is rarely complete. Rather, patients have gaps or spottiness in their memories of personal and public events. Recent evidence suggests that the retrograde amnesia is typically greater for public information (knowledge of events in the world) than for personal information (autobiographic details of the patient's life) (Lisanby et al. 2000). The emotional valence of autobiographic events—that is, memories of pleasant or distressful events—is not related to their likelihood of being forgotten (McElhiney et al. 1995).

Usually, as time since ECT increases, the extent of retrograde amnesia reduces substantially. Older memories are more likely to be recovered. The time course for this shrinkage of retrograde amnesia is often more gradual than that for resolution of anterograde amnesia. In some patients the recovery from retrograde amnesia will be incomplete, and evidence has shown that ECT can result in persistent or permanent memory loss (Lisanby et al. 2000; McElhiney et al. 1995; Sackeim et al. 2000; Sobin et al. 1995; Squire et al. 1981; Weiner et al. 1986b). Owing to a combination of anterograde and retrograde effects, many patients may manifest persistent loss of memory for some events that transpired in the interval starting several months before and extending to several weeks after the ECT course. There are individual differences, however; some patients may experience persistent amnesia extending several years before ECT, although this effect is uncommon. Profound and persistent retrograde amnesia may be more likely in patients with preexisting neurologic impairment and patients who receive large numbers of treatments using methods that accentuate acute cognitive side effects (e.g., sine wave stimulation, bilateral electrode placement, high electrical stimulus intensity).

To determine the occurrence and severity of cognitive changes during and following the ECT course, orientation and memory functions should be assessed before ECT is initiated and throughout the course of treatment (see Chapter 12 for details).

5.8.2. Subjective Effects

Shortly after ECT, most patients report that their cognitive function is improved relative to their pre-ECT baseline (Calev et al. 1991a; Coleman et al. 1996; Cronholm and Ottosson 1963a; Frith et al. 1983; Mattes et al. 1990; Pettinati and Rosenberg 1984; Sackeim et al. 1993, 2000; Shellenberger et al. 1982; Weiner et al. 1986b). Indeed, recent research has shown that 2 months after ECT the memory self-ratings of former patients are markedly improved relative to their pre-ECT baseline and are indistinguishable from those of healthy control patients (Coleman et al. 1996). In patients who have received ECT, memory self-ratings show little association with the results of objective neuropsychologic testing (Calev et al. 1991a; Coleman et al. 1996; Cronholm and Ottosson 1963a; Frith et al. 1983; Squire and Slater 1983; Squire and Zouzounis 1988; Weiner et al. 1986b). Outside the context of ECT, in both healthy individuals and neurologically impaired samples, subjective memory assessments generally have shown weak or no association with objective neuropsychologic measures (Bennett-Levy and Powell 1980; Broadbent et al. 1982; Larrabee and Levin 1986; Rabbitt 1982; Sackeim and Stern 1997). In contrast, strong associations are observed between mood state and memory self-ratings among patients who have received ECT as well as in other populations (Coleman et al. 1996; Frith et al. 1983; Mattes et al. 1990; Pettinati and Rosenberg 1984; Stieper et al. 1951; Weiner et al. 1986b). In essence, patients with the greatest symptomatic benefit from ECT typically report the greatest improvement in subjective evaluations of memory. Thus, when patients report subjective memory impairment after ECT, their mood as well as their cognition should be assessed.

A small minority of patients treated with ECT later report devastating cognitive consequences (Donahue 2000; Freeman and Kendell 1980, 1986). Patients may indicate that they have dense amnesia extending far back into the past for events of personal significance or that broad aspects of cognitive function are so impaired that the patients are no longer able to engage in former occupations. Because these subjective reports of profound cognitive deficits are rare, determination of their absolute base rates is difficult. Multiple factors likely contribute to these perceptions by former patients.

First, in some patients self-reports of profound ECT-induced deficits may reflect objective loss of function. As noted, as with the adverse effects of any medical intervention, individual differences occur in the magnitude and persistence of ECT's cognitive effects. In rare cases, ECT may result in a dense and persistent retrograde amnesia extending to years before the treatment (Sackeim 2000).

Second, some of the psychiatric conditions treated with ECT result in cognitive deterioration as part of their natural history. This deterioration may be particularly likely in young patients in their first psychotic episode (Wyatt 1991, 1995) and in older patients in whom ECT may unmask a dementing process (Chen et al. 1999; Devanand et al. 1996). Although cognitive deterioration would have occurred inevitably in such individuals, the experience of transient short-term side effects with ECT may sensitize patients to attribute the persistent changes to the ECT treatment (Sackeim 1992; Squire 1986).

Third, as noted above, subjective evaluations of cognitive function typically show poor association with objective measurements and strong association with measures of psychopathology (Coleman et al. 1996). Only one study recruited patients with long-term complaints about effects of ECT and compared them with two control groups (Freeman et al. 1980). Objective neuropsychologic differences among the groups were modest, but there were marked differences in assessments of psychopathology and medication status. Patients reporting persistent deficits due to ECT were less likely to have benefited from the treatment and were more likely to be presently symptomatic and receiving psychotropic treatment (Freeman et al. 1980; Frith et al. 1983).

Discrepancies between the results of objective neuropsychologic testing and patient perceptions of pronounced deficit may also result from various other factors, including limitations in the types of cognitive function that can be objectively measured (Kellner 1996a; Sackeim 1992, 2000), selection bias in ECT follow-up studies whereby patients with marked deficits do not participate in longitudinal testing, and intrinsic difficulties in validating a phenomenon that has a low frequency.

5.9. Other Adverse Subjective Reactions

It is estimated that, following ECT, approximately 80% of patients report that they would have the treatment again if needed (Freeman and Cheshire 1986; Pettinati et al. 1994). However, negative subjective reactions to the experience of receiving ECT may occur and should be considered adverse side effects (Sackeim 1992). Prior to ECT, as with many medical procedures, patients often are apprehensive. Rarely, some patients develop an intense fear of the procedure that escalates during the ECT course and that may become an obstacle to treatment compliance (Fox 1993). Family members are also frequently apprehensive about the effects of the treatment. As part of the consent process before starting ECT, patients and family members should be given the opportunity to express their concerns and questions to the attending physician or members of the ECT treatment team (see Chapter 8 and Appendix B). Because much of the apprehension may be based on lack of information, it is often helpful to provide patients and family members with an information sheet describing basic facts about ECT (see Chapter 8 and Appendix B). This material should be supplemental to the consent form. It is also useful to make video material on ECT available. Addressing the concerns and educational needs of patients and family members should be a continuing process throughout the ECT course. In centers that regularly conduct ECT, it has been found useful to have ongoing group sessions, led by a member of the treatment team, for patients receiving ECT and their significant others. Such group sessions, including prospective and recently treated patients and their families, may engender mutual support and serve as a forum for education about ECT.

RECOMMENDATIONS

5.1. General Issues

a. Physicians administering ECT should be aware of the principal adverse effects that may accompany its use.
b. The type, likelihood, and persistence of adverse effects should be considered on a case-by-case basis in the decision to recommend ECT and in the informed consent process (see Chapter 8).
c. Efforts should be made to minimize adverse effects by optimizing the patient's medical condition before treatment, making appropriate modifications in ECT technique, and using adjunctive medications if indicated (see also Section 4.1).

5.2. Cardiovascular Complications

a. To detect cardiac arrhythmias, hypertension, and hypotension, the ECG and vital signs (blood pressure, pulse, and respiration) should be monitored during each ECT treatment (see Section 11.8.3).
b. The ECT treatment team should be prepared to manage cardiovascular complications known to be associated with ECT. Necessary personnel, supplies, and equipment should be readily available (see Chapters 9 and 10).

5.3. Prolonged Seizures

Each facility should have policies outlining the steps to be taken to terminate prolonged seizures and status epilepticus (see Section 11.9.3).

5.4. Prolonged Apnea

Resources for maintaining an airway for an extended period, including intubation, should be available in the treatment room (see Chapters 9 and 10).

5.5. Headache, Muscle Soreness, and Nausea

Systemic side effects should be identified and symptomatic treatment considered. Headache and nausea are the most common systemic side effects of ECT.

5.6. Treatment-Emergent Mania

If patients switch from depressive or affectively mixed states to hypomania or mania during a course of ECT, a determination should be made whether to continue or suspend further ECT treatment.

5.7. Postictal Delirium

Depending on its severity, postictal delirium can be managed supportively or pharmacologically. Pharmacologic prophylaxis should be considered when patients repeatedly manifest postictal delirium.

5.8. Cognitive Side Effects

a. To detect and monitor the presence of ECT-related cognitive dysfunction, orientation and memory function should be assessed prior to ECT and periodically throughout the ECT course (see Section 12.2.1 for details). This assessment should include attention to patient self-reports of memory difficulty.
b. Based on assessment of the severity of cognitive side effects, the physician administering ECT should review the contributions of concomitant medications, ECT technique, and spacing of treatments and then take appropriate action. Potential treatment modifications include changing from bilateral to right unilateral electrode placement, decreasing the intensity of electrical stimulation, increasing the time interval between treatments, altering the dosage of medications, or, if necessary, terminating the treatment course.

CHAPTER 6

Pre-ECT Evaluation

Although components of the evaluation of patients for ECT vary on a case-by-case basis, each facility should have a minimal set of procedures that are to be undertaken in all cases (Coffey 1998). A psychiatric history and examination, including past response to ECT and other treatments, is important to ensure that an appropriate indication for ECT exists. A careful general medical history and examination, focusing particularly on neurologic, cardiovascular, and pulmonary systems as well as on effects of previous anesthesia inductions, are crucial to identify medical risks (see Chapter 3 and Section 4.1). Assessment should also include inquiry about dental problems and a brief inspection of the mouth, looking for loose or missing teeth and noting the presence of dentures or other appliances (see Sections 4.1.4 and 5.5).

The pre-ECT evaluation should be performed by an individual privileged to administer ECT as well as by the anesthesia provider. Findings should be documented in the clinical record by a note summarizing the indications for and risks of ECT and suggesting any additional evaluative procedures, alterations in ongoing medications (see Chapter 7), or necessary modifications in ECT technique (see Chapter 11). Procedures for obtaining informed consent should be implemented (see Chapter 8).

No laboratory tests are routinely required as part of the pre-ECT workup. Laboratory testing is used to confirm the presence and severity of medical risk factors identified by the medical history and examination (see also Section 4.1). Although young, physically healthy patients may not require any laboratory evaluation, common practice is to perform a minimum screening battery of tests, often including a complete blood count, measurement of serum potassium and sodium levels, and an electrocardiogram. A pregnancy test should be considered in women of childbearing age, although ECT is generally safe for both the fetus and the pregnant mother (see Section 4.3). Some facilities do not specify any specific routine laboratory testing, whereas others have protocols involving specification of testing on the basis of age or certain medical risk factors such as cardiovascular or pulmonary history (Beyer et al. 1998). Because the risk of musculoskeletal injuries with ECT has been largely obviated by the use of muscular relaxation, spinal radiographs are no longer routinely necessary; they may, however, be useful in patients with clinically significant preexisting disease affecting the spine. Similarly, an electroencephalogram, brain computed tomography scan, or brain magnetic resonance imaging scan should be considered if other data suggest that a brain abnormality may be present. Use of pre-ECT cognitive testing is discussed elsewhere (See Section 12.2.1).

Although no data exist on the optimal time interval between the pre-ECT evaluation and the first treatment, the evaluation should be performed as close as possible to the initiation of treatment. Still, the pre-ECT evaluation may have to be spread over a number of days because of the need for specialty consultations, laboratory testing, meetings with the patient and significant others, and other factors. The treatment team should be aware of pertinent changes in the patient's condition over this time interval and should initiate further evaluation as indicated.

The decision to administer ECT is based on the type and severity of the patient's psychiatric illness, the patient's treatment history, and a risk/benefit analysis of available psychiatric therapies. This decision also requires agreement among the attending physician, ECT psychiatrist, and consentor. Medical consultation is sometimes used to obtain a better understanding of the patient's medical status, or when assistance in the management of medical conditions is desirable. To ask for "clearance" for ECT, however, assumes that such consultants have the special experience or training required to assess all risks and benefits of ECT compared with treatment alternatives—a requirement that is unlikely to be met.

RECOMMENDATIONS

Local policy should determine the components of the routine pre-ECT evaluation. Although additional tests, procedures, and consultations may be indicated on an individual basis, such an evaluation should include all the following:

- A psychiatric history and examination, including an assessment of the effects of any prior ECT, to determine the indication for ECT
- A medical evaluation, including a general medical history and physical examination and an assessment of the teeth and mouth to define risk factors
- An evaluation by an individual privileged to administer ECT (ECT psychiatrist—Section 9.2), as documented in the clinical record by a note summarizing indications and risks and suggesting any additional evaluative procedures, alterations in ongoing medications, or necessary modifications in ECT technique
- An anesthetic evaluation addressing the anesthetic risk and advising of the need for modification in ongoing medications or anesthetic technique
- An informed consent (see Chapter 8)

CHAPTER 7

Use of Medications During the Course of Electroconvulsive Therapy

7.1. General Considerations

Before beginning ECT, all medications taken by the patient should be reviewed. The aim of this review is to optimize the patient's medical status and avoid potential adverse effects due to drug–drug and drug–treatment interactions. Medications prescribed for medical conditions are usually continued (see Sections 4.1 and 7.2), although the timing of administration and dosage may require adjustment. However, some medications may need to be withdrawn or changed (see Section 7.3) because of potential interference with ECT's therapeutic action or increased risk of adverse effects when combined with ECT (e.g., cognitive impairment, prolonged seizures, or cardiovascular toxicity). Some medication, when discontinued, may need to be gradually tapered to minimize withdrawal reactions.

Some medications may be taken in the morning before ECT, whereas others should be withheld until the patient recovers from the treatment session. Pre-ECT orders for each treatment should specify the medications and dose administered or withheld prior to the treatment.

7.2. Medications Typically Continued Through the ECT Course

7.2.1. Medications Administered Prior to Each Treatment

In general, medications thought to exert a protective effect with respect to ECT-induced physiologic changes and those necessary to optimize medical status should be given prior to the treatment. Examples include antihypertensive and antianginal agents; antiarrhythmics (except lidocaine or its analogues, which may block seizure elicitation [Devanand and Sackeim 1988; Hood and Mecca 1983]); antireflux agents; bronchodilators (except theophylline); glaucoma medications (except long-acting cholinesterase inhibitors); and corticosteroids. Medications given prior to the treatment can be taken with a small sip of water.

Although the intention behind pre-ECT administration of such medications is to enhance the safety of the procedure, the ECT psychiatrist and anesthesia provider should be alert to potential negative interactions. For example, the use of β-blockers as antihypertensives may increase the risk of marked hypotension or asystole during ECT (Decina et al. 1984).

7.2.2. Medications Withheld Until After Each Treatment

Other medications such as diuretics that may increase the likelihood of incontinence or, very rarely, bladder rupture, may be withheld until after the treatment (Irving and Drayson 1984; O'Brien and Morgan 1991). The nothing-by-mouth (NPO) requirement for ECT may affect patients with diabetes. Hypoglycemic medications, including insulin, are generally withheld until after the treatment. However, some practitioners advocate splitting the morning dose of long-acting insulin and administering half of it before ECT and half after the treatment when indicated (Weiner and Sibert 1996). Because insulin requirements may fluctuate substantially over the course of ECT, ongoing monitoring of glucose levels and adjustment of insulin dosing may be necessary (Finestone and Weiner 1984). When glucose control is unstable, a medical consultation may be helpful.

When possible, all psychotropic medication should be held until after the treatment. This procedure is particularly important for lithium, benzodiazepines, and anticonvulsant medications (see Section 7.3). In rare circumstances, patients are so agitated that they can comply with treatment only if they receive a pharmacologic intervention. Haloperidol or droperidol administered intramuscularly might be used in this circumstance.

7.3. Medications Often Decreased or Withdrawn Prior to or During an ECT Course

Certain medications may increase the risks of ECT. Consideration should be given to decreasing the dosage or discontinuing these agents before beginning the ECT course. When making decisions about concurrent psychotropic administration, practitioners should be aware that many agents, including sedative/hypnotics and antidepressants, may have withdrawal effects that emerge with abrupt taper or discontinuation. Some symptoms associated with this abrupt withdrawal (e.g., rebound anxiety, nausea, headache) may be mistaken by the patient or clinician as adverse effects of ECT. Thus, whenever possible, medications should be withdrawn gradually.

7.3.1. Theophylline

Even with blood levels in the therapeutic range for asthma control, theophylline has been linked to status epilepticus during ECT (Abrams 1997a; Devanand et al. 1998; Fink and Sackeim 1998; Peters et al. 1984; Rasmussen and Zorumski 1993). Thus, theophylline should be discontinued whenever possible or its dosage should be kept as low as is compatible with satisfactory pulmonary function. In recent years, a number of alternative asthma medications have been developed, making the need to use theophylline uncommon. These newer agents do not appear to elevate the risk for status epilepticus. Although theophylline increases seizure duration (Swartz and Lewis 1991), recent findings that seizure duration may not be related to the efficacy of ECT (Nobler et al. 1993; Sackeim et al. 1991, 1993, 2000) bring the need for such an effect into question.

7.3.2. Lithium

There is divergent opinion about the safety of continuing lithium during ECT (Lippmann and El-Mallakh 1994). Many patients have received lithium during ECT without incident (Jha et al. 1966; Lippmann and Tao 1993; Mukherjee 1993). However, patients receiving lithium during ECT may be at a higher risk for delirium or prolonged seizures (Ahmed and Stein 1987; El-Mallakh 1988; Rudorfer et al. 1987; Small and Milstein 1990; Small et al. 1980; Standish-Barry et al. 1985; Strömgren et al. 1980; Weiner et al. 1980a, 1980b). This risk rapidly diminishes with dosage reduction or withdrawal of the lithium.

For patients with severe and recurrent mood disorder, complete discontinuation of lithium may not be advisable, particularly when ECT is used as continuation/maintenance treatment. The decision to continue lithium during ECT should be made on a case-by-case basis, weighing possible risks of neurotoxicity against risks of relapse if the medication is withdrawn. It is possible that the risk of toxicity increases at higher serum lithium levels and that it might be reduced by keeping lithium levels in the low-to-moderate therapeutic range. Omitting the previous day's dose or doses may produce a sufficient decrease in lithium levels for many patients, particularly those receiving continuation/maintenance ECT.

7.3.3. Benzodiazepines

Many patients treated with ECT may be receiving benzodiazepines for symptoms of anxiety, agitation, or insomnia. Substantial evidence has shown that benzodiazepines reduce seizure duration in a dose-dependent fashion (Boylan et al. 2000; Krueger et al. 1993; Standish-Barry et al. 1985), and it is suspected that these agents interfere with maximal seizure expression. Given the independent amnestic effects of benzodiazepines, there is theoretical concern that negative synergism with ECT may accentuate cognitive side effects. Furthermore, some have argued that concurrent treatment with benzodiazepines diminishes the efficacy of ECT (Greenberg and Pettinati 1993; Nettlebladt 1988; Pettinati et al. 1990; Standish-Barry et al. 1985; Strömgren et al. 1980). For example, some evidence has shown that clinical outcome with right unilateral ECT is inferior in depressed patients receiving benzodiazepines compared with patients who are free of these agents (Pettinati et al. 1990). However, given differences in symptom profiles, it is possible that patients treated with concomitant benzodiazepines have an intrinsically different probability of ECT response than patients not given these medications. To have greater certainty about this issue, clinical trials are needed in which patients are randomly assigned to ECT with and without a concurrent benzodiazepine.

If clinically feasible, efforts should be made to lower the dose or discontinue benzodiazepines before an ECT course. To limit rebound anxiety and other withdrawal symptoms, attention should be paid to the rate of taper if a benzodiazepine is reduced or discontinued. If a benzodiazepine is used during ECT, it should have a relatively short half-life (e.g., lorazepam) and be withheld at least 8 hours before an ECT treatment. Also, some facilities have policies limiting the maximal dosage of benzodiazepines a patient may receive during ECT (e.g., 3 mg/day lorazepam). When continuing benzodiazepine treatment, a strategy requiring further study is to briefly reverse the action of the benzodiazepine by administering the benzodiazepine antagonist flumazenil at the time of the ECT treatment (Bailine et al. 1994; Krystal et al. 1998). When flumazenil is used in benzodiazepine-dependent patients, a short-acting benzodiazepine such as midazolam should be administered soon after the induced seizure to avoid postictal withdrawal effects.

Other options are available for treating symptoms of anxiety and insomnia in patients receiving ECT. Some agents, like chloral hydrate, may share the anticonvulsant properties of benzodiazepines and are likely to present the same concerns about their use. Other sedative/ hypnotic and antianxiety medications such as zolpidem, buspirone, antihistamines, and the antidepressant trazodone are used by some practitioners during a course of ECT. These agents differ in whether their action is primarily anxiolytic or hypnotic, and their effects on the safety and efficacy of ECT have not been studied. Still other practitioners use small doses of antipsychotic medications for this purpose.

7.3.4. Anticonvulsant Medications

Many of the considerations raised about benzodiazepines apply to the management of patients receiving anticonvulsant medications. These medications may increase seizure threshold and interfere with seizure expression (Green et al. 1982; Nobler and Sackeim 1993; Sackeim et al. 1991). Seizure expression may be particularly problematic with agents that suppress major motor seizure activity, for example, barbiturates, carbamazepine, phenytoin, primadone, and valproic acid (as opposed to ethosuximide, felbamate, gabapentin, lamotrigine, methsuximide, and vigabatrin, which may not have such effects).

Many practitioners decrease the dosage of anticonvulsant medications before ECT, whereas others prefer to reduce dosage only when it is difficult to produce adequate seizures. However, "seizure adequacy" is not well defined, and there is a concern that seizures may have long duration (suggesting adequacy) but weak expression and minimal therapeutic properties (Nobler et al. 1993; Sackeim et al. 1987a, 1993, 2000). Consequently, when anticonvulsants are prescribed for a psychiatric indication (e.g., mood stabilization) rather than for a seizure disorder, it is prudent to avoid this potential negative impact on efficacy by tapering and discontinuing these agents as rapidly as possible before an index ECT course.

For patients receiving continuation/maintenance ECT while also receiving anticonvulsant medications for mood stabilization, it is probably sufficient to withhold one or two dosages of the medication prior to each treatment, as was noted for lithium. This recommendation is particularly applicable for agents with short half-lives.

For patients receiving anticonvulsants for the treatment of a seizure disorder, the morning dosage is usually withheld before ECT. Serum level monitoring may be helpful in maintaining anticonvulsants in the low therapeutic range, thereby minimizing interference with the induction of ECT seizures. Because of the anticonvulsant properties of ECT (Sackeim 1999), some practitioners maintain patients with seizure disorders at reduced doses of anticonvulsant medications during an index ECT course.

7.3.5. Monoamine Oxidase Inhibitors

There has long been reluctance to administer anesthesia (including that given with ECT) to patients currently or recently receiving nonselective monoamine oxidase inhibitors (MAOIs). In the presence of a MAOI, there is concern that any pressor agents given to treat a hypotensive episode would not be catabolized and could precipitate a hypertensive crisis. Some ECT practitioners and anesthesia providers continue to advocate withdrawal of MAOIs for 7–14 days before starting ECT. However, despite extensive documented experience with concurrent use of MAOIs and ECT, few examples of untoward effects have been reported (Freese 1985; Imlah et al. 1965; Monaco and Delaplaine 1964; Muller 1961; Remick et al. 1987; Wells and Bjorksten 1989) and the combination is generally believed to be safe. Nonetheless, prudent practice dictates that certain precautions be observed. Hypotension in the presence of MAOIs should not be treated with an indirect-acting vasopressor (e.g., ephedrine). Rather, neosynephrine or a similar agent is recommended. Meperidine is contraindicated, and other narcotics are best avoided (Sedgwick et al. 1990).

It is unlikely that selective MAOIs (e.g., selegiline or moclobemide) pose a serious risk during ECT, particularly at moderate therapeutic dosages. However, few data on the use of these agents with ECT have been reported (Kellner et al. 1992).

7.4. Pharmacologic Augmentation of ECT

ECT is increasingly prescribed for patients who have demonstrated treatment resistance or frequent recurrence (Chanpattana et al. 1999b;

Prudic et al. 1990, 1996; Sackeim et al. 1990a, 1990b). Consequently, in the absence of evidence of increased adverse effects, even the possibility of synergistic therapeutic action between psychotropic medications and ECT may suggest consideration of combining these treatment modalities.

7.4.1. Antipsychotic Medications

The combination of ECT and antipsychotic medication may be more effective in the treatment of schizophrenia than either form of treatment alone (Fink and Sackeim 1996; Krueger and Sackeim 1995). Although this literature is characterized by a host of methodologic difficulties, it was suggested in each of the three studies in which ECT alone was compared with ECT combined with antipsychotic medication that the combination was more effective (Childers 1964; Ray 1962; Small et al. 1982). A larger number of investigations contrasted combination treatment with monotherapy using an antipsychotic medication. With the exception of the study by Janakiramaiah et al. (1982), evidence in each study indicated that treatment with an antipsychotic medication in combination with ECT was more effective than treatment with an antipsychotic medication alone (Abraham and Kulhara 1987; Childers 1964; Das et al. 1991; Ray 1962; Small et al. 1982; Smith et al. 1967; Ungvári and Pethö 1982). In some cases, a superior outcome was obtained despite an apparent lower average antipsychotic dose in the combination condition (Small et al. 1982; Smith et al. 1967; Ungvári and Pethö 1982). Few of these studies followed patients beyond the acute treatment period and none standardized continuation or maintenance treatments. Therefore, the relative persistence of any advantage for combination treatment is unknown. In this respect, the findings reported by Smith et al. (1967) were particularly intriguing, suggesting a reduced rate of relapse in patients treated acutely with antipsychotic medications and ECT relative to antipsychotics alone. When considered with the similar follow-up results of May et al. (1981), there is reason to explore whether ECT may exert a long-term beneficial effect in schizophrenia, particularly in combination with antipsychotic medication.

A key clinical question is whether ECT (alone or in combination with antipsychotic medication) is effective in treating patients with schizophrenia who are medication resistant. In almost all instances, the first-line treatment of schizophrenia is pharmacotherapy with an antipsychotic medication. Thus, the role of ECT is largely limited to patients who have not responded to one or more pharmacologic interventions.

Almost all information on this issue comes from case series. In general, these reports have documented encouraging short-term response rates for the combination treatment in patients with medication-resistant schizophrenia (Chanpattana et al. 1999b; Childers and Therrien 1961; Friedel 1986; Gujavarty et al. 1987; Milstein et al. 1990). Of note, Chanpattana et al. (1999a) studied patients with medication-resistant schizophrenia and randomized patients who responded to combination treatment with ECT plus traditional antipsychotic medication. After randomization to continuation treatment with ECT alone, antipsychotic medication alone, or combined ECT plus antipsychotic medication, patients receiving the combination treatment had substantially less relapse than either form of monotherapy.

All evidence concerning the synergistic effects of ECT and antipsychotic medications pertains to schizophrenia. It is unknown whether similar benefit would be obtained in other psychotic disorders, particularly psychotic depression. Conceptually, the synergistic action of antidepressant and antipsychotic medications in psychotic depression (Nelson et al. 1986; Parker et al. 1992; Spiker et al. 1985) would argue for a similar synergistic action with ECT. Alternatively, the response rates for ECT monotherapy in psychotic depression are high and there may be little room for improvement (Buchan et al. 1992; Parker et al. 1992; Sobin et al. 1996).

Almost all of the research on the combination of ECT and antipsychotic medications pertains to traditional antipsychotics. Information about newer, atypical antipsychotics derives only from case series (Klapheke 1993). Although there was initial concern that the combination of ECT and clozapine might result in prolonged or spontaneous seizures (Bloch et al. 1996), safe and effective use has been reported (Benatov et al. 1996; Bhatia et al. 1998; Cardwell et al. 1995; Frankenburg et al. 1993; Safferman and Munne 1992; Sedgwick et al. 1990). Reserpine is the only antipsychotic medication for which there is an established hazard when administered concurrently with ECT. Now rarely used for either its antipsychotic or antihypertensive properties, reserpine should not be given with ECT because concurrent administration has been associated with death (Bross 1957; Gaitz et al. 1956).

7.4.2. Antidepressant Medications

In many parts of the world, antidepressant medications are continued during the ECT course (Royal College of Psychiatrists 1995). Practice in the United States has typically involved withdrawing patients with depression from such medications prior to or at the beginning of the ECT course (American Psychiatric Association 1990). However, the potential value of combining ECT with antidepressant medications is undergoing reconsideration. With respect to efficacy, two essential questions arise: 1) does concomitant treatment improve the short-term antidepressant effects of ECT, and 2) does concomitant treatment reduce the rate of early relapse following ECT?

With two exceptions (Lauritzen et al. 1996; Nelson and Benjamin 1989), virtually all research on the pharmacologic augmentation of ECT in major depression was conducted during the 1950s and 1960s. In this early work, several investigators claimed that ECT combined with a tricyclic antidepressant (TCA) (Dunlop 1960a; Kay et al. 1970; Ravn 1966; Sargant 1961) or MAOI (Dunlop 1960b; Muller 1961) resulted in faster or more certain response. Although some of these claims were impressionistic, there was supportive evidence from controlled trials (Kay et al. 1970; Muller 1961). In contrast, the early literature also contained negative findings regarding synergistic effects of ECT when combined with TCAs (Seager and Bird 1962; Wilson et al. 1963) or MAOIs (Imlah et al. 1965; Monaco and Delaplaine 1964). Of note, Imlah et al. (1965), Kay et al. (1970), and Seager and Bird (1962) all found that combining ECT with an antidepressant medication and continuing the medication after response markedly reduced the relapse rate compared with continued treatment with placebo.

This early work was inconclusive and generally limited by three factors. First and foremost, patients often received ECT as a first-line treatment and were far less resistant to pharmacologic intervention than is the case today. Second, standards for pharmacologic treatment have changed (Quitkin 1985; Prudic et al. 1996; Sackeim et al. 1990b), and this early work used medication dosages now considered suboptimal. Third, much of this work had design limitations, including small sample size and nonblinded evaluation.

The two modern studies that have examined this issue both found evidence that a TCA may improve ECT outcome. Nelson and Benjamin (1989) conducted a retrospective study of 84 elderly patients with unipolar major depression. Patients were categorized as receiving ECT alone, ECT plus low-dose TCA (e.g., serum nortriptyline level 2–49 ng/mL), or ECT plus therapeutic-dose TCA (e.g., serum nortriptyline level 50–149 ng/mL). The groups were equivalent in age, gender distribution, and the rate of psychotic depression. Suprathreshold right unilateral ECT was used, and patient records were blindly evaluated for degree of clinical improvement, extent of postictal confusion, and cardiac side effects. Patients who received a combination of ECT and TCA had superior clinical outcome. This effect was graded, increasing in magnitude from the low-dose to the therapeutic-dose groups; these groups also required significantly fewer treatments than the group that received ECT alone (8.1 vs. 9.8 treatments). No differences were found among the groups in postictal confusion or cardiac side effects, with a trend for fewer cardiac side effects in the combination groups.

Lauritzen et al. (1996) recently conducted a double-blind trial in which patients with cardiac disease ($n = 35$) were randomized to treatment with ECT and paroxetine (30 mg/day) or ECT and placebo. Patients without cardiac disease ($n = 52$) were randomized to ECT and paroxetine (30 mg/day) or ECT and imipramine (150 mg/day). ECT was started with bilateral electrode placement for the first three treatments and was then switched to right unilateral ECT. At baseline, the randomized groups were equivalent in demographic and clinical features. No difference was found between the paroxetine and placebo groups (cardiac patients) in clinical ratings following ECT or in the number of treatments administered. In contrast, the group treated concurrently with imipramine (no cardiac disease) had superior outcome to the paroxetine comparison group and the other groups as reflected in significantly lower symptom severity scores. Like the retrospective findings of Nelson and Benjamin (1989), this controlled and blinded study suggested that a concurrent TCA may improve clinical outcome with ECT, and, furthermore, that this benefit may not occur with a selective serotonin reuptake inhibitor.

In summary, soon after the introduction of antidepressant medications, several attempts were made to determine whether pharmacologic augmentation of ECT improved outcome. The findings were inconsistent, and the studies were characterized by serious methodologic limitations. Foremost is the concern that, at the time of this work, ECT was used far more commonly as a first-line treatment than it is today. Among patients with major depression who have not failed an adequate medication trial, the efficacy of ECT may be so strong as to leave little room for improvement (Prudic et al. 1990, 1996). However, medication resistance is now ECT's leading indication, and it has predictive value with regard to ECT outcome. With the diminution in rates of ECT response, there is a critical need to reconsider the role of pharmacologic augmentation. The very limited recent evidence suggests that there is reason to consider concurrent treatment with an antidepressant medication and ECT, particularly among medication-resistant patients.

All prior research on the combination of ECT and antidepressants has focused on whether the combination improved response to ECT, with no information about subsequent effects on relapse. No study has randomized patients to antidepressant medication or placebo concurrent with ECT and then switched the placebo patients to active continuation therapy after response to ECT and compared their relapse rate with those patients who were continued on antidepressant medication throughout. In other words, no attempt has been made to determine whether starting antidepressant medication before or during the ECT course provides a "head start" on relapse prevention (Sackeim 1994). This dearth of applicable research is surprising, because ECT is typically discontinued abruptly after remission (no taper), and it is believed that a delay of a 4–6 weeks or longer often occurs before antidepressant medications exert their full benefit, at least during acute-phase treatment (Hyman and Nestler 1996).

Thus, particularly among patients with medication-resistant depression, concurrent treatment with an antidepressant medication and ECT should be considered. The possibility exists that this combination may improve short-term clinical outcome. In addition, patients with medication resistance relapse at a high rate (Sackeim et al. 1990a; Shapira et al. 1995), with relapse especially likely in the first few weeks after ECT (Sackeim et al. 1990b, 1993, 2000). It is possible that starting an antidepressant medication early during ECT will help sustain remission.

Before selecting a specific antidepressant medication, it may be wise to review the classes of medication that the patient has failed during the index episode using conservative criteria for the adequacy of trials (dose, duration, and compliance). Although unstudied, it would make sense to administer a different class of antidepressant medication during and after ECT rather than continuing one to which the patient has already manifested resistance.

In terms of the safety of combining antidepressants and ECT, evidence comes from only a few systematic studies (El-Ganzouri et al. 1985; Nelson and Benjamin 1989) and a more extensive case report literature (see Klapheke 1997 for a review). TCAs have generally been shown to be safe when used with ECT (Lauritzen et al. 1996; Nelson and

Benjamin 1989), at least when prescribed at recommended therapeutic doses. Particularly in patients with preexisting cardiovascular disease, the theoretical concern about cardiovascular or anticholinergic toxicity at unusually high doses should prompt caution in the prescribing of TCAs in conjunction with ECT. Caution is also advised in patients receiving complex medication regimens that may include more than one antidepressant. In both situations, increased monitoring may be indicated to detect adverse affects.

Given the frequent use of selective serotonin reuptake inhibitors, information about their safety in combination with ECT is important. One systematic study (Lauritzen et al. 1996) and several case series suggest that the combination is likely to be safe. An early report of increased seizure duration with fluoxetine (Caracci and Decina 1991) was followed by a report of decreased seizure duration (Gutierrez-Esteinou and Pope 1989), and it appears that this combination does not increase the risk for prolonged seizures (Harsch and Haddox 1990; Kellner and Bruno 1989; Zis 1992). Given the very long half-life of fluoxetine, it is likely that many patients have received ECT with substantial blood levels of this compound, and the absence of reports of adverse effects is reassuring. In their systematic study, Lauritzen et al. (1996) treated 45 patients with paroxetine and ECT. There was no indication of increased adverse effects. Nonetheless, further study of the safety of combined selective serotonin reuptake inhibitor therapy and ECT is warranted.

Given reports of slightly increased rates of spontaneous seizures in some patients on high doses of bupropion (Davidson 1989), there is a theoretical concern that this antidepressant might produce prolonged seizures when combined with ECT. The available case report materials (Figiel and Jarvis 1990; Kellner et al. 1994b) do not allow definitive conclusions to be drawn about the safety of bupropion and ECT. Caution is recommended, particularly in patients on high doses.

7.4.3. Pharmacologic Modification of Cognitive Side Effects

Electroconvulsive shock (ECS), the analogue of ECT in animal experimentation, is the most common procedure used to produce amnesia and screen compounds for protective effects on memory. A wide variety of pharmacologic agents have been found to reduce or block the amnestic effects of ECS in animals (Krueger et al. 1992). In contrast, limited clinical research has been conducted in testing pharmacologic methods to reduce the cognitive side effects of ECT. Although a scattering of positive reports are available (Andrade et al. 1995; Levin et al. 1987; Prudic et al. 1999; Stern et al. 1991), the findings are preliminary and of uncertain clinical significance. As yet, there is no accepted pharmacologic method to reduce the cognitive side effects of ECT (see Chapter 5).

RECOMMENDATIONS

7.1 General Considerations

a. All medications should be reviewed as part of the pre-ECT evaluation.
b. Medications thought to exert a protective effect with respect to ECT-induced physiologic changes should be given before each treatment.
c. Medications that may interfere with the therapeutic properties of ECT or cause other adverse effects should be decreased or withheld.
d. When applicable, medications should be discontinued gradually to reduce withdrawal symptoms.
e. Pre-ECT orders should specify which medications are to be administered and which are to be withheld before each treatment.

7.2. Medications Typically Continued Through the ECT Course

7.2.1. Medications Administered Prior to Each Treatment

Classes of agents generally given before an ECT treatment include (but are not limited to) antihypertensives (except diuretics), antianginals, antiarrhythmics (with the exception of lidocaine and its derivatives), antireflux agents, bronchodilators (except theophylline), glaucoma medications (except long-acting cholinesterase inhibitors), and corticosteroids.

7.2.2. Medications Withheld Until After Each Treatment

Classes of agents generally withheld or given at a decreased dose prior to each ECT treatment include (but are not limited to) diuretics, hypoglycemics (except insulin in certain patients), and psychotropic medications (especially benzodiazepines and anticonvulsants).

7.3. Medications Decreased or Withdrawn Prior to or During an ECT Course

a. Theophylline should be discontinued or decreased as much as is compatible with satisfactory pulmonary function because of the risk of status epilepticus.

b. Lithium should be discontinued or its levels should be kept in the low therapeutic range based on risk/benefit analysis of potential toxicity versus the risk of affective relapse.

c. When clinically feasible, patients should be tapered from benzodiazepines before the start of ECT.

d. Nonbenzodiazepine anxiolytic/hypnotic agents should be considered for patients requiring such pharmacologic intervention.

e. If benzodiazepines are necessary, dose should be minimized and a medication with a relatively short half-life used (e.g., lorazepam).

f. Anticonvulsant medications used for psychotropic (mood stabilizing) properties should be discontinued before the start of an index ECT course.

g. When anticonvulsant medications are used for treatment of a seizure disorder, the morning dosage is often withheld and blood levels kept in the low therapeutic range.

h. MAOIs generally do not need to be withheld during a course of ECT.

i. Medications contraindicated with MAOIs include indirect-acting vasopressors and meperidine.

7.4. Pharmacologic Augmentation of ECT

a. Antipsychotic medications may be continued during ECT because of the likelihood of synergistic therapeutic effects. This procedure is best established in the treatment of schizophrenia but may pertain to other psychotic conditions.

b. In patients with major depression, consideration may be given to combining an antidepressant medication and ECT to enhance antidepressant response or to reduce the risk of relapse when ECT is stopped.

CHAPTER 8

Consent for Electroconvulsive Therapy

8.1. General

"The core notion that decisions regarding medical care are to be made in a collaborative manner between patient and physician" has, over the past few decades, evolved into a formal legal doctrine of informed consent (Applebaum et al. 1987, p. 12). Such doctrine highlights a number of important questions about the nature of consent to treatment: What is informed consent? Who should provide consent, and under what circumstances? How and by whom should capacity for consent be determined? What information should be provided to the consentor and by whom? And how should consent be managed with incompetent or involuntary patients?

General reviews of informed consent issues as they relate to ECT can be found in Parry (1986), Roth (1986), Taub (1987), and Winslade (1988), whereas capacity for consent and the use of ECT in incompetent or involuntary patients is specifically addressed in Applebaum et al. (1987), Bean et al. (1996), Boronow et al. (1997), Culver et al. (1980), Gutheil and Bursztajn (1986), Levine et al. (1991), Mahler et al. (1986), Martin and Bean (1992), Martin and Glancy (1994), Reiter-Theil (1992), Roth et al. (1977), Roy-Byrne and Gerner (1981), Salzman (1977), and Wettstein and Roth (1988).

The psychiatric profession, both in the United States and elsewhere, has offered a number of practical guidelines for the implementation of consent in the clinical setting. In this regard, the conceptual requirements for informed consent proposed by the 1978 American Psychiatric Association Task Force on ECT are still applicable: 1) the provision of adequate information, 2) a patient who is capable of understanding and acting reasonably on such information, and 3) the opportunity to consent in the absence of coercion. Specific recommendations concerning consent for ECT often reflect a trade-off between preserving patient autonomy and ensuring that patients are not deprived of the opportunity to receive effective treatment (Ottosson 1992).

A hallmark of informed consent is the quality of interactions between the consentor and the physician, particularly because consent for ECT is an ongoing process. The physician's role in these interactions includes keeping the consentor abreast of what is transpiring, involving the consentor in decision making, and remaining sensitive to the consentor's concerns and feelings about these decisions.

8.2. Requirement for Consent

Because informed consent for ECT is mandated both ethically and by regulation, it is incumbent on facilities using ECT to implement and monitor compliance with reasonable and appropriate policies and procedures. Although the practitioner is legally obligated to follow state and local regulatory requirements concerning consent for ECT, judicial and political efforts should be made to correct overregulation (Taub 1987; Winslade et al. 1984). In this regard, ECT should not be considered different from other medical or surgical procedures with comparable risks and benefits. Regulations should not unduly obstruct the patient's access to treatment, because needless prolongation of procedures to provide ECT to incompetent or involuntary patients may result in unnecessary suffering, increased physical morbidity, and even fatalities (Johnson 1993; Miller et al. 1986; Mills and Avery 1978; Roy-Byrne and Gerner 1981; Tenenbaum 1983; Walter-Ryan 1985).

8.3. When and by Whom Should Consent Be Obtained?

As with consent for medical and surgical procedures, the patient should provide informed consent unless he or she lacks capacity or unless otherwise specified by law. The involvement of significant others in this process should be encouraged (Consensus Conference 1985) but not required (Tenenbaum 1983).

ECT is unusual but not unique among medical procedures because it involves a series of repetitive treatments spaced over an appreciable time period (typically 2–4 weeks for an acute ECT course). Because it is the series of treatments, rather than any single treatment, that confers both the benefits and adverse effects of ECT, consent should apply to the treatment series as a whole (unless otherwise required by law). However, consent should be obtained again if an unusually large number of treatments (as locally determined) are required in the management of an acute episode of illness (see Sections 8.4 and 11.11).

Because an ECT course generally extends over multiple weeks, the informed consent process should continue across this period. Patient recall of consent for medical and surgical procedures is commonly faulty (Herz et al. 1992; Hutson and Blaha 1991; Meisel and Roth 1983; Roth et al. 1982; Swan and Borshoff 1994). For patients receiving ECT, this recall difficulty may be exacerbated by both the underlying illness and the treatment itself (Squire 1986; Sternberg and Jarvik 1976). For these reasons, the consentor should be given ongoing feedback about clinical progress and side effects as well as any factors that may substantially influence these outcomes. Any questions or concerns should be addressed (American Psychiatric Association Council on Psychiatry and Law 1997). If the consentor expresses reluctance about receiving ECT, he or she should be reminded of the right to accept or refuse further treatment.

Continuation/maintenance ECT (see Chapter 13) differs from a course of ECT in that 1) its purpose is the prevention of relapse or recurrence, 2) the patient's clinical condition is improved compared with that preceding the index ECT course, and 3) it is characterized by both a greater intertreatment interval and a less well-defined endpoint. Because the purpose of continuation/maintenance treatment differs from that of an acute course of ECT, a new informed consent process should be initiated, including the signing of a separate consent form. Because a continuation ECT series often lasts at least 6 months, and because continuation/maintenance ECT is provided to individuals who are clinically improved and already knowledgable about the treatment, a 6-month interval is suggested before readministration of the formal consent document (unless otherwise required by law).

Ideally, the consent process involves discussions with the consentor about general aspects of ECT and information unique to the patient, as well as the signing of the informed consent document. The information essential to consent to ECT should be provided by a knowledgable physician acting individually or in concert with other professional staff.

Ideally, this physician should also have a therapeutic alliance with the patient. In practice, this requirement can be accomplished by the attending physician, treating psychiatrist, or other knowledgable physician. Consent for anesthesia may either be included in the ECT consent process or separately obtained by an anesthesia provider.

8.4. Information to Be Conveyed

Use of a formal consent document for ECT ensures the provision of essential information to the consentor. Earlier task force recommendations (American Psychiatric Association 1990; American Psychiatric Association Task Force on ECT 1978), other professional guidelines, and regulatory requirements (Mills and Avery 1978; Taub 1987; Tenenbaum 1983; Winslade 1988; Winslade et al. 1984) have encouraged the use of comprehensive written information about ECT as part of the consent process. It is advisable that the generic portions of this material—those not specific to the individual patient—be either contained within the formal consent document or included as a patient information supplement. In either case, informational material should be given to the consentor to keep. In surgical patients, patient information supplements have been shown to significantly enhance recall of information provided prior to surgery (Askew et al. 1990).

Informational material provided as part of the consent process should be sufficient in scope and depth to allow a reasonable person to understand and evaluate the risks and benefits of ECT compared with treatment alternatives. Because individuals vary considerably in education and cognitive status, efforts should be made to tailor information to the consentor's ability to comprehend such data. In this regard, the practitioner should be aware that too much technical detail can be as counterproductive as too little. Sample consent forms and supplementary patient information material are included in Appendix B. If these documents are used, appropriate modifications should be made to reflect local requirements. It is also suggested that reproductions be in large type to ensure readability by patients with poor visual acuity.

To further enhance the understanding of ECT, many practitioners now augment written materials with videotapes designed to cover the topic of ECT from the layman's perspective (Battersby et al. 1993; Baxter et al. 1986; Dillon 1995; Guze et al. 1988; Westreich et al. 1995). Potential videos should, to the extent possible, be reviewed with respect to the current accuracy of material conveyed therein. Major discrepancies from other material provided in the consent process should be conveyed to the consentor.

To rely entirely on such generic materials as the sole informational component of the informed consent process is ill advised. Even with considerable attention to readability, many patients understand less than half of what is contained in a typical medical consent form (Roth et al. 1982). In this regard, patients with psychiatric disorders do not perform worse than medical or surgical patients (Meisel and Roth 1983). Because of this situation, the consent process should also include a discussion between the consentor and a knowledgeable physician (American Psychiatric Association Council on Psychiatry and Law 1997). This discussion should summarize the main features of the consent document, provide additional individual-specific information applicable to the patient for whom ECT is considered, and allow a further opportunity for the consentor to express his or her wishes and have questions answered. Examples of individual-specific information include the rationale for ECT, reasonable treatment alternatives, specific benefits and risks, and any major alterations planned in the ECT procedure. This discussion should also be briefly summarized in the patient's clinical record.

Substantial alterations in the treatment procedure or other factors having a major effect on risk/benefit considerations should be conveyed to the consentor on a timely basis. The consentor's continued agreement to proceed with ECT in such cases should be documented in the patient's clinical record. The need for ECT treatments exceeding the typical range (see Section 11.11) and the switching of stimulus electrode placement (see Section 11.6) represent two examples of such alterations.

The consent process generally includes coverage of the topics listed below. As previously noted, it is advisable that the consent form and/ or patient information sheet contain the generic portions of this material (i.e., those portions not specific to the individual patient), including

1. Who is recommending ECT and for what reason
2. A description of applicable treatment alternatives for the patient
3. A description of the ECT procedure, including the times when treatments are given (e.g., Monday, Wednesday, Friday mornings) and the location of treatment (i.e., where treatments will take place)

4. A discussion of the relative merits and risks of different types of stimulus electrode placement and the specific choice that has been made for the patient

5. The typical range for the number of treatments to be administered and a statement that reconsent will be obtained if the number of treatments in the index course exceeds a set maximum number (for that facility)

6. A statement that there is no guarantee that ECT will be effective

7. A statement that there is generally a substantial risk of relapse after ECT and that continuation treatment of some sort is nearly always indicated

8. The likelihood (e.g., "extremely rare," "rare," "uncommon," or "common") and anticipated severity of major risks associated with the procedure (see Chapter 5), including mortality, adverse effects on cardiovascular and central nervous systems (including both transient and persistent cognitive effects), and common minor side effects

9. An acknowledgment that consent for ECT also entails consent for appropriate emergency treatment in the event that this is clinically indicated

10. A description of behavioral restrictions that may be necessary during the pre-ECT evaluation period, the ECT course, and the recuperative interval

11. An offer to answer questions at any time regarding the recommended treatment and the name(s) of the individual(s) who can be contacted with such questions

12. A statement that consent for ECT is voluntary and can be withdrawn at any time

In light of the accumulated body of data dealing with structural effects of ECT (Devanand et al. 1994), "brain damage" should not be included as a potential risk of treatment.

8.5. Capacity to Provide Voluntary Consent

Informed consent requires that a patient be capable of understanding and acting reasonably on information provided about the procedure. For the purpose of these recommendations, the term *capacity* reflects this criterion. There is no clear consensus about what constitutes the *capacity to consent*. Criteria for capacity to consent have tended to be vague, and formal "tests" of capacity are only now under active investigation (Bean et al. 1996; Grisso and Appelbaum 1995; Martin and Glancy 1994). It is suggested, instead, that the individual obtaining consent consider the following general principles in making a determination. First, capacity to consent should be assumed to be present unless compelling evidence exists to the contrary. Second, the occurrence of psychotic ideation, irrational thought processes, or involuntary hospitalization do not in themselves constitute such evidence. Third, the patient should demonstrate sufficient comprehension and retention of information, as well as adequacy of judgment and decision making, so that he or she can reasonably decide whether to consent for ECT.

Unless otherwise mandated by statute, a determination of capacity is generally made by the attending physician. Should the attending physician doubt whether capacity to consent is present, an appropriate physician consultant not otherwise associated with the patient's care may be asked to assist in this determination.

There may be concern that the attending physician is biased toward finding that capacity to consent exists when the patient's decision agrees with his or her own. In this regard, however, ECT is no different from other treatment modalities. Furthermore, fixed requirements for a priori review of capacity to consent by consultant, special committee, appointed lawyer, or judicial hearing would only impede patient access to timely, appropriate ECT treatment.

Patients who have previously been adjudicated legally incompetent for medical purposes usually have consent for ECT provided by a legally appointed guardian or conservator, although this may vary depending on jurisdiction.

For patients with capacity to consent, ECT should be administered only with their agreement. To do otherwise would infringe on their right to refuse treatment. Situations in which the patient lacks capacity to consent are generally covered by regulations that include how and from whom surrogate consent may be obtained. In such instances, all of the information typically provided regarding ECT and alternative treatment should be shared with this individual. To the extent allowable by law, consideration should be given to any opinions expressed by the patient while in a previous state of determined or presumed capacity. Opinions of major significant others should also be considered.

Informed consent is defined as voluntary when the consentor's ability to reach a decision is free from coercion or duress. Because the treatment team, family members, and friends all may have opinions about whether ECT should be administered, it is reasonable that these opinions and their basis be expressed to the consentor. In practice, the line between "advocacy" and "coercion" may be difficult to establish. Particularly susceptible to undue influence are consentors who are either highly ambivalent or are unwilling or unable to take full responsibility for the decision (neither of which are rare occurrences with patients referred for ECT). Staff members involved in the patient's treatment should keep these issues in mind.

Threats of involuntary hospitalization or precipitous discharge from the hospital because of ECT refusal clearly represent undue influence. However, consentors have the right to be informed of the anticipated effects of their actions on the clinical course and overall treatment plan. Similarly, because physicians are not expected to follow treatment plans they believe are ineffective or unsafe, an anticipated need to transfer the patient to another attending physician should be discussed in advance with the consentor.

It is important to understand the issues involved in a consentor's decision to refuse or withdraw consent. Such decisions sometimes may be based on misinformation or may reflect unrelated matters, such as anger toward the self or others or a need to manifest autonomy. In addition, a patient's mental disorder can itself limit the ability to cooperate meaningfully in the informed consent process, even in the absence of psychosis.

As with patients lacking capacity to consent, several suggestions have been offered to help guarantee the right of involuntarily hospitalized patients to accept or refuse specific components of the treatment plan, including ECT. Examples of such recommendations include the use of psychiatric consultants not otherwise involved in the patient's care, appointed lay representatives, formal institutional review committees, and legal or judicial determination. Although some degree of protection is indicated in such cases, overregulation will serve to limit unnecessarily the patient's access to treatment.

RECOMMENDATIONS

8.1. General

a. Policies and procedures should be developed to ensure proper informed consent, including when, how, and from whom consent is to be obtained and the nature and scope of information to be provided.
b. These policies and procedures should be consistent with state and local regulations.

8.2. Requirement for Consent

a. Informed consent should be obtained from the patient except when the patient lacks capacity to consent (see Section 8.5).
b. Informed consent for ECT is given for a specified treatment course (see Section 11.11) or for a period of continuation/maintenance ECT (see Sections 13.2 and 13.3).
c. Consent for future treatments may be withdrawn at any time, including between ECT treatments, by the individual providing consent.

8.3. When and by Whom Should Consent Be Obtained?

a. Informed consent for ECT, including the signing of a formal consent document, should be obtained 1) before beginning an acute ECT treatment course, 2) if an unusually large number of treatments becomes necessary during an acute ECT treatment course, and 3) before initiating a period of continuation or maintenance ECT. In the latter case, the consent process should be repeated at least every 6 months.
b. Informed consent should be obtained by the patient's attending physician, treating psychiatrist, or other physician knowledgable about both the patient and ECT (unless otherwise specified by law).
c. When separate informed consent for ECT anesthesia is required, it

should be obtained by a privileged or otherwise authorized anesthesia provider.

d. Throughout the ECT course, the consentor should receive ongoing feedback about clinical progress and side effects and any questions or concerns should be addressed.

e. If the consentor expresses reluctance about the treatment at any time before or during the ECT course, he or she should be reminded of the right to accept or refuse treatment.

8.4. Information to Be Conveyed

8.4.1. General Considerations

a. Information describing ECT (see below) should be conveyed in a written consent document. This document and/or a summary of general information related to ECT should be given to the consentor to keep (examples are provided in Appendix B). The use of a separate consent document may be required for anesthesia with ECT in certain settings.

b. In addition to the written consent document, the consent process should also include an overview of general information on ECT as well as information specific to the individual patient. Such information should be presented orally to the consentor by the attending physician, treating psychiatrist, or other knowledgeable physician. Further information may also be provided by other staff members.

c. It is advisable that the consent form and/or patient information sheet contain the generic portions of the material (i.e., those portions not specific to the individual patient).

d. Other supplementary patient information material (e.g., videos) may be helpful.

e. The consentor should be informed if substantial alterations in the treatment procedure arise that may have a major effect on risk/benefit considerations. These discussions should be documented in the clinical record.

f. All information should be provided in a form understandable to the consentor and should be sufficient to allow a reasonable person to understand the risks and benefits of ECT and to evaluate the available treatment options.

g. The consentor should have an opportunity to ask questions relevant to ECT or treatment alternatives.

8.4.2. Specific Information Provided

The consent process should include coverage of the following topics:

- Who is recommending ECT and for what reason
- A description of applicable treatment alternatives
- A description of the ECT procedure, including the times when treatments are given and the location where treatments will occur
- A discussion of the relative merits and risks of the different stimulus electrode placements and the specific choice that has been made for the patient
- The typical range for number of treatments to be administered as well as a statement that reconsent will be obtained if the number of treatments in the index course exceeds a set maximum number (for that facility)
- A statement that there is no guarantee that ECT will be effective
- A statement concerning the need for continuation treatment
- A description of the likelihood and severity (in general terms) of major risks associated with the procedure (see Chapter 5), including mortality, cardiopulmonary dysfunction, confusion, and acute and persistent memory impairment. In addition, the common minor side effects of ECT should be delineated (e.g., headaches and musculoskeletal pain).
- A statement that consent for ECT also entails consent for appropriate emergency treatment in the event that this is clinically necessary during the time the patient is not fully conscious
- A description of any restrictions on patient behavior likely to be necessary before, during, or after ECT
- An offer to answer questions at any time regarding the recommended treatment and the name(s) of the individual(s) who can be contacted with such questions
- A statement that consent for ECT is voluntary and can be withdrawn at any time

8.5. Capacity to Provide Voluntary Consent

8.5.1. General Considerations

a. Use of ECT requires voluntary consent from an individual with capacity to make such a decision.

b. Individuals with mental illness are considered to have the capacity to consent to ECT unless evidence to the contrary is compelling. The presence of psychosis, irrational thinking, or involuntary hospitalization can impair capacity but does not constitute proof that capacity is lacking.
c. Unless otherwise specified by statute, the determination of capacity to consent should generally be made by the patient's attending physician. If the attending physician is uncertain whether capacity to consent is present, an appropriate physician consultant, not otherwise associated with the patient's care, may be used.
d. In the event of refusal or withdrawal of consent to ECT, the attending physician and/or treating psychiatrist should inform the consentor of anticipated effects of this action on clinical course and treatment planning.

8.5.2. Patients Having the Capacity to Provide Consent

For patients with the capacity to consent, ECT should be administered only in the presence of voluntary patient agreement, including signing of a formal consent document.

8.5.3. Patients Lacking the Capacity to Provide Consent

a. For patients lacking the capacity to provide consent, state and local law covering consent to treatment should be followed, including statutes pertinent to emergency situations in which a delay in treatment may lead to death or serious impairment in health.
b. Surrogate decision makers should be provided with the information described above.
c. To the extent allowable by law, consideration should be given to any positions previously expressed by the patient when in a state of determined or presumed capacity as well as to the opinions of major significant others.

CHAPTER 9

Staffing

9.1. Responsibility of Facility

Facilities offering ECT should designate a psychiatrist privileged in administering ECT to develop and oversee compliance with policies and procedures for ECT, including those related to staffing, equipment, and supplies. Furthermore, facilities should implement an ECT quality improvement program. Examples of activities include monitoring occurrences of major adverse effects and ensuring adherence to policies and procedures. Any observed deficiencies should be corrected.

9.2. The ECT Treatment Team

9.2.1. Members

ECT is a complex procedure that requires a well-trained, competent staff of professionals if it is to be administered in a safe and effective fashion. The ECT treatment team functions as a unit and typically consists of a psychiatrist (termed here *ECT psychiatrist*), an anesthesia provider, one or more ECT treatment nurses or assistants, and one or more recovery nurses, with responsibilities and qualifications as delineated below. When properly qualified, the ECT psychiatrist may also perform the duties of the ECT treatment nurse or, rarely, the anesthesia provider. However, because of the need for at least two health care professionals in the treatment area during the administration of ECT, the ECT psychiatrist may not subsume all three of these roles simultaneously. For each position on the treatment team, the pool of available staff members should be kept as small as possible to maximize continuity of care and to ensure that each individual has sufficient ongoing experience to maintain proficiency in his or her work.

ECT should not be delivered by unskilled trainees acting without proper supervision. All physicians administering ECT should be privileged in the performance of their ECT-related duties by the organized medical staff of the facility under whose auspices ECT will be delivered (see Chapter 16). The need to ensure competence of the ECT staff is sufficiently important that practitioners operating outside of an organized medical staff (e.g., individual or small group practice) should be privileged for ECT-related duties by another facility with an organized medical staff. All anesthesia providers should be privileged to deliver general anesthesia. ECT programs are encouraged to develop local procedures for ensuring that nursing staff members involved in ECT have received adequate training and assessment of competency before assuming ECT-related duties. Psychiatric, anesthetic, and nursing trainees may assist in the performance of ECT-related duties only under the direct supervision of appropriately privileged attending physicians or credentialed staff and only at a level commensurate with the level of relevant training they have received.

9.2.2. Responsibilities

9.2.2.1. ECT Psychiatrist

Because his or her training and experience in ECT is the most comprehensive, the ECT psychiatrist should maintain overall responsibility for the administration of ECT. The ECT psychiatrist is also responsible for 1) assessing the patient prior to beginning ECT, 2) ensuring that the pre-ECT evaluation has been completed (see Chapter 6), 3) determining that ECT is still indicated prior to each ECT treatment, 4) ensuring that the delivery of ECT is compatible with established policies and procedures (see Chapter 11), 5) instituting appropriate ECT modifications as indicated, and 6) making sure that evaluation and treatment results are properly documented (see Chapter 14).

Practice varies as to whether the ECT psychiatrist oversees all other aspects of the patient's mental health care during the ECT course or whether this latter function is fulfilled by a separate attending physician. The same individual may function as both ECT psychiatrist and attending physician. When such functions are separate, it is important for both physicians to agree on treatment decisions such as the rationale for ECT and the number and type of ECT treatments. However, the ECT psychiatrist should maintain overall responsibility for the conducting of ECT, including determination of how each treatment is administered (except for anesthetic considerations). The concept of the ECT psychiatrist as a "button-pusher" is incompatible with quality care.

9.2.2.2. Anesthesia Provider

Even for a procedure as brief as ECT, the administration of anesthesia requires skill in airway management, use of ultra-brief anesthetic and relaxant agents, cardiopulmonary resuscitation, and management of acute adverse events. The anesthesia provider must be capable of managing acute medical emergencies that could occur during and immediately after ECT (see Chapter 5) and must also be familiar with relevant emergency medications and emergency life support. A nurse anesthetist or, rarely, the ECT psychiatrist may serve in this capacity if trained to the competencies described above and appropriately privileged (see Chapters 15 and 16) (Moscarillo 1989; Pearlman et al. 1990). However, high-risk patients needing more complex anesthetic management require the presence of a qualified anesthesiologist.

The provision of anesthetic care often has an impact on the safety and efficacy of ECT. Thus, it is critical that the ECT psychiatrist and anesthesia provider agree on the patient's medical management, including type and dosage of medications and intervention for adverse events. Nonetheless, the anesthesia provider has primary responsibility for emergency management of cardiopulmonary function and maintaining life support.

9.2.2.3. ECT Treatment Nurse or Assistant

The role of the ECT treatment nurse or the assistant varies from location to location (Burns and Stuart 1991; Froimsin et al. 1995; Gunderson-Falcone 1995; Halsall et al. 1995). Typically, he or she is a registered nurse whose responsibilities include assisting the ECT psychiatrist and anesthesia provider in duties such as coordinating treatment logistics, readying the treatment area for ECT, helping patients to and from the treatment area, applying stimulus and monitoring electrodes, and monitoring vital signs. It is important that the responsibilities of such staff be consistent with their training and clinical competence. Especially when ECT is delivered on an ambulatory basis (see Section 11.1), additional nursing duties are relevant and may include assessment before each treatment and delivery of postrecovery care. Many facilities have provided an even more comprehensive role for the ECT treatment nurse or assistant, again, compatible with the training and competency of available staff. Such roles include providing clinical or financial case management, assisting with patient and family education and informed consent procedures, assisting in pre-ECT evaluation and documentation, and overseeing the availability of ECT-related equipment and supplies.

9.2.2.4. Recovery Nurse

The recovery nurse, a registered nurse, provides care for patients in the recovery area (now often termed the "postanesthesia care unit" or PACU). Duties include monitoring vital signs, pulse oximetry, electrocardiogram (ECG), and mental status. The recovery nurse should be capable of administering oxygen and intravenous fluids, providing suctioning, and delivering supportive care for postictal disorientation and agitation. These duties should be supervised by the anesthesia provider or a comparably qualified professional. Recovery area staffing should be sufficient to ensure adequate performance of these duties at all times.

RECOMMENDATIONS

9.1. Responsibility of Facility

a. The director of each such facility, or his or her designee, should appoint a psychiatrist privileged to administer ECT to be responsible for maintaining up-to-date policies and procedures regarding ECT, for ensuring that these policies and procedures are met, and for seeing that appropriate staffing, equipment, and supplies are available.
b. Each such facility should implement an ECT quality improvement program.
c. All persons involved in the delivery of ECT should be privileged in the performance of clinical ECT-related duties by the organized medical staff of the facility under whose auspices ECT will be administered (see Chapter 16) or be otherwise authorized to carry out such duties. In the event that no such organized medical staff exists (e.g., solo or small group practice), the individual should be privileged in the ECT-related duties by another facility having an organized medical staff.

9.2. The ECT Treatment Team

9.2.1. Members

a. The ECT treatment team consists of at least an ECT psychiatrist, an anesthesia provider, and one or more recovery nurses.
b. The additional use of at least one ECT treatment nurse or assistant in the treatment room or area is strongly encouraged.
c. Psychiatric, anesthetic, and nursing trainees may assist attending-level practitioners in performing ECT-related duties only under direct supervision and only at a level commensurate with the level of relevant training they have received.

9.2.2. Responsibilities

9.2.2.1. ECT Psychiatrist

a. The ECT psychiatrist should maintain overall responsibility for the proper administration of ECT.

b. The ECT psychiatrist should assess the patient before the first treatment, confirm that the pre-ECT evaluation has been completed and documented satisfactorily (Chapter 6), determine that ECT is indicated before each treatment, and ensure that the delivery of ECT is compatible with established policies and procedures (Chapter 11).

9.2.2.2. Anesthesia Provider

a. Each facility should determine whether and under what circumstances individuals from specific disciplines, including anesthesiology, nurse anesthesia, and psychiatry, may serve as anesthesia provider for ECT (see Chapter 16).
b. The anesthesia provider should be responsible for the maintenance of an airway and oxygenation and, with the assistance of the ECT psychiatrist, the delivery of anesthetic, relaxant, and adjunctive agents and the management of emergent adverse reactions.
c. The anesthesia provider should be capable of managing foreseeable medical emergencies until other appropriate personnel are available.

9.2.2.3. ECT Treatment Nurse or Assistant

a. The ECT treatment nurse or assistant should be responsible for selected tasks delegated by the ECT psychiatrist or anesthesia provider and compatible with his or her training and competencies.
b. Examples of such tasks include the following: education of patients and their families regarding ECT, assisting the physician with the informed consent process, providing clinical or financial case management, logistically coordinating treatments, readying the treatment area for administration of ECT, assisting patients to and from the treatment area, applying the stimulus and monitoring electrodes, placing the bite-block, monitoring vital signs, documenting any treatment-related data, and ensuring that ECT-related supplies, including those necessary for handling medical emergencies, are kept in stock and that relevant equipment is properly maintained.
c. For patients receiving ambulatory ECT, additional duties may be assumed, including assessing patients before each ECT treatment and delivering postrecovery care.

9.2.2.4. Recovery Nurse

a. The recovery nurse should be a registered nurse who is responsible for monitoring vital signs and mental status during the acute postictal/postanesthetic period. The recovery nurse should also be capable of monitoring and adjusting the flow of intravenous fluids, administering oxygen, suctioning oropharyngeal secretions, behaviorally managing postictal disorientation and agitation, and determining when intervention by the anesthesia provider or ECT psychiatrist is indicated.

b. If multiple patients will be in the recovery area simultaneously, it is preferable to have more than one recovery nurse available.

CHAPTER 10

Location, Equipment, and Supplies

10.1. Characteristics of the Treatment Site

An optimal treatment site should include three separate functional areas for waiting, treatment, and recovery and should not be used concomitantly for purposes other than ECT administration. Logistically, the various areas should be as close to each other as possible. However, they should be sufficiently distinct as to isolate patients in one area from patients and staff in other areas. Facilities administering outpatient ECT should also provide space for conducting pretreatment assessments and an area (or areas) where patients and those accompanying the patient can stay before and after the treatment session (see Sections 11.1, 11.2.2, and 11.10.4). It is helpful if this area is near the treatment area so that significant other(s) may remain with the patient before ECT.

The treatment environment should be comfortable for patients and their families, giving consideration to the need for confidentiality. Facilities should also ensure that space, ventilation, and lighting are sufficient to conduct treatments and recovery in a safe, unencumbered fashion. Adequate space should also be present for storing ECT-related records, equipment, and supplies.

The treatment site should be readily accessible to the resources needed to treat medical emergencies while maintaining proximity to inpatient psychiatric units. Facilities providing outpatient ECT should also consider the ease of treatment site access to ambulatory patients. Because of the need for ready availability of emergency equipment, supplies, and personnel, some facilities locate the treatment site in, or adjacent to, intensive care units or outpatient or inpatient surgical areas. Although such arrangements may be logistically necessary, the use of a surgical operating theater is suboptimal in other ways and should be avoided.

10.2. Equipment

Both the treatment and recovery areas should contain equipment to monitor patient vital signs and provide initial management of medical emergencies. In addition to a stethoscope, this equipment should include either a manual sphygmomanometer or an automatic device for blood pressure measurement. Both areas should also contain devices for electrocardiographic (ECG) and oxygen saturation of hemoglobin (pulse oximetry) monitoring as well as an oxygen delivery system capable of providing intermittent positive pressure oxygen and suction capability. To maintain an adequate airway, equipment in the treatment area should include an intubation set and equipment for managing patients with difficult airways (Caplan et al. 1993; Crosby et al. 1998; Wilson and Benumof 1998). The oxygen delivery system should be capable of providing intermittent positive-pressure oxygen by endotracheal tube as well as by mask. Treatment area beds or stretchers should have firm mattresses and side rails and be able to elevate both the head and the feet easily.

The treatment area should contain an ECT treatment device. Access to a backup ECT device and additional stimulus and physiologic monitoring cables is useful in the event of equipment malfunction. To determine the extent of muscle blockade prior to stimulus delivery, a reflex hammer should be present. In this regard, some practitioners also find a peripheral nerve stimulator useful. In determining seizure adequacy and detecting prolonged seizures, ictal electroencephalographic (EEG) monitoring is essential (Section 11.8.2 and 11.9). The treatment area should also have a sphygmomanometer or other means of monitoring ictal motor duration (Section 11.8.1.2). A defibrillator should be readily accessible.

10.3. Medications

Essential medications for administering ECT include anesthetic and muscle-relaxing agents (see Section 11.4). The primary anesthetic agent is generally methohexital, with succinylcholine used as a muscle relaxant. It is often useful to have alternative anesthetic agents available (e.g., etomidate, ketamine, propofol, or thiopental). Specific clinical situations may require alternative or supplementary nondepolarizing muscle relaxing agents such as curare, atracurium, mivacurium, rocuronium, or rapacuronium that in turn require reversing agents such as physostigmine, neostigmine, or edrophonium. To potentiate ictal responses, some practitioners coadminister caffeine sodium benzoate or flumazenil with ECT (see Chapter 7). To terminate prolonged or spontaneous seizures (see Section 11.9.3) and/or treat postictal delirium (see Section 11.10.3), agents such as diazepam, midazolam, or lorazepam should be on hand. Alternatively, the primary anesthetic can be used. Although lorazepam is the drug of choice for status epilepticus, fosphenytoin or phenytoin should also be available for use as a secondary treatment (American Academy of Neurology 1998; Treiman et al. 1998).

To minimize the cardiovascular impact of ECT, several other medications are commonly given and should be available in the treatment site. For example, anticholinergic agents (atropine or glycopyrrolate) are used to diminish secretions or decrease the risk of vagally mediated bradyarrhythmias (see Section 11.4.1). Several agents, including adrenergic blockers and vasodilators, have been of value in minimizing the sympathetic effects of ECT. Medications for treating cardiovascular emergencies such as arrhythmias, uncontrolled hypertension, hypotension, or cardiac arrest should also be available. These drugs include pressor agents, antiarrhythmic agents, and specific agents used in advanced cardiac life support (ACLS) protocols (Cummins 1994). For initial management of severe bronchospasm or anaphylactic shock, other medications that must be available immediately include epinephrine, diphenhydramine, aminophylline, and methylprednisolone as well as β-adrenergic agonists such as isoetharine or albuterol for administration via nebulizer.

Nausea, headache, and muscle soreness may occur after ECT (see Section 5.6). To manage these side effects, antinausea agents and nonnarcotic analgesics should be present at the treatment site. At times, narcotic analgesics may also be indicated. Nonparticulate antacids or histamine-2 selective histamine blocking agents are sometimes given before ECT to decrease gastric acidity and minimize the risk of aspiration.

Medications should be stored securely, particularly controlled drugs that must also be inventoried and verified according to hospital policy and other applicable regulations.

10.4. Supplies

The treatment site should have the supplies needed to induce anesthesia, provide ventilation, monitor physiologic functions (including seizure activity), and perform resuscitation. Sufficient quantities should be present to handle all anticipated needs.

Whenever possible, items that come into contact with body fluids should be disposable. Items such as bite-blocks may be designated for use by an individual patient and stored in a labeled plastic bag after sterilization. All procedures for sterilization and disinfection of reusable items should conform to relevant standards (Centers for Disease Control 1987; Centers for Disease Control and Prevention 1993; Rutala 1996).

- Sphygmomanometer or other method to monitor ictal motor duration
- Pulse oximeter
- Oxygen delivery system capable of providing intermittent positive pressure oxygen by mask or endotracheal tube
- Suction apparatus
- Intubation set and equipment for managing difficult airways
- Reflex hammer

e. A defibrillator should be readily accessible.

f. Access to a backup ECT treatment device and additional stimulus and physiologic monitoring cables is encouraged.

g. Availability of a peripheral nerve stimulator is also encouraged.

10.3. Medications

a. The treatment site should contain pharmacologic agents that are sufficient to induce anesthesia and muscle relaxation, modulate the parasympathetic and sympathetic effects of the ECT seizure, and provide first-line management of uncontrolled hypertension, hypotension, cardiac arrhythmias, cardiopulmonary arrest, anaphylaxis, prolonged seizures, or status epilepticus.

b. Specific medications that should be present include

- A primary anesthetic agent (methohexital sodium)
- A primary muscle relaxant (succinylcholine)
- An anticholinergic agent (glycopyrrolate and/or atropine sulfate)
- Agents for first-line management of arrhythmias, hyper- and hypotension, and cardiac arrest, such as

  - β-adrenergic blocking agents such as labetalol and esmolol
  - α-adrenergic blocking agents such as prazocin and clonidine
  - Pressor agents such as epinephrine, dopamine, norepinephrine, and phenylephrine
  - Vasodilators such as hydralazine, phentolamine, and nitroglycerin (tablets, paste, and/or sublingual spray)
  - Antiarrhythmics such as bretylium, digoxin, lidocaine, verapamil, and procainamide
  - Other agents for cardiopulmonary resuscitation

- Agents for the initial management of severe bronchospasm or

RECOMMENDATIONS

10.1. Characteristics of the Treatment Site

a. The treatment site should consist of a well-lit and well-ventilat treatment area and separate recovery and waiting areas.

b. It is desirable for waiting patients to be isolated from auditory a visual contact with treatment and recovery areas.

c. Facilities administering outpatient ECT should provide space f conducting pretreatment assessments and an area (or areas), pre erably near the treatment area, where the patient and those a companying the patient can stay before and after the treatmen session.

d. Dedicated space should be available within the treatment site fc ECT-related equipment, supplies, and records.

10.2. Equipment

a. Equipment should be available in both the treatment and recovery areas to provide suction; deliver intermittent positive-pressure oxygen; and monitor vital signs, cardiac rhythm, and hemoglobin oxygen saturation.

b. Additional equipment should be present in the treatment area for intubation, seizure induction, physiologic response monitoring, and resuscitation in case of cardiovascular or respiratory difficulty.

c. The recovery area should contain ECG monitoring and pulse oximetry devices.

d. The treatment area should contain the following equipment:

- Stretcher or bed with a firm mattress, side rails, and the capacity to elevate both the head and the feet
- Automatic blood pressure monitoring device or manual sphygmomanometer
- Stethoscope
- ECT treatment device with EEG monitoring capability
- ECG monitoring equipment

anaphylactic shock, such as epinephrine, diphenhydramine, methylprednisolone, aminophylline, and the β-adrenergic agonists for administration via nebulizer (e.g., isoetharine or albuterol)

- Other agents for managing status epilepticus, such as lorazepam or diazepam, fosphenytoin or phenytoin, and phenobarbital
- Antinausea agents such as prochlorperazine, promethazine, and ondansetron
- Nonnarcotic analgesics such as ibuprofen, ketorolac, and acetaminophen

c. Suggested additional medications include:

- Alternative anesthetic agents such as etomidate, ketamine, propofol, or thiopental
- Alternative or supplementary nondepolarizing relaxant agents such as curare, atracurium, mivacurium, rocuronium, or rapacuronium
- Acetylcholinesterase inhibitors such as edrophonium, neostigmine, and physostigmine
- A nonparticulate antacid such as bicitrate
- Narcotic analgesics
- Narcotic antagonists such as naloxone
- Miscellaneous agents such as the benzodiazepine antagonist flumazenil

d. Medications should be stored securely in a room with restricted access.
e. Controlled drugs need to be inventoried and verified according to hospital policy and other applicable regulations.

10.4. Supplies

a. The treatment site should have sufficient quantities of supplies to induce anesthesia, monitor physiologic functions (including seizure activity), and provide ventilation and resuscitation.
b. Necessary supplies include

- Bite-blocks (mouthguards)
- Infusion sets
- Intravenous fluids
- Masks for oxygen delivery
- Oro- and nasopharyngeal airways

- Endotracheal tubes
- Suction catheters
- Syringes and syringe needles in assorted sizes
- Electrode gel or paste
- Monitoring electrode pads and leads
- Stimulus and monitoring cables for ECT device
- Recording paper for monitoring use
- Alcohol pads
- Material to prepare stimulus and monitoring electrode sites
- Gauze pads in assorted sizes
- Tape in assorted sizes
- Disposable gloves
- Containers for disposal of sharps and clinical waste

c. It is also useful to have access to butterfly needles in assorted sizes and heparin locks and flush solution.

d. Gowns, masks, and face shields for universal precautions should be readily available.

e. Whenever possible, items that come into contact with body fluids should be disposable. Bite-blocks and face masks may be also designated for use by an individual patient and stored in a labeled plastic bag after cleaning.

f. All procedures for sterilization and disinfection of reusable items should conform to relevant standards.

CHAPTER 11

Treatment Procedures

11.1. Determining Whether ECT Should Be Administered on an Inpatient or Outpatient Treatment Basis

The decision to treat on an inpatient or outpatient basis should be considered during the pre-ECT evaluation. In practice, this choice depends on a number of criteria, including patient preference, and should be viewed as a dynamic, ongoing process throughout the ECT course. Certain situations will indicate a switch from inpatient to outpatient setting and others will suggest a switch in the opposite direction.

In making this decision the same indications, relative contraindications, consent requirements, and components of the pre-ECT evaluation hold for both inpatient and ambulatory ECT. The inpatient setting should be used whenever the patient's psychiatric condition precludes safe and effective management on an outpatient basis. For example, patients at high risk of suicide should not be treated as outpatients until such risk is sufficiently diminished that they can be discharged from the inpatient setting. Psychotic ideation, severe preexisting cognitive impairment, or inanition may raise doubt about the patient's capacity to receive ambulatory ECT (Fink et al. 1996).

Likewise, patients at high risk of serious medical complications or who present with anticipated risks that may be difficult to detect or manage on an outpatient basis should initially receive ECT treatments as inpatients. Once it can be shown that these risks are sufficiently diminished to allow safe outpatient management, a change in the treatment setting can be considered. Examples here include individuals who are at substantially increased risk to develop a post-ECT delirium (e.g., preexisting neurologic impairment, history of ECT-induced organic brain syndrome from previous courses of treatment [see Sections 4.1.2 and 5.5]) or patients with serious medical conditions that greatly increase other risks of ECT (e.g., unstable aneurysm [see Chapter 3]). The Association for Convulsive Therapy Task Force concluded that patients in American Society of Anesthesiologists (1963) categories 4–5 (rated on the basis of medical condition and history prior to treatment on a 1 to 5 scale, where 1 is lowest risk and 5 is highest) should receive ECT while hospitalized. For patients in category 3, which represents an intermediate degree of risk, this decision should be made on an individual basis depending on type and extent of risk as well as the effects of other factors (Fink et al. 1996; Ross and Tucker 1990). Patients at high risk and in need of ECT should be treated in facilities with a wide range of medical capabilities.

Patients should not be referred for outpatient ECT unless they are willing and able to comply with the requirements of this setting. In addition to avoiding oral intake for several hours before each treatment, such requirements include the ability to reliably adjust medication intake in conjunction with each treatment as well as follow specific directions on bowel, bladder, and grooming behavior before each treatment. Attention should also be paid to ensuring safe transit from the facility after treatment. To help ensure compliance with these requirements, it is necessary that outpatients have a responsible person available who will assist in this process. The absence of such an individual will make outpatient ECT impossible unless these "care-taking" functions can be provided by temporary transfer to a structured environment (such as a nursing home or day hospital program) for the duration of the acute ECT course. When travel hardship is substantial, inpatient treatment may be necessary.

Patients, significant others, and caregivers should be informed of these behavioral requirements on an ongoing basis. Instructions should be supplemented by a standardized information sheet given after each treatment on discharge from the facility. Because the patient's condition may change with time, compliance with behavioral requirements should be assessed before each treatment and suitability for inpatient or outpatient setting should be regularly reevaluated. It should be noted that in some patients rapid symptomatic improvement may be associated with a greater need for hospitalization—for example, individuals whose newly increased energy affords them the drive to act on suicidal urges. When the degree of risk and the extent of the patient's ability to comply with behavioral requirements are difficult to assess prior to an index ECT course, it may be prudent to initiate treatments on an inpatient basis. This situation appears to be particularly common with elderly patients (Fink et al. 1996).

During and shortly after an index ECT course and for patients receiving continuation/maintenance ECT at short (e.g., weekly) intervals, activities that are likely to be impaired by the adverse cognitive effects of ECT should generally be avoided, including driving. Because marked individual differences occur in the severity and duration of cognitive side effects, and because these adverse effects vary with treatment parameters (see Chapter 5), limitations on such activities should be tailored to the individual patient and adjusted as indicated. With long intervals between treatments, as is typical with continuation/ maintenance ECT, adverse cognitive side effects usually do not persist beyond the day of the treatment. At a minimum, patients receiving outpatient index ECT should be specifically instructed to refrain from making major life decisions, including those related to matters of business, personal finances, and interpersonal relations, until the ECT course is completed and residual cognitive side effects have cleared. Patients should also be strongly cautioned that ECT may impair driving ability during and shortly after an index course of treatment.

To ensure that an overall treatment plan is properly implemented over a course of ECT (either index or continuation/maintenance), an attending physician should be designated who maintains overall responsibility for patient management during and immediately after the outpatient ECT course. In some cases, this individual is the ECT psychiatrist, whereas in other situations a separate provider fulfills this role. In the latter case, it is important that this provider coordinate the overall plan of care with the ECT treatment team, including matters such as inpatient versus outpatient setting, stimulus electrode placement, number of treatments, and choice of continuation treatment. Patients and significant others should be instructed to inform the attending physician or the ECT treatment team of any adverse effects of ECT or changes in medical condition before the next treatment.

11.2. Preparing the Patient

11.2.1. Before the First Treatment

As described in Chapter 6, a pre-ECT psychiatric and general medical evaluation should be completed before the first treatment. The ECT psychiatrist should ensure that this evaluation has been performed.

11.2.2. Before Each Treatment

Before each treatment, nursing staff should ascertain compliance with pretreatment orders. Patients should have had nothing to eat or drink by mouth for several hours prior to the treatment, except for necessary medications with a small sip of water. Typical recommendations are a fasting period of 6–8 hours for solid food and 2 hours for clear liquids (American Society of Anesthesiologists Task Force on Perioperative Fasting 1999). Patients with cognitive impairment or psychosis may have difficulty remembering food and water intake restrictions and may require supervision. When patients arrive for ECT they should be asked if they have taken anything by mouth over the past several hours. The nursing staff should have patients void, check the patients' heads and hair for pins and jewelry, and ensure that the patients' hair is clean and dry. Hair spray or cream can produce shorting of the electrical current through the hair, singeing the hair and interfering with seizure induction. Eyeglasses, contact lenses, and hearing aids should be removed. Dentures should also be removed unless specially indicated (e.g., loose and isolated teeth that need protection). Finger rings need not be removed. The fingernail or toenail used for pulse oximetry should be free of nail polish. Vital signs should be recorded.

Prior to the treatment, the ECT psychiatrist should interview the patient to determine whether any significant changes in mental status or clinical symptoms have occurred since the last treatment. The ECT psychiatrist should review orders in the patient's medical record since the last ECT. Both the ECT psychiatrist and anesthesia provider should be aware of any change in medications since the last treatment and any change in medical status. The patient's mouth should be checked for the presence of foreign bodies and loose or sharp teeth. When the patient is ready for ECT, intravenous access should be established. This access often involves maintaining an intravenous line with a saline or lactated Ringer's drip, although some practitioners prefer to inject medications directly into a lockable indwelling catheter. In either case, the intravenous line should be adequate to handle emergency needs, and care should be taken to ensure that all intravenously administered medications are flushed. Intravenous access should be maintained at least until the patient is conscious and vital signs are stable. For patients with difficult intravenous access, options include leaving a lockable indwelling catheter in place between treatments or using a peripherally inserted central catheter (PICC) line or portacath (MacKenzie et al. 1996).

For inpatients, at least some of these activities usually occur on the inpatient unit, whereas for outpatients, additional potential locations include an area adjacent to the recovery area, an ambulatory surgery suite, or a day hospital. Using the recovery area space itself is not desirable because it exposes alert patients to those who are emerging from the postictal, anesthetized state. With outpatients, it is also helpful to provide a waiting area for individuals who accompany them to the facility. Optimally, this area should be convenient to the location where the patients are being prepared for treatment so that the significant other(s) can stay with the patient and help keep them comfortable during the pre-ECT period (during which time some patients are anxious). Attention to such patient satisfaction issues facilitates the development and maintenance of a positive relationship among patients, their significant others, and the ECT team.

Particularly for patients receiving ambulatory ECT, the ECT psychiatrist should ascertain whether any unexpected or severe adverse effects took place after the previous treatment, whether any change in medical conditions or alteration in medication regimen or compliance has occurred over the interval between treatments, and whether any further evaluation or alteration in treatment technique is indicated. Given the relative lack of privacy as well as the level of distraction generally present in the actual treatment room, such assessments should occur in a separate allocated space if at all possible.

11.3. Airway Management

The anesthesia provider is responsible for airway management during the entire ECT procedure. Before the first ECT treatment of each day, the anesthesia provider should verify that relevant equipment is functioning adequately and that supplies for resuscitation are available.

11.3.1. Establishing an Airway

For each patient, the ability to provide adequate ventilation should be verified before the muscle relaxant is administered. Patients who may require particular attention include those who are obese or in the third trimester of pregnancy and those with pulmonary disease or congestion. Unless specifically indicated, as may occur in late stages of pregnancy (see Section 4.3), routine use of intubation should be avoided.

11.3.2. Oxygenation

Oxygenation (100% O_2, positive pressure, and a respiratory rate of 15–20 breaths per minute) should be maintained from the onset of anesthesia until adequate spontaneous respiration is resumed, except during application of the electrical stimulus. Several minutes of preanesthetic oxygenation may be useful for patients at risk for myocardial ischemia and for patients with weakly expressed or short seizures (Bergsholm et al. 1984; Chater and Simpson 1988; Holmberg 1953; Räsänen et al. 1988). Preoxygenation is also an important component of the management of patients at risk for rapid hemoglobin oxygen desaturation after anesthetic induction. This group includes morbidly obese patients and those with pulmonary disease. A minimum of 2–5 minutes of ventilation with 15–20 breaths per minute of 100% oxygen at 5 L/min is recommended (Gold et al. 1981; Valentine et al. 1990). Oxygen delivery should be resumed during the seizure (Lew et al. 1986; McCormick and Saunders 1996; Swindells and Simpson 1987) because cerebral oxygen consumption increases on the order of 200% (Davis et al. 1944; Ingvar 1986; Kreisman et al. 1983; Saito et al. 1996). Care should be taken to avoid inducing electroencephalographic (EEG) artifact during this ventilatory process. Because of the effects of the muscle relaxant and the seizure, patients remain apneic during the immediate postictal state and require oxygenation until the recovery of spontaneous respiration. To monitor adequacy of oxygenation, oximetry should be used in all patients (see Section 11.8.3).

11.3.3 Protecting Teeth and Other Oral Structures

Before applying the electrical stimulus, a flexible protective device (bite-block) should be inserted in the mouth. Use of a plastic airway (e.g., Guedel-type) as a bite-block is not recommended because of the increased risk of tooth fracture or jaw injury (Abrams 1997a). The electrical stimulus results in direct stimulation of pterygoid, masseter, and temporalis muscles, which produces a clamping action of the jaw muscles that is not blocked by the muscle relaxant (Minneman 1995). Use of a flexible material that extends across the mouth, with maximal cushioning in the molar area, absorbs the force of this clamping action and protects the teeth and other oral structures. Bite-blocks should allow passage of air, because nostrils may become blocked by secretions. It is useful to have different-sized bite-blocks to accommodate patients with different mouth sizes. In the uncommon circumstance of patients with only one or a few fragile teeth, use of a bite-block may contribute to dental complications. It may be preferable to leave dentures in place and to use gauze padding between the gums to absorb the force of the jaw clamping. Regardless, it is always necessary to use some form of protection to absorb the clamping force. To prevent or limit potential trauma with passage of the electrical stimulus, the patient's chin should be manually supported, keeping the jaw tight against the bite-block.

11.4. Medications Used with ECT

11.4.1. Anticholinergic Agents

Immediately after the electrical stimulus, a short period of bradycardia frequently occurs that then converts to tachycardia during the seizure. Bradyarrhythmias are also common during the postictal period. Premedication with an anticholinergic agent prior to anesthetic induction reduces the risk of vagally mediated bradyarrhythmias or asystole (Shettar et al. 1989). Not all practitioners routinely use such medications, because evidence of their utility in moderating the cardiovascular effects of ECT is limited (Bouckoms et al. 1989; Miller et al. 1987; Rich et al. 1969; Wyant and MacDonald 1980; Zielinski et al. 1993). However, the controlled studies largely excluded patients with preexisting cardiac illness, limiting the relevance of their conclusions for patients believed to be at greatest risk for cardiovascular complications (Miller et al. 1987). Furthermore, if the electrical stimulus fails to elicit a seizure (subconvulsive administration), bradycardia immediately after the stimulus is of graver concern. The protection afforded by the ictal tachycardia (due to seizure-related catecholamine release) is absent, and the probability of asystole is greater (Decina et al. 1984; McCall 1996). Because administration of subconvulsive stimuli is intrinsic to empirical titration for identifying seizure threshold (Sackeim et al. 1987c), many practitioners routinely administer an anticholinergic agent at treatment sessions in which titration is planned. Many practitioners believe that use of an anticholinergic agent is especially indicated for patients receiving sympathetic blocking agents (e.g., β-blockers) or any other circumstance in which it is medically important to prevent the occurrence of a vagal bradycardia (Zielinski et al. 1993). On the other hand, in some patients an anticholinergic agent may aggravate preexisting tachycardia and result in increased cardiac workload (rate pressure product) (Mayur et al. 1998). Other potential adverse effects of anticholinergics include constipation/fecal impaction and urinary retention.

Traditionally, anticholinergic agents have been administered either intravenously, 2–3 minutes prior to anesthesia, or intramuscularly, 30–60 minutes prior to anesthesia. The latter technique has the advantage of maximizing reduction of secretions, thus potentially improving airway management. However, the intravenous route is preferred because it guarantees that the anticholinergic has been administered, obviates the need for an additional injection, and avoids increased dryness of the mouth at a time when the patient cannot drink fluids (Kramer 1993, Kramer et al. 1992). Perhaps most importantly, the action of the anticholinergic medication in increasing heart rate can be observed prior to the anesthetic induction, thus ensuring adequacy of anticholinergic dosage. Given individual differences in distribution and duration of action, intramuscular administration 30–60 minutes prior to anesthesia may not offer protection for some patients. Subcutaneous administration of the anticholinergic agent should not be used.

The typical anticholinergic agents used are atropine, 0.4–0.8 mg iv (or 0.3–0.6 mg im) or glycopyrrolate, 0.2–0.4 mg iv or im. Glycopyrrolate has the theoretical advantage of being less likely to cross the blood-brain barrier. However, controlled comparisons of glycopyrrolate and atropine in ECT have not revealed differences in effects on cognition, cardiac function, or postictal reports of nausea (Greenan et al. 1985; Kelway et al. 1986; Kramer et al. 1986; Simpson et al. 1987; Sommer et al. 1989; Swartz and Saheba 1989). Relative to glycopyrrolate, atropine may have greater consistency in producing the desired vagal-blocking effect. The practitioner should take into account the muscarinic properties of any other pharmacologic agents that have been administered.

11.4.2. Anesthetic Agents

ECT should be performed using only ultra-brief general anesthesia (Drop and Welch 1989; Gaines and Rees 1986). The purpose of anesthesia is to produce unconsciousness throughout the period of muscle relaxation, including the seizure. Therefore, unconsciousness should last only several minutes. Excessive anesthetic dosage may prolong unconsciousness and apnea, raise seizure threshold, shorten seizure duration, increase the risk of cardiovascular complications, and intensify amnesia (Boylan et al. 2000; Krueger et al. 1993; Miller et al. 1985). However, if dosage is too low, loss of consciousness may be incomplete, autonomic arousal may occur, and a frightening period of pre-ECT paralysis may be recalled after the procedure. Thus, the aim is to produce a "light level" of anesthesia.

Methohexital is the preferred anesthetic agent for ECT because of its established safety record, effectiveness, and low cost. The typical dose of methohexital is 0.5–1.0 mg/kg given as a single intravenous bolus. Alternative agents are etomidate, ketamine, propofol, and thiopental. Thiopental may be associated with a higher incidence of postictal arrhythmias compared with methohexital (Pitts 1982), although this difference has been questioned (Pearlman and Richmond 1990).

Despite the recent increase in propofol use, evidence of its effects on the relative safety and efficacy of ECT is still preliminary. Numerous studies have shown that propofol (0.75–1.5 mg/kg iv) results in a reduction in the magnitude of hemodynamic changes that accompany ECT as well as a reduction in seizure duration (Avramov et al. 1995; Boey and Lai 1990; Bone et al. 1988; Dwyer et al. 1988; Fear et al. 1994; Fredman et al. 1994; Kirkby et al. 1995; Lim et al. 1996; Malsch et al. 1994; Martensson et al. 1994; Martin et al. 1998; Matters et al. 1995; Mitchell et al. 1991; Rampton et al. 1989; Rouse 1988; Simpson et al. 1988; Villalonga et al. 1993). The initial finding of decreased seizure duration with propofol led some researchers to question the advisability of its routine use for ECT (Swartz 1992). However, it has become increasingly clear that seizure duration has limited relevance to the efficacy of ECT (Nobler et al. 1993; Sackeim et al. 1991, 1993, 2000). Furthermore, randomized trials have not shown a difference in therapeutic outcome when propofol was used as the anesthetic agent compared with either methohexital or thiopental. Pain on injection may be more frequent with propofol. In other medical contexts, propofol seems to be associated with particularly rapid and "smooth" recovery from anesthesia. However, propofol does not appear to differ from other anesthetic agents in the speed of postictal recovery or the magnitude of postictal cognitive deficits after ECT (Martensson et al. 1994; Matters et al. 1995).

Use of etomidate (0.15–0.30 mg/kg) (Greenberg et al. 1989; Ilivicky et al. 1995; Trzepacz et al. 1993) or ketamine (2–3 mg/kg) (Lunn et al. 1981; Rasmussen et al. 1996) is typically considered for patients who are resistant to seizure elicitation or who manifest brief or abortive seizures with other anesthetic agents. Across their respective dosing ranges, seizure duration is longer with etomidate than methohexital or propofol (Avramov et al. 1995; Saffer and Berk 1998; Trzepacz et al. 1993). Etomidate may be more frequently associated with pain on injection and a longer recovery period than methohexital. Etomidate may be particularly considered for patients with congestive heart failure and related conditions because it is less likely to result in hypotensive effects compared with alternatives. Ketamine can be sympathomimetic and occasionally may produce altered states of consciousness in the postictal period, including hallucinations. Its use is usually reserved for instances in which adequate seizure elicitation cannot be accomplished with maximal device settings. Regardless of the anesthetic medication used, the appropriateness of dosage should be determined at each treatment and adjustments made at subsequent treatments.

11.4.3. Muscle Relaxants

A skeletal muscle relaxant should be used to modify convulsive motor activity and enhance airway management. The preferred relaxant agent is succinylcholine (0.5–1.0 mg/kg) administered as an intravenous bolus. Before administering the muscle relaxant, the anesthesia provider should ensure that a patent airway is present and that the patient will be unconscious prior to the onset of respiratory paralysis. The relaxant may be administered either immediately after the anesthetic agent or after initial signs of unconsciousness. The latter method is generally preferable because of treatment-to-treatment variability in anesthetic response within patients. Otherwise, patients may recall a frightening experience of paralysis without unconsciousness, despite the subsequent elicitation of a generalized seizure.

The purpose of the muscle relaxant is to produce sufficient modification of the convulsive movements to minimize the risk of musculoskeletal injury. Complete paralysis is neither necessary nor desirable. However, for some patients, such as those with osteoporosis or a history of spinal injury, complete relaxation may be indicated and dosage may be adjusted upward. Adequacy of muscle relaxation should be determined at each treatment session and dosage should be modified at successive sessions to achieve the desired effect.

Use of a nondepolarizing muscle relaxant may be indicated in patients with pseudocholinesterase deficiency, cholinesterase inhibition (e.g., secondary to some antiglaucoma medications or exposure to organophosphate pesticides), hypercalcemia, severe neuromuscular disease or injury (e.g., quadriplegia, amyotrophic lateral sclerosis, muscular dystrophy), severe osteoporosis, severe muscular rigidity, or personal or family history of malignant hyperthermia (American Medical Association 1990; Book et al. 1994). Succinylcholine should also be avoided in patients with severe and widespread burns, because it may result in excessive potassium release (Dwersteg and Avery 1987). Atracurium, 0.3–0.5 mg/kg (Burnstein and Denny 1993; Hickey et al. 1987; Hicks 1987; Messer et al. 1992; Stack et al. 1988); mivacurium, 0.15–0.2 mg/kg (Gitlin et al. 1993; Janis et al. 1995; Kelly and Brull 1994); rocuronium, 0.45–0.6 mg/kg (Motamed et al. 1997; Pino et al. 1998; Tsui et al. 1998); and rapacuronium, 1.0–2.0 mg/kg (Fisher et al. 1999; Szenohradszky et al. 1999) are alternatives to succinylcholine (Savarese et al. 1994). Relative to succinylcholine, atracurium, mivacurium, rocuronium, and rapacuronium produce more prolonged paralysis and are more expensive. Because of their duration of effect, their action should be reversed by administering an anticholinesterase agent such as neostigmine or physostigmine combined with atropine after seizure induction (Kramer and Afrasiabi 1991; Savarese 1998). Both the onset and offset of action of these agents should be monitored with a nerve stimulator.

Before the electrical stimulus is applied, the adequacy of muscle relaxation is ascertained by the diminution or loss of knee, ankle, or plantar withdrawal reflexes, loss of muscle tone, and/or the diminution or failure to respond to a nerve stimulator. A nerve stimulator is especially useful for patients in whom the extent of relaxation is uncertain and who are at heightened risk for musculoskeletal complications, or in whom nondepolarizing muscle relaxants are used on an exclusive basis. With a depolarizing muscle relaxant such as succinylcholine, it is unlikely that maximal effect has taken place until after muscle fasciculations have disappeared. The electrical stimulus is usually applied following the disappearance of fasciculations. The last body part to fasciculate is usually the legs. Elderly patients often take longer to reach full relaxation than younger patients (Beale et al. 1994a).

Routine determination of pseudocholinesterase levels or dibucaine number is not recommended. Such determinations should be reserved for patients with a personal or family history of prolonged apnea following exposure to muscle relaxants (Berry and Whittaker 1975; Viby-Mogensen and Hanel 1978). In such cases, dibucaine number may be more informative. In the event of a positive test or prolonged apnea at a previous treatment, succinylcholine in very low doses (e.g., initial dose of 1–5 mg iv) or an alternative agent such as atracurium or rocuronium should be considered (Hickey et al. 1987; Kramer and Afrasiabi 1991). The anesthesia provider should be aware of the medical conditions and medications that may influence the action of muscle relaxant agents (American Medical Association 1990; Marco and Randels 1979).

After the first ECT treatment, some patients report deep muscle pain. If the convulsive movements were well modified, this phenomenon may be caused by intense fasciculations after succinylcholine administration. The intensity of succinylcholine-induced fasciculations may be diminished by administering curare (3–4.5 mg iv) or atracurium (3–4.5 mg iv) prior to the succinylcholine. If these medications are used, it may be necessary to increase the succinylcholine dose by 10% to 25% to achieve the same degree of muscle relaxation as at the previous treatment, because succinylcholine and curariform agents are competitive in their action. It should be noted, however, that complaints of muscle soreness are often not reported at subsequent treatments despite no change in technique.

11.4.4. Agents Used to Modify the Cardiovascular Response to ECT

Cardiovascular complications are the most common cause of medical morbidity and mortality with ECT (see Section 5.1), especially in the elderly (Sackeim 1998) and in those presenting with cardiovascular disease (Zielinski et al. 1993) (see Section 4.1.3). It is surprising, therefore, that little prospective controlled research has been done to evaluate the possible protection afforded by pharmacologically modifying the acute hemodynamic effects of ECT. In recent years, prophylactic use of β-adrenergic blocking agents such as labetalol or esmolol has become more common, with the goal of lessening the hypertensive and tachycardic effects of seizure induction (Figiel et al. 1993, 1994; Howie et al. 1990; Kovac et al. 1991; McCall et al. 1991; Stoudemire et al. 1990). Other agents that are used with similar aims include nitrates (Ciraulo et al. 1978), hydralazine (Abrams 1991), calcium channel blockers (Wells et al. 1989), diazoxide (Kraus and Remick 1982), and ganglionic blockers (e.g., trimethaphan) (Petrides et al. 1996). Likewise, in recent years, a growing number of centers have begun using propofol as the anesthetic instead of methohexital or thiopental, despite its anticonvulsant action, because propofol results in a smaller magnitude of hemodynamic changes

(Avramov et al. 1995; Boey and Lai 1990; Bone et al. 1988; Dwyer et al. 1988; Kirkby et al. 1995).

Driving this practice is the belief that the frequency or severity of arrhythmias, cardiac ischemia, and other cardiovascular adverse events are reduced by minimizing the ECT-induced increases in heart rate and blood pressure (Figiel et al. 1994; Maneksha 1991; O'Connor et al. 1996). However, in patients with preexisting cardiac illness, few studies have compared rates of cardiac complication with or without such an intervention (Castelli et al. 1995; Stoudemire et al. 1990). Thus, whether any of these approaches is effective in limiting cardiovascular morbidity has not been well documented. Indeed, when Castelli et al. (1995) compared esmolol (1.3 or 4.4 mg/kg) and labetalol (0.13 or 0.44 mg/kg) with placebo in patients at elevated cardiac risk, the β-blockers successfully reduced ECT-induced hemodynamic elevations, but no evidence of benefit was found with respect to cardiac complications. The findings were negative because no adverse events, including significant ST-segment changes, were noted in any treatment group, including placebo.

When to use such a strategy requires judgment, and three major considerations suggest that indiscriminant use should be avoided. First, asystole during ECT can be an unintended side effect of administering agents that decrease heart rate, particularly β-blockers (Decina et al. 1984; Kaufman 1994; McCall 1996). The application of the electrical stimulus results in vagal stimulation regardless of whether a seizure is induced. This parasympathetic discharge almost invariably results in decreased heart rate unless patients are premedicated with an anticholinergic agent such as atropine or glycopyrrolate (McCall et al. 1994). Seizure induction produces a sympathetic discharge with an outpouring of catecholamines and a subsequent conversion from bradycardia to tachycardia. At or after the end of the seizure, reflex bradycardia may occur. For various reasons, subconvulsive stimulation (the administration of an electrical stimulus below the seizure threshold) can happen at any time during ECT. In this case, the parasympathetic discharge is unopposed, and in the presence of a β-blocker, asystole may result (Decina et al. 1984; McCall 1996). Similarly, medications that limit heart rate increases can exaggerate postseizure reflex bradycardia.

Second, one of the most common circumstances for considering the use of an agent to limit hemodynamic change is when patients are tachycardic or hypertensive before receiving ECT. The concern here is that further increases in heart rate or blood pressure will not be tolerated. However, two studies examined predictors of the magnitude of the peak hemodynamic changes during ECT and consistently found that patients with baseline tachycardia or hypertension (or elevated rate pressure product) showed the smallest absolute increases after seizure induction (Prudic et al. 1987; Webb et al. 1990). In other words, the patients of most concern often show the least dramatic increases in hemodynamic variables without any procedural alterations. In part, this relationship may be due to the fact that sympathetic discharge may occur with pre-ECT anxiety, and ceiling effects limit further sympathetic activity with seizure induction.

Finally, there is a theoretical concern that pretreating to limit hemodynamic changes may be counterproductive with respect to other side effects. During electrically induced seizures, cerebral blood flow increases markedly, on the order of 300%. Oxygen use and glucose metabolism also increase, with estimates on the order of 200% (Ackermann et al. 1986; Siesjö et al. 1986). Given the magnitude of the hemodynamic changes associated with ECT, autoregulation of cerebral blood flow is not maintained (Saito et al. 1995, 1996). Thus, the increased cardiac output and peripheral hypertension associated with the seizure may be necessary to sustain the profound ictal increase in cerebral blood flow. In turn, the enhanced cerebral blood flow provides the transport of the oxygen and carbohydrate supplies that are necessary to sustain the large ictal increase in cerebral metabolic rate. Speculatively, limiting the peripheral hemodynamic surge may reduce the supply of oxygen and carbohydrates to the brain. This relative ischemia could account for the reduced seizure duration seen with a variety of these agents, including β-blockers (Howie et al. 1990; Kovac et al. 1991; McCall et al. 1991; O'Flaherty et al. 1992) and propofol (Avramov et al. 1995; Kirkby et al. 1995) and theoretically could worsen cognitive side effects.

In this light, judgment is needed about when to use pharmacologic modifications to blunt the cardiovascular effects of ECT (see also Section 4.1.3). In patients who are unequivocally at increased risk for vascular complications, such as those with unstable aneurysms, it is wise to fully block the hemodynamic changes that accompany seizure induction, and such modifications should be used prophylactically at all treatments (Devanand et al. 1990). In patients with unstable hypertension or other cardiac conditions, an attempt should be made to stabilize the medical condition before beginning ECT. In most patients, with or without preexisting cardiac illness, many practitioners will forego prophylaxis and monitor cardiovascular changes closely at the initial treatments. The occasional sustained hypertension or significant arrhythmia after seizure induction is then treated acutely, and prophylaxis is considered for subsequent treatments. Following these guidelines, one study documented that 38 of 40 patients with prospectively determined serious cardiac illness successfully completed an ECT course (Zielinski et al. 1993). A strong working relationship with the anesthesia provider and an informative cardiology consultation are helpful in optimizing the management of patients with significant cardiac illness.

11.5. ECT Devices

A variety of devices to administer ECT is in use. Appendix C provides a list of the devices presently used in clinical treatment in the United States, as well as a partial description of their features. These devices generate either a unidirectional or a bidirectional pulse stimulus or a bidirectional sine wave stimulus. Some ECT devices are capable of delivering more than one type of waveform, as specified by the user.

11.5.1. Waveform Characteristics

Figure 11–1 illustrates the waveforms in current use. Waveforms differ markedly in their efficiency in eliciting seizures (Sackeim et al. 1994). Generally speaking, a less intense stimulus, in units of charge (milli-Coloumb [mC] or milliampere-second [mA-sec]) or energy (joules or watt-second), is needed to produce a seizure with a brief pulse stimulus than a sine wave stimulus (Weiner 1980). This difference may be on the order of threefold. It is believed that the leading edge of each phase of the waveform is responsible for neuronal depolarization and seizure induction. Through the process of accommodation, the firing threshold of neurons can be increased by applying a slow-rising current, as occurs with a sine wave stimulus. In contrast, a fast-rising current (e.g., brief pulse) will result in cell firing at lower current intensity (Koester 1985). The optimal current duration to produce central neuronal depolarization may be on the order of only 0.1–0.2 ms (Sackeim et al. 1994). Continuing to stimulate a neuron immediately after it has fired is inefficient because there is a refractory period before it can again be depolarized.

As shown in Figure 11–1, the traditional sine wave stimulus is slow to reach maximum intensity and has a long phase duration. Therefore,

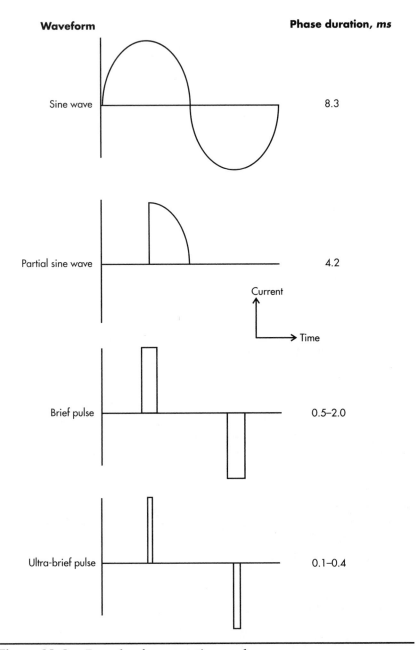

Figure 11–1.   *Examples of representative waveforms.*
A single cycle of each waveform is shown, with current on the vertical axis and
time on the horizontal axis.

at the beginning of each phase, stimulation intensity is too low to produce effective depolarization and the neuronal threshold will increase. After peak intensity is reached with the sine wave, the long-phase duration results in stimulation during neuronal refractory periods. In contrast, the brief pulse waveform reaches peak intensity virtually instantaneously. The duration of each pulse is relatively short, with rapid return to baseline. Therefore, this configuration is more electrically efficient in eliciting seizures.

Comparative studies of sine wave and brief pulse waveforms have shown that short-term cognitive side effects are considerably more severe with sine wave stimulation (Carney et al. 1976; Valentine et al. 1968; Weiner et al. 1986a). Likewise, there is evidence that disruption of the EEG is more profound with sine wave stimulation (Weiner et al. 1986b). These differences are likely due to the greater electrical efficiency of brief pulse stimulation. It had been suggested that some patients who did not respond to treatment with a brief pulse stimulus may benefit from treatment with a sine wave stimulus (Price and McAllister 1986; Price et al. 1986). However, comparative studies have generally found that sine wave and brief pulse stimulation are equivalent in efficacy (Andrade et al. 1988a; Carney et al. 1976; Scott et al. 1992; Valentine et al. 1968; Weiner et al. 1986a). Consequently, the continued use of sine wave stimulation in ECT is not justified. Sine wave stimulation is inherently inefficient in electrical dosing, results in more severe cognitive side effects, and has no advantages with respect to efficacy.

An unresolved issue in the use of brief pulse stimulation concerns the optimal pulse width. As indicated, the chronaxie or optimal duration of a pulse to produce neuronal depolarization may be on the order of 0.1–0.2 ms (Sackeim et al. 1994). In accordance with this, some evidence indicates that pulse widths on the order of 0.5–0.75 ms are more efficient in seizure elicitation than pulse widths of longer duration (e.g., 1.5 ms) (Rasmussen et al. 1994; Swartz and Larsen 1989). Nonetheless, the range of brief pulse duration (pulse width) available with currently marketed ECT devices is between 0.25 and 2 ms, considerably longer than the chronaxie for neuronal depolarization. Indeed, with some devices the shortest pulse width that can be delivered is 1.0 ms. In contrast, ultra-brief pulse widths (less than 0.5 ms) may be particularly efficient at seizure elicitation (Lisanby et al. 1997). Several studies have established that ultra-brief pulse configurations can reliably elicit generalized seizures in animals (Hovorka et al. 1960; Hyrman et al. 1985;

Liberson 1945, 1947) and humans (Cronholm and Ottosson 1963a; Goldman 1949; Liberson 1948; Pisvejc et al. 1998; Robin and de Tissera 1982) at substantially lower absolute electrical dosage than is the case with standard brief pulse stimulation. There had been reluctance in the field to consider the use of ultra-brief pulse configurations (American Psychiatric Association 1990), largely based on the findings of Cronholm and Ottosson (1963a) and Robin and de Tissera (1982) that this type of stimulation may have reduced efficacy or require additional treatments to produce therapeutic response. However, it is also likely that ultra-brief pulse stimulation was not optimized in these studies, either in terms of the particular characteristics of the waveform, such as pulse frequency and peak current, or in terms of overall intensity relative to threshold. At the time, it was not known that stimulus intensity with respect to seizure threshold had an impact on the efficacy of the treatment (McCall et al. 2000; Sackeim et al. 1987a, 1993, 2000). Therefore, the aim was only to use a highly efficient waveform that minimized absolute stimulus dosage. It was not recognized that ensuring that stimulation was substantially suprathreshold had implications for efficacy. Ongoing research is examining the possibility that the use of ultra-brief pulses combined with suprathreshold stimulation may preserve the efficacy of ECT while further reducing cognitive side effects.

11.5.2. Mode of Stimulus Delivery

ECT devices also differ in whether they operate on principles of constant current, constant voltage, or constant energy. With constant current devices, the peak current is either fixed or set by the user. The device adjusts the voltage administered during the stimulation to keep the current at the desired level. By Ohm's law (voltage = current × resistance), voltage varies as a function of the impedance (or resistance) to the passage of the current. Thus, an increase in impedance requires an increase in voltage to keep the current constant.

Because the quality of contact at the interface between the electrodes and the skin is a major determinant of impedance, inadequate contact results in increased impedance. In such circumstances, as illustrated in Figure 11–2, constant current devices deliver the predetermined stimulus current to the patient by increasing the output voltage. Highly excessive output voltage may result in burns to the skin. For this reason, constant current devices should be equipped with voltage limiters that prevent delivery of excessive voltage under abnormally high impedance conditions. However, the user should be aware that when the device limits the voltage because of excessive impedance, the current will not be maintained at the set level. Thus, the patient may fail to have a seizure or, if a seizure occurs, the stimulus intensity may be close to threshold with reduced therapeutic effects.

With constant voltage devices, the current varies inversely with impedance. By Ohm's law, an increase in impedance will result in a decrease in the intensity of the delivered current. This phenomenon is also illustrated in Figure 11–2. It has been suggested that current intensity (charge, mC) relative to the area of neural tissue through which it passes (current density, mC/cm^2) is the critical factor in both seizure induction and other neurobiologic effects of the ECT stimulus (Agnew and McCreery 1987; Offner 1942, 1946; Pudenz et al. 1975; Sackeim et al. 1987c, 1994; Woodbury and Davenport 1952). This relationship raises concern about the rationale for the use of constant voltage principles in ECT devices. The user may not have access to information about the current intensity administered. In addition, with greatly increased impedance due to relatively poor contact or skin conditions, the resulting decrease in current intensity with constant voltage devices may not permit induction of an adequate seizure. Thus, no conceptual justification exists for the use of a constant voltage device in ECT.

Another approach to stimulus delivery is to keep the output energy constant. With such a device, the user selects the energy to be administered in units of joules (watt/second). To keep the energy constant, the device will vary the duration of the stimulus. The theoretical justification for such a design is also not self-evident. To deliver the user-determined energy, a shorter stimulus duration will be given to patients with higher impedances than to those with lower impedances. With a constant energy device, as with a constant voltage device, the delivered charge will be inversely proportional to the impedance in the circuit. Yet, as indicated earlier, it is unlikely that variation in impedance is relevant to therapeutic properties or adverse effects. Furthermore, doubt has been raised about the usefulness and validity of quantifying the ECT stimulus in units of energy (joules) as opposed to units of charge (mC) (Sackeim et al. 1987c, 1994; Weiner et al. 1987). Thus, there is no conceptual justification for the use of a constant energy device in ECT.

With a constant current device, the clinician typically manipulates the total dosage by varying the time of exposure to the current—that is, the total charge. With most brief pulse devices, this dosage adjustment

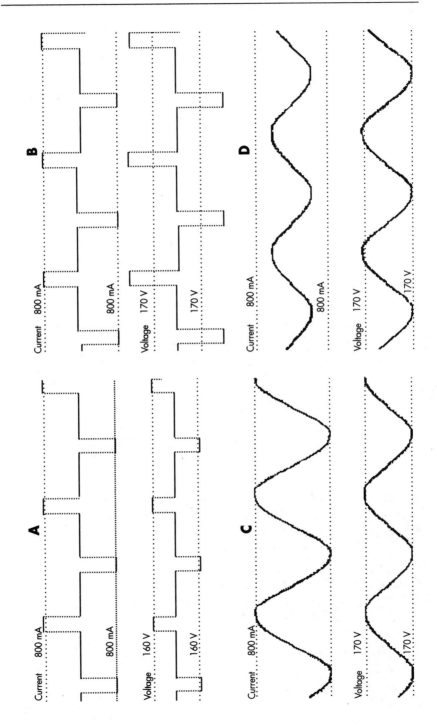

Figure 11–2. *An example of constant current and constant voltage principles.*

In **A**, a constant current, brief pulse stimulus was administered with a fixed and known circuit resistance of 200 Ω. The stimulus settings were 60 Hz, 2 ms, 1 second, and 800 mA. In **B**, the same stimulus was delivered with a circuit resistance of 400 Ω. Note that the current levels during each pulse were unchanged but that the voltage was doubled. In **C**, a constant voltage sine wave stimulus was administered with a circuit resistance of 200 Ω. The stimulus settings were 120 V (RMS, or 170 V peak) for 0.3 seconds (60 Hz). In **D**, the resistance was increased to 400 Ω. Note that voltage was now maintained but that current decreased to one half of its previous value. For stimulations **A–D**, the horizontal lines on the current tracing indicate (**B**) ±800 mA. The horizontal lines for the voltage channel indicate ±160 V for the brief pulse stimulus (**A**) and ±170 V for the brief pulse stimulus (**B**) and the sine wave stimulus (**C** and **D**).

Source. From Sackeim HA, Long J, Luber B, et al.: "Physical Properties and Quantification of the ECT Stimulus, I: Basic Principles." *Convulsive Therapy* 10(2):93–123, 1994. Used with permission of Lippincott Williams & Wilkins.

may be done by varying the frequency of pulses, the width of pulses, or the duration of the pulse train. Each of these manipulations alters the time of exposure to a fixed current. With some devices one can also adjust the amplitude of the peak current. Whether varying the time of exposure to the current or the current amplitude, the use of a constant current mode of delivery has the advantage that the clinician is guaranteed delivery of a predetermined charge, independent of fluctuations in impedance.

11.5.3. Stimulus Parameters

Within a waveform, several features of the stimulus may be varied. With constant current brief pulse devices, the clinician may alter some or all of the following parameters: the frequency of pulses, the width of pulses, the amplitude of peak current during pulses, and the duration of the pulse train (Figure 11–3). There may also be the option of whether pulses are unidirectional or bidirectional and whether pulses are uniformly or intermittently distributed in the pulse train. A summary measure of overall stimulus intensity (charge or energy) may be constant, despite radically different configurations of stimulus parameters. For example, the charge of a bidirectional brief pulse stimulus delivered with a pulse frequency of 40 Hz, a pulse width of 1.4 ms, a pulse amplitude of 800 mA, and a train duration of 2 seconds will be 179.2 mC. An identical charge would be delivered by doubling the frequency to 80 Hz, decreasing the pulse width to 1.0 ms, and shortening the train duration to 1.4 seconds.

Evidence of how different stimulus configurations impact on the therapeutic and other effects of ECT is limited. Preliminary evidence indicates that increasing the train duration of a brief pulse constant current stimulus is somewhat more efficient in seizure elicitation than increasing pulse frequency (Devanand et al. 1998; Swartz and Larson 1989). In general, it appears that extending the pulse width of the ECT stimulus beyond 1.0 ms is the least efficient method when incrementing stimulus intensity. Investigation of the relative efficiency of manipulations of pulse amplitude (current) has not been reported.

11.5.4. Maximal Device Output

The constant current brief pulse devices currently marketed in the United States have a maximal output of 504–576 mC or approximately 100 J

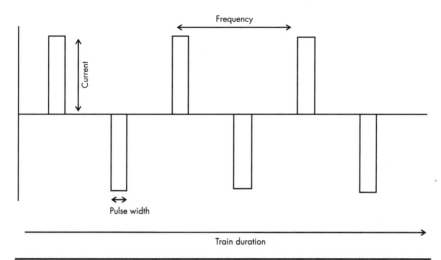

Figure 11–3. *Representation of the parameters in a bidirectional brief pulse stimulus.*

The amplitude or height of each pulse reflects the current administered and is measured in milliamps (mA). With constant current stimulation, this amplitude will be consistent across all pulses. ECT devices vary in using pulse currents ranging from 500 to 900 mA. The duration of each pulse is the pulse width and typically varies between 0.25 and 2.0 ms. The number of pulse pairs (bidirectional pulses) per second determines the frequency of the stimulus. A total of 80 pulses or 40 pulse pairs per second is equivalent to a frequency of 40 Hz. Depending on the device, frequency may vary from 20 to 120 Hz. The total duration of the pulse train determines the stimulus duration. Depending on the device, this may vary from 0.5 to 8.0 seconds.

at a 220-Ω impedance. Versions of these same devices marketed in Europe, Canada, and elsewhere have at least double this maximal output.

Marked variability exists among psychiatric patients in the minimal stimulus intensity necessary to produce a seizure (i.e., seizure threshold). Some have estimated that, with constant current brief pulse stimulation, the range in seizure threshold in routine clinical practice is as much as 50-fold (Boylan et al. 2000; Sackeim 1997b). Rare patients with markedly high seizure threshold will be encountered in whom elevated thresholds are not attributable to concurrent medications, excessive anesthetic dosage, or other modifiable factors that could compromise the treatment (Krystal et al. 2000; Lisanby et al. 1996). In such circumstances, stimulation at maximal device settings may be insufficient to produce a seizure. In addition, it has become increasingly evident that the dosage of right unilateral ECT must be substantially suprathreshold (e.g., more than 150% above or 2.5 times threshold) for optimal therapeutic effects (McCall et al. 2000; Sackeim 1997b; Sackeim et al. 1987a, 1993, 2000). There is also reason to suspect that a small number of patients respond to bilateral ECT only when electrical intensity is at least moderately suprathreshold (i.e., 50%–150% above threshold) (Sackeim 1991). Thus, in patients with high seizure threshold, delivery of maximal device output may not be sufficient to achieve therapeutic response (Abrams 2000; Krystal et al. 2000; Lisanby et al. 1996).

When maximal device output is insufficient to produce a seizure at all or provides an insufficient dose relative to seizure threshold, and reversible causes of the elevated threshold have been ruled out (see Section 11.9), the practitioner may have to use the technique of "double stimulation." This technique involves delivering two electrical stimuli as close in time as possible to provide summation (Andrade 1991). If the interval between the stimuli is too great (e.g., more than a few seconds), it is unlikely that the two stimuli will summate to produce an effective seizure. Although occasionally necessary, the use of double stimulation is a less optimal solution than the use of an ECT device with a higher maximal output capability.

11.5.5. Device Operation and Maintenance

Device manufacturers should provide detailed descriptions of testing procedures and preventative maintenance instructions. Prior to the first use of an ECT device, the practitioner should be familiar with the principles that underlie operation of the instrumentation. It is also important that biomedical engineering or other qualified staff ascertain and document that the stimulus output characteristics and all other controls, parameters, and features are functioning properly and are appropriately calibrated. Shipping and handling of the device can result in malfunction or miscalibration and users should not rely solely on the calibration performed by the manufacturer. The device manual provided by the manufacturer should outline the steps necessary to ensure adequate functioning, including the tolerance level for departure of parameters from exact values (e.g., ±10%).

As with other medical devices, a regular schedule of retesting or recalibration by biomedical engineering or otherwise qualified staff should be implemented, particularly in terms of electrical safety considerations. The intervals between retesting should minimally meet those stipulated in device manuals or local facility requirements. At minimum, it is suggested that retesting be conducted annually. The results of retesting should also be documented. Experience with ECT devices indicates that it is relatively rare to observe drift in stimulus output characteristics with standard use. However, if unusual conditions occur that may affect the integrity of the device (e.g., electrical malfunction, fire, spillage), immediate retesting should be carried out prior to subsequent clinical use.

11.5.6. Electrical Safety Considerations

Several electrical safety considerations exist when administering ECT. The ECT device should come equipped with a three-pronged, grounded electrical plug and must be connected to a three-pronged, grounded outlet approved for medical devices. Under no circumstances should the grounding be defeated, for example, by plugging the device into a two-pronged outlet. Unless battery operated, any electrical device in contact with the patient should be connected to the same electrical circuit as the ECT device. This configuration may be accomplished by having all electrical equipment connected through the same power strip to an approved, grounded outlet or wiring the ECT suite so that all electrical outlets share a common ground. The adequacy of this common ground should be verified at regular intervals. It is advisable that this circuit have automatic ground fault interruption.

Generally speaking, patient contact with other devices should be avoided, except when required for physiologic monitoring. Contact of the patient with other devices or other conducting media increases the chances of alternative ground paths for the ECT stimulus. This unlikely event can occur only if there is a ground fault in the ECT or other device and both do not share the same ground. Under such conditions, a portion of the ECT stimulus current may pass through the heart, with potentially lethal effects. Under no circumstances should any individual other than the patient be in contact with the metal portion of the ECT electrodes during the passage of the stimulus.

For safety purposes, the device should indicate to the user that a stimulus is being delivered. Ordinarily this may be a tone or light that occurs only during the passage of current. The auditory mode is preferred as it does not require that the operator look away from the patient during the initiation of stimulation. It is also useful for devices to be equipped with a distinct warning signal, to alert all members of the treatment team that a stimulus is about to be delivered. This feature helps ensure that the stimulus is delivered only after preparation of the patient is complete and the staff involved in the procedure are ready. Likewise, for safety purposes, the ECT device should be equipped so that the practitioner can abort the delivery of stimulus on an instantaneous basis (by release of the treatment button) if malfunction or other untoward events become apparent during stimulus delivery.

11.6. Stimulus Electrode Placement

11.6.1. Choice of Electrode Placement

Electrode placement affects the breadth, severity, and duration of cognitive side effects. Bilateral ECT produces more short- and long-term adverse cognitive effects than right unilateral ECT (d'Elia 1970; Fromholt et al. 1973; McElhiney et al. 1995; Sackeim et al. 1986, 1993; Squire 1986; Weiner et al. 1986a). In addition, the likelihood of developing a transient delirium, at times requiring interruption or premature discontinuation of the ECT course, is considerably greater with bilateral than with right unilateral ECT (Daniel and Crovitz 1982, 1986; Miller et al. 1986; Sackeim et al. 1993). Months after the treatment course, the extent of amnesia for autobiographical events may be greater in patients who received bilateral compared with right unilateral ECT (Lisanby et al. 2000; McElhiney et al. 1995; Sackeim et al. 2000; Sobin et al. 1995; Weiner et al. 1986a).

Electrode placement may also affect efficacy. In the treatment of major depressive disorder, when stimulus intensity is very low and just above seizure threshold, the efficacy of right unilateral ECT is markedly reduced (Letemendia et al. 1993; Krystal et al. 1995; Sackeim et al. 1987b, 1993, 2000). Although the efficacy of right unilateral ECT notably improves when stimulus intensity is moderately suprathreshold (e.g., 150% above or 2.5 times the initial threshold), this form of right unilateral ECT may still be inferior in clinical outcome to low- or higher-dosage bilateral ECT (Sackeim et al. 1993, 2000). However, recent evidence suggests that when markedly suprathreshold stimulation (e.g., 500% above or 6 times the threshold) is used with right unilateral ECT, its efficacy is fully equivalent to bilateral ECT (McCall et al. 2000; Sackeim 1997b; Sackeim et al. 2000). This finding coincides with evidence that right unilateral ECT is particularly efficacious when a high fixed electrical dosage is used (Abrams et al. 1991; d'Elia 1992; McCall et al. 1995, 2000). Furthermore, preliminary evidence indicates that markedly suprathreshold right unilateral ECT retains clinically significant advantages over moderately dosed (150% above the threshold) bilateral ECT in terms of the breadth, magnitude, and persistence of adverse cognitive effects (Sackeim 1997b; Sackeim et al. 2000).

When treating major depressive disorder, right unilateral ECT should be used with a minimum electrical dosage that exceeds initial seizure threshold by 150% (i.e., 2.5 times the threshold) or more. An even higher intensity relative to threshold (up to 500% above or six times threshold) may exert greater efficacy with relatively little difference in cognitive side effects (Sackeim et al. 2000). In contrast, for most patients the maximal dosage administered with bilateral ECT should be, at most, moderately suprathreshold (i.e., 50%–150% above threshold). Increasing the stimulus dosage above this value with bilateral ECT only rarely enhances efficacy and is likely to accentuate cognitive side effects (Ottosson 1960; Sackeim et al. 1993). This line of reasoning suggests that the minimum dosage for right unilateral ECT should be at least 2.5 times the initial seizure threshold, which for most patients should be the maximal dosage administered with bilateral ECT (Crimson et al. 1999).

Given the maximal electrical output of ECT devices in the United States (504–576 mC), instances will occur in which it is not possible to administer substantially suprathreshold stimulation with right unilateral ECT. In a large multisite study, Boylan et al. (2000) reported that approximately 90% of patients treated with right unilateral ECT had initial seizure thresholds less than 100 mC. Thus, most patients can be treated with a stimulus dose that is at least five times the initial threshold. To avoid coupling marginally suprathreshold stimulation with right unilateral ECT, exceptional patients with very high seizure thresholds may need to be treated with bilateral ECT.

In terms of cognitive side effects, the advantages of right unilateral compared with bilateral ECT are presumably maintained across psychiatric diagnoses (Sackeim 1992). Information is limited, however, on the impact of electrode placement on the efficacy of ECT in diagnostic groups other than major depressive disorder. It has been suggested that bilateral electrode placement is particularly indicated for patients with acute mania (Milstein et al. 1987), although evidence on this point is contradictory (Black et al. 1986, 1989a; Mukherjee et al. 1988). In schizophrenia, comparative trials of unilateral and bilateral ECT have not detected a difference in efficacy (Bagadia et al. 1988; Doongaji et al. 1973; el-Islam et al. 1970; Wessels 1972). However, this issue is still unresolved because these studies had small samples and other methodologic problems (Krueger and Sackeim 1995). A reasonable conclusion is that the relative efficacies of unilateral and bilateral ECT are not established in psychiatric conditions other than major depressive disorder.

Even in major depressive disorder, a small subgroup of patients may respond only to bilateral ECT (Price and McAllister 1986; Sackeim et al. 1993). Although controversy exists in this regard (Strömgren 1984), some practitioners do not consider patients resistant to ECT until they have failed to respond to an adequate course of moderately suprathreshold bilateral treatment (Abrams 1986, 1997a; Crimson et al. 1999; Sackeim et al. 1993, 2000).

The extent to which practitioners use unilateral or bilateral ECT varies considerably (Farah and McCall 1993). Some practitioners use unilateral or bilateral ECT exclusively. Others start patients with unilateral ECT and switch to bilateral ECT if patients fail to respond or if response is excessively slow (Abrams and Fink 1984). For example, patients are often switched to bilateral ECT if they have not shown sufficient improvement after six right unilateral treatments. Alternatively, in the face of inadequate response, some practitioners increment the dosage of right unilateral ECT before switching to bilateral ECT. Another policy is to initiate bilateral ECT in patients whose psychiatric or medical status requires a greater assurance of rapid clinical response. A further alternative strategy is to start all patients with bilateral ECT, switching to right unilateral ECT when cognitive side effects become severe, particularly in cases of sustained delirium.

Practitioners should be skilled in administering both unilateral and bilateral ECT. Given the intricacies involved in choosing between bilateral and unilateral ECT, practitioners should have a clear understanding of the variations in therapeutic and adverse effects with electrode placement. In addition, they should appreciate that other factors interact with electrode placement and modify clinical or adverse effects. Of particular concern, the combination of bilateral electrode placement, grossly suprathreshold stimulus intensity, and sine wave stimulation is likely to maximize cognitive deficits without conferring additional therapeutic advantage. In contrast, an accumulating amount of evidence suggests that, at sufficient electrical intensity, right unilateral

ECT has significant advantages over bilateral ECT with respect to cognitive side effects and yet exerts comparable therapeutic effects (Sackeim et al. 2000). These findings should encourage greater use of right unilateral ECT by practitioners and also emphasize that decisions about electrode placement should be made in concert with decisions about stimulus intensity. Furthermore, because electrode placement impacts on therapeutic and adverse effects, decisions about electrode placement should be discussed with the consentor and the attending physician.

11.6.2. Electrode Positioning

One method of electrode positioning, the bifrontotemporal position, has been commonly used to administer bilateral ECT. This positioning involves estimating, on each side of the head, the midpoint of the line connecting the external canthus and the tragus. The midpoint of the stimulus electrode is then placed approximately 1 inch above this point (see Figure 11–4). Therefore, with a 2-inch electrode, the bottom of the electrode is tangential to the line connecting the external canthus and the tragus. In recent years, two other bilateral placements have been proposed. After an early study with closely spaced bifrontal stimulus electrodes demonstrated decreased memory effects but limited efficacy compared with traditional bifrontotemporal placement (Abrams and Taylor 1973), a more recent investigation using a wider bifrontal placement found that this technique may be associated with both fewer cognitive side effects and greater efficacy than traditional bifrontotemporal placement (Lawson et al. 1990; Letemendia et al. 1993). An even more recent replication study has provided some corroborative data supporting the efficacy and safety of this technique (Bailine et al. 2000). A clinical series has also been reported using an asymmetric placement, with a frontal position on the left side and the standard frontotemporal position on the right side (Swartz 1994). However, further research is needed regarding these alternative bilateral electrode placements.

Although various placements have been used for unilateral ECT, a configuration that maximizes interelectrode distance may be optimal with regard to efficacy and seizure elicitation (Pettinati et al. 1986). Among the unilateral placements, the d'Elia (1970) location is recommended. This placement involves determining the intersection of the lines connecting the two auditory tragi and the nasion and inion. The midpoint of the parietal electrode is then placed approximately 1 inch lateral to this point (see Figure 11–4). The frontotemporal electrode is in

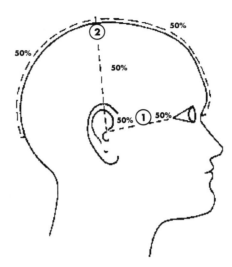

Figure 11–4.   *Location of stimulus electrodes with bilateral and right unilateral electrode placement.*

With bilateral ECT, stimulus electrodes are placed in Position 1 on both sides of the head, with midpoints approximately 1 inch above the center of a line connecting the tragus and external canthus. When using 2-inch-diameter electrodes, the bottom of the electrode will be tangential to the line, as illustrated above. With right unilateral ECT, one electrode is placed in Position 1 and the other is located in Position 2 at the intersection of the midpoints of the lines going from left to right tragus and from inion to nasion. The midpoint of these lines defines the vertex, and with 2-inch electrodes the top of the electrode is adjacent to the vertex.

the same position as in traditional bilateral ECT. A prefrontal unilateral placement should be avoided because of difficulties in seizure elicitation (Erman et al. 1979). Whether using unilateral or bilateral ECT, care should be taken to avoid stimulating over or adjacent to a skull defect.

Stimulus electrode placement in left-handed patients is uncertain. It is estimated that approximately 70% of left-handed patients are lateralized for language functions in a manner similar to that of right-handed patients, 15% have bilateral representation of language, and 15% have reversal of the typical pattern, with right hemisphere superiority for language functions (Bryden 1982; Bryden and Steenhuis 1991; Peters 1995; Rasmussen and Milner 1977). In right-handed patients, right unilateral ECT produces less disruption of verbal functions than left unilateral ECT or bilateral ECT (Daniel and Crovitz 1983b). The same relation may hold for most left-handed patients. Although its use has been uncommon, one method used to discern whether left or right unilateral ECT is less likely to disrupt language functions involves alternating the laterality of unilateral placement over the first few treatments and then determining which placement is associated with less severe acute confusion and verbal amnesia (Pratt et al. 1971).

If handedness is considered in determining electrode placement, it is important to recognize that the hand used in writing and the patient's report of handedness are fallible indicators (Peters 1995). Many strongly left-handed individuals write with the right hand. Individuals who are basically right handed may report being ambidextrous or left handed (or vice versa) because of inconsistencies in hand usage for different activities. Inquiries should be made concerning a set of specific activities, such as throwing a ball, use of a knife and fork, use of scissors, and so on. Standardized sets of items are readily available (e.g., Oldfield 1971; Porac and Coren 1981; Rackowski et al. 1976). Predominant hand usage should determine assignment of handedness. Assessment of asymmetry in other domains (e.g., eyedness or footedness) is not germane.

Considerable evidence indicates that lateralization of function pertains to affective as well as cognitive realms (Davidson 1995; Sackeim et al. 1982). For instance, some data suggest that, in most individuals, the right hemisphere plays a greater role in the development or maintenance of depressed mood than the left hemisphere, regardless of handedness. This hypothesis may account for some limited evidence that right unilateral ECT is more efficacious than left unilateral ECT in treating major depression (Flor-Henry 1986; Lisanby and Sackeim 2000; Small et al. 1993), although these findings have been questioned (Abrams 1989; Abrams et al. 1989). In this light, most practitioners prefer to administer right unilateral ECT independent of handedness.

11.6.3. Stimulus Electrode Site Preparation

Careful attention should be paid to the preparation of the scalp stimulus electrode sites and to the contact between the electrodes and the scalp. Inadequate preparation or poor coupling results in increased impedance. With constant current devices, high impedance results in delivery of excessive voltage or failure to maintain the current at the prescribed level. In the latter case the patient may fail to have an adequate seizure (see Section 11.9), and the intensity of the stimulation administered may be unknown. With constant voltage devices, high impedance will produce a decrease in the intensity of the administered current and may also result in missed or abortive seizures.

A standard procedure for electrode site preparation should be developed by each facility. One method involves cleansing the skin with a solvent such as rubbing alcohol. After the site has dried, an abrasive conductant is rubbed into the scalp to lower site impedance. Conductant gel is then applied to the electrodes to ensure an adequate interface. If the electrode site is covered by a significant amount of hair, as is likely to be the case for the rostral (upper) electrode with unilateral placement, it is usually sufficient to simply part the hair prior to rigorous application of the solvent and abrasive conductant. Routine clipping of the hair is unnecessary. Use of saline-soaked pads as the conductant on electrodes is discouraged. If such pads are used, particular care must be taken that saline is not dripped across the surface between electrodes. Indeed, smearing of any conducting medium across the scalp between the electrodes will produce an alternate path for the stimulus current. Because the smeared conducting medium has a low impedance, a greater proportion of current will pass across the scalp instead of entering the brain. This shunting of current results in a lessened ability to elicit a seizure.

Generally speaking, a larger electrode surface area will result in lower impedance to the passage of the current. The metal electrodes may be coupled to the scalp using a snugly fitting band or handheld electrodes. Adhesive (disposable) pad electrodes are also in use; like the snugly fitting band, disposable adhesive electrodes have the advantage of not requiring an operator to hold them in place when bilateral ECT is performed. Problems with proper positioning of adhesive electrodes arise at times, however, because of extensive hair at the bifrontotemporal sites. Furthermore, a handheld electrode for the rostral (parietal) site typically is required to conduct unilateral ECT. In general, firm pressure of the electrode against the scalp helps minimize impedance. Handheld electrodes must be insulated so that the user is not in contact with the electrode or with exposed wiring connecting the stimulus cable to the electrode. The use of tongs as electrode holders is discouraged. It is difficult to adjust tongs relative to asymmetries in skull anatomy, preventing proper electrode placement.

11.6.4. Impedance Testing

Some ECT devices can assess the integrity of the ECT circuit prior to the administration of the stimulus. Use of such a static impedance testing procedure is strongly encouraged. During this procedure, an imperceptible current is passed, and the impedance in the total circuit is assessed. This information is used to determine whether the impedance to the current passage is too low or too high. The most common source of abnormally low static impedance is smearing of a conductive medium between the electrodes. Low impedance may also result if the patient has administered a cream, gel, or spray to the hair or has heavy perspiration. Excessively high impedance may be due to poor contact between an electrode and the scalp, incomplete or improper preparation of the electrode sites, poor contact between the electrodes and the stimulus cable, a break in the stimulus cable, or poor connection or disconnection of the stimulus cable from the device. Some devices provide a continuous readout of impedance values prior to stimulation. Even if static impedance values are in a generally acceptable range (e.g., less than 3,000 Ω depending on the device), a marked increase in static impedance prior to stimulation should alert the practitioner to the fact that electrode contact at the sites may not be optimal.

In the case of an abnormal static impedance value, the cause of the low or high impedance should be ascertained and remedied before proceeding with the treatment. Administration of another testing procedure (or the continuous readout from devices so equipped) should determine whether the steps taken have been effective. In extremely rare circumstances, patients may have skin properties that result in low static impedance test results regardless of the integrity of the circuit. Some devices will explicitly alert the user to an abnormal static impedance value and will automatically disengage stimulus delivery. Some devices may have override options so that the stimulus can be delivered despite the static impedance failure if it is believed that the static impedance failure was caused by intrinsic patient factors that cannot be altered. Such an override should be used only in extremely rare cases of low static impedance attributable to the patient's skin condition. Other devices indicate the static impedance value determined from the test procedure without disengaging stimulus delivery for abnormal values. Devices that feature automatic disengagement of stimulus delivery provide an extra margin of safety. In some cases in which stimulation is given despite abnormally high impedance, the stimulus output may not match the parameters set by the operator, the stimulus dose given to the patient will be unknown, and a seizure may not be produced. It should be emphasized that with appropriate methods for electrode and scalp preparation and placement, one should rarely need to administer the stimulus despite an abnormal static impedance value.

11.7. Stimulus Dosing

Several factors should be weighed in determining the dosage of the ECT stimulus. As noted, patients have marked variability (as much as 50-fold) in the electrical threshold for eliciting an adequate seizure (Boylan et al. 2000; Coffey et al. 1995a; Colenda and McCall 1996; Enns and Karvelas 1995; Lisanby et al. 1996; Sackeim 1997b; Sackeim et al. 1987c; Shapira et al. 1996). If the same electrical intensity is used to elicit seizures in all patients, it must be disproportionately high to allow for patients with high thresholds. In patients with low thresholds, such a high intensity will be many times more than that needed to produce an adequate seizure and may be associated with unnecessary cognitive side effects. Children and adolescents are particularly likely to have very low thresholds for seizure elicitation.

In addition, stimulus intensity can affect efficacy and cognitive side effects. Regardless of electrode placement, the speed of clinical response with barely suprathreshold stimuli may be slower than with higher intensity stimuli (Robin and de Tissera 1982; Nobler et al. 1997; Sackeim et al. 1993, 2000). With right unilateral electrode placement, stimuli barely above threshold will be therapeutically weak (Letemendia et al. 1993; Sackeim et al. 1987b, 1993, 2000). However, higher-intensity stimulation is associated with more severe short-term cognitive deficits (Cronholm and Ottosson 1963b; McCall et al. 2000; Ottosson 1960; Sackeim et al. 1993; Valentine et al. 1968).

Patients treated with bilateral ECT generally should receive moderately suprathreshold stimulation, defined as between 50% and 150% above seizure threshold (1.5–2.5 times threshold). The efficacy of unilateral ECT requires a dosage that exceeds threshold to a greater extent than in bilateral ECT (McCall et al. 2000; Sackeim 1997b; Sackeim et al. 1987b, 1993, 2000). Patients treated with right unilateral ECT generally should receive moderately to markedly suprathreshold stimulation, defined as between 150% and 500% above seizure threshold (2.5–6 times threshold).

In general, three methods are in use for determining stimulus intensity (Farah and McCall 1993). First, many practitioners use an empirical titration procedure (Sackeim et al. 1987a) because they prefer to be cognizant of the degree to which stimulus dosage exceeds seizure threshold. Second, some practitioners use a formula to specify electrical dosage that accounts for one or more of the factors that predict seizure threshold (Petrides and Fink 1996b). Factors such as electrode placement, gender, age, anesthetic dosage, and concomitant medications have some predictive value with respect to seizure threshold (Beale et al. 1994b; Boylan et al. 2000; Coffey et al. 1995a; Colenda and McCall 1996; Enns and Karvelas 1995; Gangadhar et al. 1998; Krueger et al. 1993; Sackeim et al. 1987c, 1991; Shapira et al. 1996). Third, some practitioners prefer to administer a fixed electrical dosage (Abrams 1997a).

Because of limited success in predicting the wide individual differences in seizure threshold on the basis of patient or treatment factors, empirical titration provides the most precise method for quantifying seizure threshold. A titration procedure is usually conducted at the first treatment. An initial dosage that is expected to result in an adequate seizure in only a minority of patients is selected. Once it is established that the stimulus was subconvulsive and did not elicit sustained motoric or EEG manifestations of a seizure, the stimulus intensity is increased and the patient is restimulated. The interval between restimulations should be approximately 20 seconds to account for delayed seizures that may occur with barely suprathreshold stimuli and to allow for clearing of the residual effects of the previous subconvulsive stimulus. The distribution of seizure threshold values is such that most patients have an adequate seizure by the second or third stimulation. Each facility should adopt a policy on the maximal number of restimulations permitted during a session; four or five stimulations is a common cutoff.

The last step in a titration schedule should incorporate a much higher increment in stimulus intensity. Failure to elicit a seizure can occasionally result in a prolonged confusional state and in no therapeutic benefit. Restimulation procedures after subconvulsive (missed) or abortive seizures are described in more detail in Section 11.9. The stimulus parameters administered and the number of stimulations should be documented at each treatment.

With empirical titration, it is uncommon to need additional anesthetic medications. Although the subconvulsive stimulus prolongs unconsciousness, a half-dose of muscle relaxant should be administered if behavioral observations suggest that muscle relaxant effects are wearing off (e.g., spontaneous movements or respiration). Some anesthesia providers believe that the patient should be pretreated with an anticholinergic agent if a second dose of a muscle relaxant is administered. Because subconvulsive stimuli result in vagal stimulation and parasympathetic-mediated bradycardia (Decina et al. 1984; McCall et al. 1994), some practitioners also require premedication with an anticholinergic agent (atropine or glycopyrrolate) when empirical titration is used (Zielinski et al. 1993). Use of an anticholinergic agent may be particularly important if patients are also pretreated with a β-blocking agent (Decina et al. 1984; McCall 1996). Limited evidence suggests that the administration of subconvulsive stimuli followed by convulsive stimuli does not intensify cognitive side effects compared with convulsive stimuli alone (Prudic et al. 1994).

To limit the possibility or number of subconvulsive administrations, some practitioners prefer to use a formula to determine stimulus intensity. The simplest formulas adjust stimulus intensity to the patient's age (Abrams and Swartz 1989) or to half the patient's age (Petrides and Fink 1996b). More complex formulas can also be used that account for additional predictive factors such as electrode placement and gender. In general, the most complex formulas account for only 40% or less of the variability in initial seizure threshold (Boylan et al. 2000; Coffey et al. 1995a; Colenda and McCall 1996; Enns and Karvelas 1995; Krueger et al. 1993; Sackeim et al. 1991; Shapira et al. 1996). Error in the formula-based estimate may result in administration of either barely suprathreshold stimulation, which may be ineffective with right unilateral ECT, or markedly suprathreshold threshold stimulation, which aggravates short-term cognitive side effects with either right unilateral or bilateral ECT (Enns and Karvelas 1995; Shapira et al. 1996). In addition, when the value obtained from a formula grossly underestimates seizure threshold, a subconvulsive stimulus will be administered and the practitioner will engage in a form of empirical titration. Nonetheless, because the use of a formula-based dosing procedure involves some individualization of stimulus intensity to patient and/or treatment factors, its use can be justified.

The third method of stimulus dosing is to administer a fixed stimulus intensity independent of patient or treatment factors. The argument can be made that high fixed-dosage stimulation maximizes the probability of response to right unilateral ECT (Abrams 1997a; Abrams et al. 1991; McCall et al. 1995, 2000). The problems in the use of formula-based dosing apply even more so to the use of a high fixed dose. Given the marked individual differences in seizure threshold, with a high fixed dose some patients may be treated with an electrical intensity that exceeds seizure threshold by 10- or 20-fold. Such a dosing strategy is likely to aggravate cognitive side effects without gains in efficacy relative to more moderate dosing. Alternatively, in rare patients with exceptionally high initial seizure threshold, use of a fixed dosing strategy can result in barely suprathreshold stimulation. Use of a high fixed dosing strategy should be reserved only for patients with sufficiently serious concomitant medical conditions in which avoidance of subconvulsive stimulation is a priority.

The determination of stimulus dosage should also consider that seizure threshold changes over the treatment course, with many patients manifesting large increases—for example, 25%–200% (Coffey et al. 1995b; Sackeim 1999; Sackeim et al. 1987d). Because of this phenomenon, dosage may be adjusted upward to maintain a consistent suprathreshold level. In patients who show slow or inadequate clinical response and no more than mild cognitive side effects, an even further dosage increase may be considered. In patients for whom a level of stimulation has consistently produced adequate seizures and severe cognitive side effects, a decrease of stimulus intensity, switch to a right unilateral placement, or spacing of treatments over longer intervals may be considered.

The use of glissando techniques, in which the intensity of the stimulus is progressively increased during delivery from a subconvulsive to convulsive level, has not been justified. Glissando was introduced prior to the use of general anesthesia in ECT as a means to produce unconsciousness and to prevent musculoskeletal injuries. With the introduction of general anesthesia, this technique is now of only historical interest.

11.8. Physiologic Monitoring

11.8.1. Seizure Monitoring

11.8.1.1. General Considerations

In recent years, it has become evident that seizure duration, whether measured at an individual treatment or cumulatively across the treatment course, has little bearing on efficacy (Nobler et al. 1993; Kales et al. 1997; Sackeim 1999; Sackeim et al. 1987c, 1991). Furthermore, seizure duration displays a complex association with stimulus intensity. When stimulus intensity is extremely close to the seizure threshold, the patient may manifest a brief or "abortive" seizure. Motor manifestations of these seizures are typically 15 seconds or less. With a small increment in stimulus intensity to a barely suprathreshold level, the patient often manifests a long seizure with low-amplitude EEG expression and an absence of postical EEG suppression. When stimulus intensity is substantially above threshold, seizure duration decreases, but EEG seizure expression is more robust (higher amplitude) and the probability of postical EEG suppression is greater (Krystal et al. 1993, 1995; Luber et al. [in press]; Nobler et al. 1993, [in press]; Riddle et al. 1993; Sackeim et al. 1991; Zis et al. 1993).

Given this information, it is unlikely that knowledge of seizure duration alone is sufficient to determine that patients have had an adequate treatment. However, when seizure duration is less than 15 seconds in both motor (convulsive) and EEG manifestations, the likelihood is high that the seizure was limited by insufficient electrical stimulation (or by other factors described in Section 11.9) and that the treatment was inadequate. Likewise, seizures are likely to be inadequate if they do not show bilateral generalization in motor and EEG manifestations. It should be appreciated that some seizures of long duration may also be therapeutically ineffective if stimulus intensity is barely suprathreshold.

Practitioners should also be alert to marked changes in seizure duration. For example, if seizure duration decreases from 100 to 40 seconds between successive treatments, the later treatment may have been problematic, particularly if the extent to which stimulus intensity exceeded threshold is unknown. Although seizure duration typically decreases over the treatment course, the magnitude of this drop between successive treatments is atypical and could be due to marginally suprathreshold stimulation or other limiting factors (see Section 11.9). In contrast, elderly patients usually have shorter seizure duration than younger patients (Boylan et al. 2000; Krueger et al. 1993; Sackeim et al. 1991; Strömgren and Juul-Jensen 1975). Moderately or markedly suprathreshold treatment may result in motor or EEG manifestations between 15 and 30 seconds and occasionally less, particularly in the elderly. These patients may be receiving fully effective treatment, and further increments in stimulus intensity may result in decreased seizure duration and accentuation of cognitive side effects.

11.8.1.2. Ictal Motor Activity

The duration of the seizure and the method of measurement should be documented at each treatment. The simplest and most reliable method for assessing seizure duration is timing the duration of motor (convulsive) movements. However, these movements are much attenuated or absent with the use of muscle relaxants (succinylcholine). Therefore, regardless of muscle relaxant dosage, it is recommended that distribution of such an agent to the hand or foot be blocked. Before the muscle relaxant is administered, a blood pressure cuff should be inflated to a pressure above the expected peak systolic pressure during the seizure (e.g., 250 mm Hg). This cuff should differ from the one used to monitor blood pressure. To observe seizure generalization, the limb used to block the distribution of the muscle relaxant should be on the same side as the electrode placement if a unilateral electrode placement is used. Use of the "cuff" procedure allows for timing of unmodified convulsive movements without risk to the patient. It should be noted that even with such a procedure, convulsive movements may be visible for longer duration in other body regions, particularly in the neck and face. The motor seizure endpoint should be taken as the disappearance of all such movements.

Another reason for use of the cuff technique is that on rare occasions the anesthetic dose will be insufficient and patients may retain consciousness while paralyzed (see Section 11.4.2). Movement in the cuffed limb will alert the treatment team to this occurrence and should be promptly followed by administration of additional anesthetic agent.

Immediately after the seizure, the cuff should be deflated to prevent a prolonged ischemic period. Furthermore, particular care is necessary in use of this technique in patients at risk for skin or musculoskeletal complications or who have severe peripheral vascular disease, deep vein thrombosis, or sickle cell disease (Beyer et al. 1998). In such patients, the cuff technique may be omitted. Optimal placement is on the distal portion of a limb (ankle is generally preferable to wrist), because it has been documented that full limb convulsive movements in patients with severe osteoporosis can lead to fracture (Levy 1988).

Occasionally, patients may have adequate seizures without motor manifestations (Mayur et al. 1999; Scott and Riddle 1989). This event may occur because the cuff is inflated too late, the ictal blood pressure increase exceeds the restriction in circulation, or for other reasons. EEG seizure activity is commonly of longer duration than motor convulsive movements (Warmflash et al. 1987). Also, patients rarely may have prolonged cerebral seizures or return of seizure activity (tardive seizures) that do not manifest in motor movements. For these and other reasons, seizures should also be monitored with EEG.

Some ECT devices allow the use of electromyography (EMG) or motion detection to time and record the ictal motor response. Although such techniques provide documentation of the motor response, they have not been shown to be more reliable than visual observation. In addition, they detect movement in only one body part, which may not correspond to the place of seizure offset.

11.8.1.3. Ictal EEG Activity

At minimum, one channel of EEG activity should be monitored with a paper record or auditory output. Recording a hard copy output is preferred. No consensus has been reached on the need to retain hard copy output. Before administering anesthetic and muscle relaxing agents, the adequacy of the EEG record should be ascertained. The clinician should be familiar with the range of artifacts that may result in apparent EEG seizure activity when none is present (anesthetic effects, movement, ECG artifact) and the different manifestations of seizure expression and termination. EEG monitoring should continue until the clinician is certain that seizure activity has terminated. Termination is most often indicated by a period of markedly attenuated activity (suppression) following the high-amplitude sharp and slow wave activity that occurs during the seizure.

The most common sites for recording EEG during ECT involve either a frontal-mastoid montage or a frontal-frontal montage. A frontal-mastoid montage is preferred (Weiner et al. 1991); the frontal-frontal montage is likely to show diminished EEG activity because an EEG channel records the voltage difference between two electrodes and synchronous voltage changes at both electrodes will cancel. In contrast, a mastoid reference is more likely to approximate a relatively inactive site, maximizing EEG seizure expression. Use of a left-sided montage assists in determining seizure generalization with right unilateral ECT. Thus, if only one EEG channel is used, common practice is to record from the left frontal and left mastoid regions.

The frontal site can be visually identified as an area at least 1 inch above the midpoint of the eyebrow. Placing this electrode higher on the forehead (i.e., 1–3 inches) can increase the amplitude of EEG seizure expression. The mastoid site is the bony prominence behind the ear. Placing the electrode high on the mastoid site will reduce contamination of the EEG with pulse artifact. It is good practice to maintain a consistent protocol for EEG site determination and preparation.

Careful attention should be paid to the preparation of the EEG sites. Poor contact and other causes of excessive impedance at EEG sites are by far the most common reason for poor EEG recordings. Such artifact interferes with determining seizure occurrence, the quality of seizure expression, and the time point and extent of suppression at seizure termination. The steps involved in preparing EEG sites are similar to those used in preparing sites for ECT electrodes.

Both the frontal and mastoid sites should be cleaned with a solvent such as rubbing alcohol and then patted dry. An abrasive conductant should be rubbed into the skin with a cotton swab or other applicator, restricted to the area corresponding to the active portion of the electrode. Restricting the area of the abrasive conductant helps ensure that the electrode adheres well to the skin. Alternatively, a wider area may be vigorously abraded and the abrasive conductant wiped dry from the skin. The electrodes are then placed in the proper positions. A disposable pediatric ECG electrode or similar disposal design is commonly used to record EEG in ECT. If alternative metal electrodes are used (gold cup, silver-silver chloride) the same steps in preparation should be employed. However, the electrode should be filled with a conductant and taped to the skin.

When the EEG leads are connected to the EEG electrodes, the practitioner should check the quality of the EEG recording. The gain or sensitivity of the EEG amplifiers should be adjusted so that low-voltage fast-frequency activity is clearly discernible. Too low a sensitivity with suppressed EEG activity at baseline or too high a sensitivity with excessive baseline amplitude may interfere with determining the occurrence and termination of the seizure. When two channels of EEG are recorded, it is important to determine which channel reflects left-sided and which reflects right-sided activity, and it is useful to record this information on the hard copy output. The configuration is easily discerned, because tapping the frontal EEG electrodes should produce a high-amplitude artifact in the relevant channel (Parker et al. 2000).

11.8.2. EEG Seizure Adequacy Measures

Recently, some ECT devices have included measures that convey information about EEG changes during and after the seizure. Preliminary evidence indicates that better clinical outcome is associated with seizures that are accompanied by higher amplitude spike-and-wave activity and followed by greater postictal EEG suppression (Folkerts 1996; Krystal et al. 1995; Luber et al. [in press]; Nobler et al. 1993, [in press]; Suppes et al. 1996). However, various factors are likely to impinge on ictal and postictal EEG expression independent of treatment outcome, including patient age, treatment number, initial seizure threshold, and medication status (Krystal et al. 1993, 1995, 1996; McCall et al. 1996a, 1996b; Nobler et al. 1993, [in press]). In addition, none of the measures incorporated in ECT devices has, as yet, been validated in a manner that supports their clinical utility. Nonetheless, among patients who show inadequate or slow response to ECT, low-amplitude ictal EEG expression or an absence of postictal EEG suppression can be taken as further evidence for the need to increment stimulus dosage or switch electrode placement from unilateral to bilateral ECT.

11.8.3. Other Physiologic Monitoring

11.8.3.1. Cardiovascular Monitoring

The morbidity and mortality associated with ECT are largely cardiovascular in origin, with the greatest such risk occurring in patients who have a history of cardiac illness (Drop and Welch 1989; Prudic et al. 1987; Rice et al. 1994; Zielinski et al. 1993). Because this risk is greatest at the time of treatment, vital signs (blood pressure and pulse) and cardiac rhythms (ECG) should be monitored at frequent intervals from immediately before anesthesia administration until several minutes after seizure termination or until these measures are stable. Oscilloscopic or polygraphic ECG monitoring is required because transient postictal arrhythmias are often observed after seizure and may require intervention. Automated noninvasive blood pressure monitoring has become routine in ECT. Such automated readings should be set at the highest frequency (e.g., every minute) after anesthetic administration and until resumption of spontaneous respiration. When vital signs have stabilized, subsequent measurements may be obtained at less frequent intervals (e.g., every 5 minutes).

The capacity to provide a hard copy of the ECG should be readily available in order to document cardiac changes, provide an informed basis for consultation, and assist in the management of complications at future treatments. Some ECT devices provide ECG hard copy output at nonstandard chart speeds. If such output is entered in the patient's clinical records, the chart speed should be indicated or labeled timing marks provided. The treatment team should be cognizant of the variety of ECG changes observed during ECT, with an appreciation of those that usually do not require medical intervention (e.g., benign atrial arrhythmia or unifocal premature ventricular contractions [PVCs]) as opposed to those that typically do require intervention (e.g., ventricular tachycardia).

11.8.3.2. Oximetry

Standards of anesthetic practice require routine use of pulse oximetry to assess the adequacy of oxygenation. Oximetry is particularly valuable in patients with baseline ventilatory dysfunction, those in whom there is difficulty in maintaining an adequate airway, those at risk for prolonged apnea or seizures of long duration, or those with other conditions that raise the risk of hypoxia.

11.8.4. Electrical Safety Considerations Regarding Monitoring

For safety reasons described earlier, connection of a malfunctioning electrical monitoring device can present a hazard to the patient, particularly if there is a ground fault. Furthermore, the proper functioning of EEG, ECG, and oximetry devices is necessary to enhance the safety of the ECT procedure. Accordingly, prior to initial use, a biomedical engineer or other qualified person should be consulted to ensure the adequate functioning and safe use of physiologic monitoring devices. Maintenance and recalibration of devices should follow manufacturer recommendations and any pertinent medical standards. Adequacy of the ground in the electrical circuit should be verified.

11.9. Management of Missed, Abortive, and Prolonged Seizures

11.9.1. Missed Seizures

A "missed" seizure or subconvulsive stimulation occurs when there is no subsequent motor (tonic or clonic movements) or EEG seizure activity after electrical stimulation. There may be, however, a brief immediate contraction of some muscle groups in response to stimulation. In addition to insufficient stimulus intensity, factors that lead to missed seizures include excessive dynamic impedance resulting from poor contact at the skin–electrode interface, premature stimulus termination, hypercarbia from inadequate ventilation, hypoxia, dehydration, and the anticonvulsant actions of medications (including benzodiazepines and barbiturate anesthetic agents).

Following a missed seizure, the practitioner should determine whether dynamic impedance was excessive, if such information is available. If the impedance value is excessive, the preparation of the electrode sites, adequacy of electrode positioning, and integrity of the electrical circuit should be examined and corrective measures should be taken. If excessive impedance was not an issue, the patient should be re-stimulated at a higher stimulus dosage.

In the case of missed seizures, it is preferable to wait at least 20 seconds between stimulations (See Section 11.7) because some seizures may, rarely, be delayed by 20 seconds or more. This interval may also allow the effects of prior stimulation to dissipate. It is common practice to restimulate at 50%–100% above the original stimulus dosage.

After successful seizure elicitation, it is important to review the causes of the missed seizure, particularly when there is repeated difficulty in producing an ictal response. If possible, any medications with anticonvulsant properties should be reduced in dosage or discontinued. There is evidence that larger doses of barbiturate anesthetics increase seizure threshold and/or decrease seizure duration (Boylan et al. 2000; Krueger et al. 1993; Miller et al. 1985). Anesthetic dosage should be reviewed and possibly reduced. Flumazenil (0.5–1.0 mg iv) can be administered at the time of anesthetic induction in patients receiving high-dose benzodiazepines (Bailine et al. 1994; Berigan et al. 1995; Doering and Ball 1995; Krystal et al. 1998). Vigorous hyperventilation should be attempted. Dehydrated patients should be examined for electrolyte imbalance and any indicated corrective measures should be taken. If the source of the problem is still unclear and increased stimulus intensity fails to elicit a seizure, then the practitioner may switch from a barbiturate anesthetic agent to etomidate (0.15–0.30 mg/kg iv) (Christensen et al. 1986; Saffer and Berk 1998; Trzepacz et al. 1993) or ketamine (2–3 mg/kg iv) (Rasmussen et al. 1996).

In the context of missed or abortive seizures, some clinicians have used the adenosine antagonist caffeine sodium benzoate (500–2,000 mg iv, equivalent to 250–1,000 mg of pure caffeine) to produce or lengthen generalized seizures (Calev et al. 1993; Coffey et al. 1987c, 1990; Hinkle et al. 1987; Shapira et al. 1985, 1987). This preparation is administered a few minutes before anesthetic induction. A less common strategy has been the use of intravenous theophylline at the time of ECT (Girish et al. 1996; Leentjens et al. 1996) or the administration of a single dose of oral sustained-release theophylline (200–400 mg) the night before ECT administration (Swartz and Lewis 1991). Each of these techniques will reliably increase seizure duration, perhaps by modulating seizure termination processes (Francis and Fochtmann 1994). However, most evidence suggests that caffeine or theophylline administration will not decrease seizure threshold and thereby facilitate seizure induction in patients with repeated missed seizures (McCall et al. 1993). Furthermore, standing regimens of theophylline may be associated with an especially high incidence of status epilepticus when combined with ECT, even when plasma levels are in the therapeutic range for the treatment of pulmonary disorder (10–20 ng/mL) (Devanand et al. 1988a; Fink and Sackeim 1998; Peters et al. 1984). Case reports also have described cardiac complications associated with combining ECT and caffeine (Acevedo and Smith 1998; Beale et al. 1994c; Jaffe et al. 1990b). In addition, a recent rodent study raised the possibility that the combination of ECT and caffeine may result in neuropathologic changes not observed with ECT alone (Enns et al. 1996). These concerns and the evidence that seizure duration per se has little, if any, relationship to ECT clinical outcome limit the circumstances in which caffeine and theophylline might be considered as augmentation agents in ECT.

11.9.2. Abortive or Brief Seizures

At times, seizures will be elicited that are abortive—that is, too short in duration (typically, less than 15 seconds by motor or EEG criteria). If, for instance, a policy is adopted that adequate seizures must be at least 15 seconds in duration, a 12-second seizure would be considered inadequate. In such circumstances, procedures may be implemented that are similar to those following a missed seizure. The same factors that result in missed seizures can produce abortive seizures. Brief seizures, however, may be due to either insufficient or markedly suprathreshold stimulus intensity (Riddle et al. 1993; Sackeim et al. 1991). Therefore, short seizures may occur when stimulus parameters are either too low or too high and the practitioner may need to estimate where they are likely to be on the relative stimulus intensity versus seizure duration curve. After an abortive seizure, the practitioner should make a clinical judgment about whether restimulation will be conducted. On the one hand, abortive seizures caused by low stimulus dosage are likely not to have therapeutic properties and restimulation may contribute to therapeutic benefit. On the other hand, short seizures related to high stimulus intensity may be effective. Particularly in frail patients with medical complications, the practitioner may prefer to have only one seizure induction at the session.

After an abortive seizure, a sharp, transient increase in seizure threshold is likely. Because of this threshold increase, restimulation immediately after an abortive seizure often produces a missed seizure or another abortive seizure. To partially overcome this "refractory period" it is advisable to use a longer time interval before restimulation than that used after a missed seizure. An interval of at least 45 seconds is generally sufficient. In addition, some practitioners believe that restimulation after an abortive seizure may require a relatively greater increase in stimulus intensity than is used after a missed seizure. Before restimulation, the patient should be examined and the need for additional anesthetic and muscle relaxant agents determined as based, for example, on return of consciousness or of spontaneous respiration. As in the case of missed seizures, the possible causes of abortive seizures should be reviewed before the next treatment session, and particular attention should be paid to factors that may increase seizure threshold and/or decrease seizure duration. A common cause of abortive seizures is excessive dose of the anesthetic agent.

In determining whether patients have had an adequate treatment, some practitioners calculate total seizure time from multiple stimulations. No empirical justification exists for this practice. A patient who has had two abortive seizures in a session, each of 11 seconds, should not be considered to have had an adequate treatment because the total seizure time exceeded a 15-second criterion. However, it is highly unusual to make a third attempt in a given treatment session. It should also be emphasized that some patients consistently display short seizures (e.g., 15 seconds in motor manifestations), regardless of the adequacy of technique. This pattern is particularly likely to occur in older patients with high initial seizure thresholds (Sackeim et al. 1991) as well as later in the ECT course, because seizure duration declines and seizure threshold rises with progressive treatment (Kales et al. 1997; Sackeim 1999; Sackeim et al. 1986). There is no evidence that such patients do not benefit from these treatments. Rather, concern about abortive seizures centers on the patient who is capable of manifesting a fully adequate seizure but has one of short duration because of factors such as concomitant medication, inadequate ventilation, inadequate stimulus intensity, or poor electrical contact.

11.9.3. Prolonged Seizures

Rarely, some patients experience prolonged seizures after ECT or may have a return of seizure activity after the initial seizure terminates (tardive seizures). As defined here, a *prolonged seizure* is one that is longer than 3 minutes by motor or EEG manifestations. Some practitioners use a more stringent definition of 2 minutes (Abrams 1997a; Royal College of Psychiatrists 1995). Each facility should develop standard protocols describing the steps to be taken in response to prolonged seizures, tardive seizures, and status epilepticus.

Because prolonged or tardive seizure activity may not be expressed in motor movements and may develop into nonconvulsive status epilepticus, EEG monitoring is invaluable in such cases (Mayur et al. 1999; Parker et al. 2000; Scott and Riddle 1989). If the seizure is prolonged or hypoxia is evident, intubation may be needed to maintain an adequate level of oxygenation. Usually after 3 minutes of seizure activity, the seizure should be aborted pharmacologically using an anesthetic agent with anticonvulsant properties or a benzodiazepine. Generally, the seizure can be terminated by administering the same barbiturate anesthetic agent (e.g., methohexital) at half or at the same dosage used for ECT anesthesia. An alternative approach is intravenous administration of a single dose and, if necessary, repeated and increasingly higher doses of a benzodiazepine such as diazepam (5–10 mg) or midazolam (1–2 mg). In the event that these steps prove unsuccessful, a standardized protocol should be followed for treating patients in status epilepticus (Aminoff 1998; Lowenstein and Alldredge 1998; Treiman et al. 1998; Walker 1998).

Patients should be monitored closely during this period, particularly for cardiovascular instability and respiratory depression, until consciousness returns and vital signs are stable. After the acute situation resolves, further evaluation may be advisable to determine the cause of the prolonged seizure, the steps that may be useful to prevent recurrence, and the presence of any sequelae. The practitioner should be familiar with the circumstances that are likely to give rise to prolonged or tardive seizures, as described in Chapter 5.

When stimulus dose titration is used at the first treatment, patients often have the longest seizure of their ECT course. With an increment in stimulus intensity at subsequent treatments, seizure duration typically decreases.

11.10. Postictal Recovery Period

11.10.1. Management in the Treatment Area

Physiologic monitoring should continue until patients are ready to be transferred from the treatment area to the recovery area. Patients should not be released from the treatment area until spontaneous respiration has resumed with adequate tidal volume and return of pharyngeal reflexes. Vital signs and ECG should be sufficiently stable so that the patient can return to a lower level of observation.

11.10.2. Management in the Recovery Area

Management of patients in the recovery area should be supervised by the anesthesia provider, who should be readily available in case of emergency. The recovery nurse should provide continuous observation and supportive care. Patients should be gently reoriented. Vital signs should be assessed at a minimum of 15-minute intervals starting with arrival in the recovery area. Patients are ready to leave the recovery area when awake with stable vital signs and otherwise prepared to return to ward care or, for outpatients, to the care of responsible significant others. Before the patient leaves the recovery area, the recovery nurse should inquire about nausea, headache, and other adverse states. The ward staff or significant others should be informed of special conditions or the need for additional monitoring or supervision. If not contraindicated, patients can be fed after leaving the recovery area.

11.10.3. Postictal Delirium

At one or more treatments, a minority of patients develop postictal delirium or excitement, characterized by motor agitation, disorientation, and poor response to commands (Devanand et al. 1989). Recovery may take from 5 to 45 minutes, usually with amnesia for the episode. Postictal delirium may result in physical injury if the patient thrashes against hard objects or in injury to staff members attempting to protect the patient. In addition, patients may dislodge the intravenous line, complicating management. Depending on severity, postictal delirium may be managed supportively or pharmacologically.

If supportive intervention is used, the patient should be continuously reassured and gently restrained to protect against physical injury and intravenous line loss. Excessively firm restraint may aggravate the condition. Environmental stimulation should be minimized, with recovery taking place in a quiet area. Pharmacologic management typically involves intravenous administration of the agent used to produce anesthesia or a benzodiazepine sedative/hypnotic agent (e.g., diazepam or midazolam). Such agents should be administered after return of spontaneous respiration, and, if possible, before the patient leaves the treatment area. Suggested starting doses are 20 mg of methohexital, 2.5–5 mg of diazepam, 0.5–2 mg lorazepam, or 0.5–1 mg midazolam, with readministration as needed. If intravenous access has been lost, intramuscular lorazepam (0.5–2 mg) may be used. If benzodiazepines are ineffective, intravenous haloperidol (2–10 mg) or droperidol (1.25–10 mg) may be administered.

Postictal delirium may occur at a single treatment, never to recur, or it may occur at each treatment in the course. Prophylaxis is recommended when postictal delirium is believed to be recurrent, having occurred at two or more consecutive treatments. Prophylaxis involves administering the anesthetic agent or benzodiazepine before the emergence of the syndrome but after the return of spontaneous respiration. It has also been suggested that administration of higher doses of anesthetic agent (Devanand and Sackeim 1992) or muscle relaxant (Swartz 1990, 1993) prior to ECT prevents the emergence of postictal agitation.

11.10.4. Postrecovery Care

Patients cleared to leave the recovery area must continue to receive some level of postrecovery care for a time period (usually at least 1 hour) commensurate with their needs and established on discharge from the recovery area. The scope of this care varies depending on the patient but generally includes observation of vital signs, reorientation (if needed), treatment of any systemic side effects, feeding, and, if appropriate, bed rest. Postrecovery care may be accomplished in various locations, including an area within or adjacent to the recovery area, an inpatient unit, an ambulatory surgery suite, or a day hospital. Whatever the choice, the location must be compatible with the performance of postrecovery monitoring functions. For outpatients, the postrecovery functions may use the same space used to provide pretreatment assessment on the day of treatment (see Section 11.2), although it is preferable to separate pretreatment assessment and postrecovery care to maximize patient satisfaction.

It is suggested that facilities providing outpatient ECT have a space near the recovery or treatment areas where outpatients and family members can wait prior to release from the facility. Observation in the waiting area may be provided either by facility nursing staff or by the individual accompanying the patient to the treatment. Criteria should be established for the release of outpatients from the facility. Outpatients usually have to return home and should be capable of independent locomotion. It is advisable that outpatients be accompanied by a responsible person when released from the facility, and practitioners should consider making this a requirement. If this procedure is not followed, a member of the treatment team or designee should evaluate the patient's psychomotor and cognitive status prior to release from the facility. The level of functioning should be compatible with a safe journey home without assistance. Patients should not drive or operate equipment for the remainder of the day of ECT treatment.

11.11. Frequency and Number of Treatments

11.11.1. Frequency of Treatments

In the United States, ECT is most commonly performed at a schedule of three times per week regardless of electrode placement. Some practitioners have suggested administration of unilateral ECT at a schedule of four or five treatments per week in the belief that more frequent treatment may speed recovery (Strömgren 1975). Some practitioners also believe that daily ECT, regardless of electrode placement, may be useful early in the treatment course when a particularly rapid response is necessary, as in cases of severe mania, catatonia, high suicidal risk, or severe inanition. Particularly with bilateral ECT, prolonged use of daily treatments increases the risk of cognitive dysfunction. No justification exists for the use of more frequent treatment regimens (Cameron et al. 1962; Exner and Murillo 1973, 1977). If severe cognitive dysfunction or delirium develops, a reduction in the frequency of treatment should be considered. Relative to a schedule of three times per week, evidence has shown that twice-weekly treatment results in the same degree of final clinical improvement, but possibly at a slower rate of response (Gangadhar et al. 1993; Lerer et al. 1995; McAllister et al. 1987; Shapira et al. 1998). Treatment twice per week may result in less severe short-term cognitive effects than a schedule of three treatments per week (Lerer et al. 1995; McAllister et al. 1987; Shapira et al. 1998). In some cases, reducing the schedule to once per week or interrupting the ECT course may be necessary, although treating once per week throughout the ECT course may limit efficacy (Janakiramaiah et al. 1998).

Multiple monitored ECT (MMECT) is a form of treatment in which more than one adequate seizure is produced in the same treatment session under continuous anesthesia. Proponents of this technique suggest that a smaller number of treatment sessions, and therefore a shorter time interval, is required to produce the same quality of remission as with conventional ECT (Maletzky 1981). Critics of the method contend that MMECT is associated with a higher risk of neurologic and cardiovascular morbidity and adverse cognitive effects (Abrams 1997a). A minority of practitioners in the United States currently use MMECT on at least an occasional basis, and few controlled comparisons of MMECT and conventional ECT have been reported (Maletzky 1986). Some practitioners reserve use of MMECT for patients who have a high anesthetic risk or an urgent need for rapid onset of therapeutic response. Others limit the number of seizures in a treatment session to two (Roemer et al. 1990). Given the concerns about the safety of eliciting multiple adequate seizures in the same treatment session and the absence of evidence about putative advantages, routine use of MMECT is not recommended. Occasionally, with urgent clinical circumstances, producing two adequate seizures in the same session may be justified. It has been suggested that this practice is useful in the treatment of patients with neuroleptic malignant syndrome (McKinney and Kellner 1997) and intractable seizure disorder (Griesemer et al. 1997). Eliciting three or more adequate seizures in the same treatment session is not recommended.

11.11.2. Number of Treatments

Patients vary widely in the number of treatments necessary to achieve a full clinical response. The total number administered should be a function of the patient's degree and rate of clinical improvement as well as the severity of cognitive adverse effects. For those patients who achieve clinical remission, the treatment course should end as soon as maximal improvement is reached. There is no evidence that additional acute phase treatment—beyond that necessary to achieve remission—has an impact on relapse rates (Barton et al. 1973; Snaith 1981). If it is decided that treatment technique has been optimal (e.g., use of bilateral electrode placement and increased stimulus intensity), termination of ECT should also be considered in patients who have shown substantial but incomplete clinical improvement yet remain unchanged after two additional treatment sessions.

During the index course of ECT, evaluation of response should focus on changes in target symptoms, with assessment made between each ECT treatment (see Section 12.1). Although the typical ECT course is between 6 and 12 treatments in patients with mood disorder, some patients manifest complete remission after only a few treatments. Other patients may not begin to show substantial clinical change until they have received 10 or more treatments (Nobler et al. 1997; Sackeim et al. 1990b, 1993; Segman et al. 1995). Larger numbers of treatments may be needed when a change in ECT technique has taken place because of lack of response and may also be needed in some cases of schizophrenia. In patients with slow or minimal clinical improvement, the indication for continued ECT should be reassessed after 6 to 10 treatments. At such time, modifications of ECT technique can be considered, including increasing stimulus intensity levels, switching from unilateral to bilateral ECT, and using medications to augment efficacy (e.g., addition of an antipsychotic medication with psychotic patients).

Each facility should have a policy regarding the number of treatments that may be given in an acute treatment course before documenting a formal assessment of the need to continue ECT. This number typically is between 12 and 20 treatments. The recommendation to administer additional ECT should be discussed with the consentor and a new consent should be obtained (Section 8.3). When an unusually large number of treatments is considered, consultation with another psychiatrist with privileges in ECT may be helpful.

Repeated courses of ECT are sometimes necessary because of relapse or recurrence of the psychiatric condition. The decision to readminister a course of ECT should take into account the quality of the previous response to the treatment, including occurrence of adverse effects. In particular, the presence and severity of persistent cognitive deficits should be considered, especially if bilateral electrode placement was used previously or is planned in the upcoming course (McElhiney et al. 1995; Sackeim et al. 2000; Weiner et al. 1986a).

There is no evidence that repeated courses of ECT lead to permanent structural brain damage (Devanand et al. 1994; Weiner 1984) or that a limit on the maximum lifetime number of treatments with ECT is appropriate (Devanand et al. 1991; Lippman et al. 1985). However, frequent relapses suggest that attempts at continuation or maintenance therapy are ineffective (Sackeim 1994; Sackeim et al. 1990a). In patients who require repeated treatment of acute episodes with ECT, attention should be given to the adequacy of post-ECT pharmacotherapy in terms of the type, dosage, and duration of medication. If adequate pharmacotherapy is ineffective in preventing relapse or cannot be tolerated because of side effects, or if the patient prefers it, ECT should be considered as a continuation or maintenance treatment (see Chapter 13).

Unlike pharmacotherapy, ECT is often stopped abruptly when remission is achieved. A significant proportion of patients who initially respond to ECT show clinical deterioration or relapse within 1 or 2 weeks of ECT termination and return for another course of treatment. If continuation pharmacotherapy will be used for relapse prevention following response to the second ECT course, a tapered termination of the second ECT course should be considered (Sackeim 1994). Although not yet empirically tested, provision of ECT on a weekly basis during the first few weeks of continuation pharmacotherapy may provide protection from relapse during the period when pharmacologic effects are building. Strategies for using ECT to prevent relapse and recurrence are discussed in Chapter 13.

RECOMMENDATIONS

11.1. Determining Whether ECT Should Be Administered on an Inpatient or Outpatient Treatment Basis

11.1.1. General Statement

a. An index ECT course may be administered on either an inpatient or an outpatient basis, or a combination thereof, as clinically indicated.
b. An intermediary setting, such as a nursing home or intermediate care facility, can be used in situations where the ambulatory setting is contraindicated but an inpatient level of care is not otherwise indicated.
c. The same indications, relative contraindications, consent requirements, and components of the pre-ECT evaluation apply for inpatient and outpatient ECT.
d. The decision on treatment setting should be made on a treatment-by-treatment basis using specific criteria.

11.1.2. Criteria for Determining the Setting for an Index ECT Course

a. ECT should be administered on an inpatient basis unless all of the following criteria are met:

- The type and seriousness of the patient's mental illness at the time of ECT do not present a significant risk to management on an outpatient basis. Patients for whom ECT should be administered on an inpatient basis include those with high suicide risk, psychosis, substantial cognitive impairment, and those who are otherwise severely incapacitated.
- Anticipated risks associated with the ECT course are detectable and manageable either during the ECT session or on an outpatient basis. Patients at high risk for serious complications are not appropriate for index ECT treatments on an ambulatory basis.

American Society of Anesthesiologists category is one factor that should be considered in risk determination.

- One or more significant others or caregivers should be available throughout the index ECT course to help ensure patient safety and compliance with the treatment plan.
- The patient is willing and able, with the assistance of specified significant others or caregivers, to comply with the behavioral requirements that are expected over this time interval (see Section 11.1).
- A physician is designated who will maintain overall responsibility for the patient during the period over which ECT treatments are administered. This individual, who may be the ECT psychiatrist, should assess the patient at frequent intervals (see Chapter 12) and should be readily available to the patient, pertinent significant others or caregivers, and the ECT treatment team.

b. ECT may be continued on an ambulatory basis when the conditions that indicated inpatient status change during the ECT course, as may occur with substantial clinical improvement. Similarly, a switch from outpatient to inpatient ECT may be prompted by worsening symptoms, increase in severity of risk factors, or other considerations.

11.1.3. Limitations on Patient Behavior

a. Before beginning outpatient ECT, each patient, significant other, or caregiver should be instructed by the treatment team about the type and duration of behavioral limitations.
b. The use of a supplementary written instruction sheet is encouraged in providing instruction about behavioral limitations during the ECT course.
c. After each ECT, reinstruction should be provided before the patient is discharged from the facility.
d. The patient's compliance with behavioral requirements should be assessed on an ongoing basis.
e. Behavioral limitations include the following:

- Patients should be instructed to avoid activities that are likely to be substantially impaired by the anticipated adverse cognitive effects of ECT, particularly if they involve a significant level of risk and especially on the day of each treatment. Patients should be strongly discouraged from driving during an index ECT course.
- Patients must follow prescribed dietary, bowel, bladder, and

grooming instructions before each ECT treatment.

- Patients must comply with the specified medication regimen, including any medication adjustments to be made on the day of each treatment.
- Any adverse effects of ECT and/or apparent changes in medical condition should be reported to the attending physician and/or ECT treatment team before the next treatment.

f. Because cognitive effects vary greatly among patients and as a function of ECT technique, limitations in activities should be tailored to each individual and adjusted as indicated. Fewer limitations in activities may be needed with the relatively long intervals between treatments typically used in continuation/maintenance ECT, because adverse cognitive effects may not persist beyond the day of treatment.

11.2. Preparing the Patient

11.2.1. Before the First Treatment

The ECT psychiatrist should examine the medical record to ensure that the pre-ECT evaluation and informed consent are complete. A standardized summary sheet for such information is useful.

11.2.2. Before Each Treatment

a. Nursing staff is responsible for the following:

- Verifying that the patient has had nothing by mouth for several hours prior to a treatment except necessary medications that may be given with a small sip of water, and observing the patient as needed to ensure that nothing is taken by mouth
- Asking the patient to void
- Checking the patient's head and hair for pins and jewelry and to ensure that the hair is clean and dry
- Removing or asking the patient to remove eyeglasses, contact lenses, hearing aids, and dentures unless otherwise indicated
- Removing or asking the patient to remove chewing gum and other foreign bodies from the mouth
- Ensuring that the fingernail or toenail used for recording pulse oximetry is free of nail polish
- Recording vital signs

- Completing a standardized checklist/reporting form, which is useful in documenting compliance with these procedures

b. The treatment team is responsible for the following:

- The ECT psychiatrist should interview the patient to determine whether significant changes have occurred in mental status or clinical state since the last treatment.
- Prior to anesthesia, the ECT psychiatrist should check that treatment orders have been recorded and followed.
- Both ECT psychiatrist and anesthesia provider should review the medical record since the last ECT treatment.
- A member of the treatment team should check the patient's mouth for foreign bodies and for loose or sharp teeth.
- The treatment team should determine whether there are any adverse effects from earlier ECT treatments.
- The treatment team should also determine whether any changes have occurred in the status of ongoing medical conditions that may affect the risks or benefits associated with ECT; this assessment of adverse effects of ECT and ongoing medical conditions is particularly important for patients receiving ECT on an ambulatory basis.

c. Intravenous access should be established and maintained, at least until the patient is conscious and vital signs are stable.
d. Space requirements for outpatient preparation include

- Easily accessible space for assessment of changes in medical or psychiatric conditions as well as adverse effects of ECT that may have occurred since the last ECT treatment
- Accessible space for those accompanying patients to the facility; when possible, it is useful to allow a significant other to wait with the patient during at least part of the time between the patient's arrival at the facility and treatment

11.3. Airway Management

a. Airway management is the responsibility of the anesthesia provider.
b. Prior to the first ECT of the day, the anesthesia provider or designee should verify that relevant equipment (e.g., oxygen delivery system, suctioning system, and intubation set) is functioning adequately and that necessary supplies for resuscitation are available.

11.3.1. Establishing an Airway

a. For each patient, the ability to provide adequate ventilation should be verified before the muscle relaxant is administered.
b. Intubation should be avoided unless specifically indicated.

11.3.2. Oxygenation

a. Except during stimulus delivery, oxygenation using positive-pressure ventilation should be maintained from the onset of anesthetic induction until adequate spontaneous respiration resumes.
b. A concentration of 100% O_2 at a flow rate of at least 5 L/min and a respiratory rate of 15–20 breaths per minute using positive pressure is suggested.
c. Up to several minutes of preanesthetic oxygenation is helpful for patients at risk of myocardial ischemia or rapid hemoglobin oxygen desaturation after induction of anesthesia.
d. Supplementary oxygen should be available in the recovery area.

11.3.3. Protecting Teeth and Other Oral Structures

a. To protect the teeth and other oral structures, a flexible protective device (bite-block) should be inserted prior to stimulation. At times, additional materials may be indicated, such as the use of dentures to protect fragile remaining teeth.
b. During the passage of the stimulus, the patient's chin should be manually supported to keep the jaw closed and the teeth tight against the bite-block.
c. It is desirable to have bite-blocks or mouth guards of different sizes available to accommodate patients with structurally different oral cavities.

11.4. Medications Used with ECT

11.4.1. Anticholinergic Agents

a. No consensus has been reached as to whether anticholinergic pre-medications should be given routinely.
b. Atropine or glycopyrrolate is used by many practitioners to mini-

mize the risk of vagally mediated bradyarrhythmias or asystole. Anticholinergic agents should be considered, especially for patients receiving sympathetic blocking agents or when the electrical stimulation is likely to be subconvulsive, as during a titration procedure. To guarantee maximum cardiovascular protection from vagal outflow, intravenous administration is preferred. Atropine may be more reliable than glycopyrrolate in preventing bradyarrhythmias.

c. Many practitioners also use atropine or glycopyrrolate to diminish oral secretions. When this is the primary aim of anticholinergic use, intramuscular administration is preferable.

d. When used, anticholinergic premedication should be administered intravenously 2–3 minutes before anesthesia or, alternatively, intramuscularly 30–60 minutes prior to anesthesia induction. Subcutaneous administration should not be used.

e. Typical dosages for atropine are 0.3–0.6 mg im or 0.4–0.8 mg iv, and for glycopyrrolate they are 0.2–0.4 mg im or iv.

11.4.2. Anesthetic Agents

a. ECT should be carried out using ultra-brief, light general anesthesia.

b. Regardless of agent, doses should be adjusted at successive treatments to provide the desired anesthetic effect.

c. Methohexital is the most commonly used anesthetic agent, typically at a dose of 0.5–1.0 mg/kg given intravenously as a single bolus.

d. Etomidate, ketamine, propofol, and thiopental are alternative anesthetic agents.

11.4.3. Muscle Relaxants

a. A skeletal muscle relaxant should be used to minimize convulsive motor activity and to improve airway management.

b. Succinylcholine, 0.5–1.0 mg/kg (as an intravenous bolus), is the preferred relaxant agent. Patients requiring complete relaxation may need higher doses.

c. When a nondepolarizing muscle relaxant is indicated, atracurium, mivacurium, rocuronium, and rapacuronium are alternative agents.

d. Doses of muscle relaxants should be adjusted at successive treatment sessions to achieve the desired effect.

e. The relaxant should be administered either after the onset of unconsciousness or immediately after injection of the anesthetic agent. However, given treatment-to-treatment variability in time to onset of unconsciousness and muscle paralysis, it is preferable to observe the onset of the anesthetic action before administering the muscle relaxant. In any event, the anesthesia provider should ensure that the patient is unconscious and that a patent airway is present prior to respiratory paralysis.

f. The adequacy of skeletal muscle relaxation should be ascertained prior to stimulation. Muscle relaxation can be assessed by the diminution or disappearance of knee, ankle, or withdrawal reflexes; loss of muscle tone; or failure to respond to electrical stimulation delivered by a peripheral nerve stimulator. With a depolarizing muscle blocking agent such as succinylcholine, it is unlikely that maximal relaxation has been achieved until after muscle fasciculations have disappeared. A screening assay for pseudocholinesterase levels or determination of the dibucaine number should be reserved for patients with a significantly elevated likelihood of enzyme deficiency; if needed, the preferred method is determination of dibucaine number.

g. In patients at increased risk for prolonged apnea because of inability to rapidly metabolize succinylcholine, relaxation during ECT can be achieved either with very low doses of succinylcholine or by using alternative nondepolarizing agents that are not metabolized by pseudocholinesterase, such as atracurium and rocuronium.

h. In patients at increased risk for succinylcholine-induced hyperkalemia, any of the alternative nondepolarizing muscle relaxant agents may be used.

11.4.4. Agents Used to Modify the Cardiovascular Response to ECT

a. Anesthesia providers and ECT psychiatrists should be familiar with pharmacologic strategies to prevent or treat adverse cardiovascular responses to ECT, including excessive hypotension, hypertension, and various arrhythmias.

b. In patients who are unequivocally at increased cardiovascular risk, consideration should be given to using prophylactic pharmacologic modification at all treatments.

c. In patients with unstable hypertension and other cardiac conditions, an attempt should be made to stabilize the medical condition before beginning ECT.

d. Pharmacologic modifications of the cardiovascular response to ECT have their own risks, and judgment is needed about when to use such strategies.

e. A strong working relationship with the anesthesia provider, a consultation with a physician with expertise in the assessment and treatment of cardiac disease, and an understanding of the cardiovascular effects of ECT are helpful in optimizing the management of patients with such conditions.

11.5. ECT Devices

11.5.1. Waveform Characteristics

a. A brief pulse stimulus is recommended.

b. Because of the potential aggravation of cognitive side effects and the lack of evidence of any therapeutic advantage, the continued use of sine wave stimulation is not justified.

11.5.2. Mode of Stimulus Delivery

a. A constant current stimulus is recommended.

b. No conceptual justification exists for ECT devices to operate on constant voltage or constant energy principles.

11.5.3. Stimulus Parameters

a. Stimulus intensity controls should allow sufficient flexibility in at least one parameter to treat patients with both low and high seizure thresholds.

b. Manipulations of train duration and pulse frequency appear to be the most efficient methods of altering stimulus intensity (see Section 11.7).

11.5.4. Maximal Device Output

Present output limitations on existing ECT devices in the United States make it difficult to treat patients with exceptionally high seizure threshold and, in some cases, to use right unilateral ECT with a substantially suprathreshold stimulus intensity. Therefore, it is desirable for such ECT devices to have a higher maximal electrical output.

11.5.5. Device Operation and Maintenance

a. Before initial use of a new device, qualified personnel should test the operation of controls, parameters, and features and calibrate the device output characteristics.
b. Device manufacturers should provide a description of testing procedures and suggested preventive maintenance instructions.
c. If device malfunction is suspected, the device should be retested or removed for servicing. Worn cables and connectors should be replaced.
d. Facilities should establish a policy regarding the frequency with which ECT devices undergo assessment of proper function and calibration. At least annual retesting is suggested.

11.5.6. Electrical Safety Considerations

a. Electrical safety testing procedures should be performed and documented prior to first use and at the intervals prescribed by pertinent standards or local requirements regarding medical devices involving patient contact.
b. Devices should allow control over the passage of the electrical stimulus, including the ability to abort the stimulus instantaneously.
c. Passage of the electrical stimulus should be accompanied by an auditory or visual indicator.
d. A means of ensuring that stimulus cables are properly connected to the ECT device and that contact with the scalp is adequate is encouraged. Methods of accomplishing this task include a pretreatment static impedance test feature to measure load impedance and an automatic stimulus abort feature that is triggered by excessively low or high load impedance.
e. ECT devices should be connected to the same electrical supply circuit as all other electrical devices in contact with the patient, including monitoring equipment (see Section 11.8.4).
f. Electrical grounding of devices should not be bypassed.

11.6. Stimulus Electrode Placement

11.6.1. Choice of Electrode Placement

a. ECT psychiatrists should be skilled in administering both unilateral and bilateral ECT.
b. Practitioners should have a clear understanding of the variations in therapeutic and adverse effects with differing electrode placements.
c. The choice of unilateral versus bilateral electrode placement should be based on an ongoing analysis of applicable risks and benefits.
d. The choice of electrode placement should be decided by the ECT psychiatrist in consultation with the consentor and the attending physician.
e. Decisions about electrode placement should be made in concert with decisions about stimulus intensity. For example, if stimulus dosages are markedly above seizure threshold, there is increasing evidence that right unilateral ECT is as effective as bilateral ECT in treating major depression but results in less cognitive impairment.
f. Evidence supporting the efficacy of right unilateral ECT for the treatment of conditions other than major depressive disorder is unclear.

11.6.2. Electrode Positioning

a. With standard bilateral (bifrontotemporal) ECT, electrodes should be placed on both sides of the head, with the midpoint of each electrode approximately 1 inch above the midpoint of a line extending from the tragus of the ear to the external canthus of the eye.
b. To minimize verbal memory impairment, virtually all unilateral ECT is administered over the right cerebral hemisphere. The preferred configuration involves one electrode in the standard frontotemporal position used with bilateral ECT, with the midpoint of the second electrode 1 inch lateral to the vertex of the scalp (d'Elia placement).
c. Stimulus electrodes should be placed far enough apart so that the amount of current shunted across the scalp is minimized.
d. Care should be taken to avoid stimulating over or adjacent to a skull defect.

11.6.3. Stimulus Electrode Site Preparation

a. Adequate contact between stimulus electrodes and the scalp should be ensured.

b. Scalp areas in contact with stimulus electrodes should be cleansed and gently abraded.

c. Before each use, the contact area of the stimulus electrodes should be coated with a conducting gel, paste, or solution.

d. Conducting gel or solution should be confined to the area under the stimulus electrodes and should never spread across the hair or scalp between stimulus electrodes.

e. When stimulus electrodes are placed over an area covered by hair, a conducting abrasive medium should be rubbed into the scalp and the hair beneath the electrodes should be parted. Clipping the underlying hair is unnecessary.

f. Stimulus electrodes should be applied with sufficient pressure to ensure good contact during stimulus delivery.

11.6.4. Impedance Testing

a. A means of ensuring the electrical continuity of the stimulus path, such as a static impedance test, is encouraged (see Section 11.5.6).

b. In the case of an abnormal static impedance value, the cause of the low or high impedance should be ascertained and remedied before proceeding with the treatment. Abnormally low static impedance values commonly result from smearing of conductive medium between the electrodes and may also occur if the patient has heavy perspiration or has administered a cream, gel, or spray to the hair. Excessively high impedance may be caused by poor contact between an electrode and the scalp, incomplete or improper preparation of the electrode sites, poor contact between the electrodes and the stimulus cable, a break in the stimulus cable, or poor connection or disconnection of the stimulus cable from the device. A marked increase in static impedance prior to stimulation should alert the practitioner to the fact that electrode contact at the sites may not be optimal.

11.7. Stimulus Dosing

a. The primary consideration with stimulus dosing is to produce an adequate ictal response (see Sections 11.8.1 and 11.8.2).

b. Regardless of the specific dosing paradigm used, restimulation at a higher stimulus intensity should be considered whenever seizure monitoring (see Sections 11.8.1 and 11.8.2) indicates that an adequate ictal response has not occurred.

c. Practitioners should have a strategy for selecting stimulus dosage that individualizes the electrical dosage to the patient. Empirical titration is the most precise method for identifying seizure threshold at the beginning of the ECT course. At subsequent treatments, dosing is adjusted relative to this empirically determined estimate of seizure threshold. Facilities using empirical titration should adopt a policy on the maximal number of restimulations permitted during a session, with four or five stimulations being a common cutoff. Formula-based procedures adjust electrical intensity for factors such as electrode placement, gender, age, anesthesia dosage, and concomitant medications. A high fixed dose strategy should be reserved for rare situations in which serious concomitant medical conditions preclude the safe use of subconvulsive stimulation.

d. The choice of a stimulus dosing strategy should consider that initial seizure threshold may vary widely among patients and generally increases over the treatment course.

e. The choice of a stimulus dosing strategy should also consider that therapeutic and adverse effects may vary depending on the extent to which the stimulus intensity exceeds the seizure threshold. A "moderately" suprathreshold dosing strategy is recommended, with a dosage range for right unilateral ECT between 150% and 500% above initial seizure threshold (i.e., 2.5–6.0 times initial seizure threshold) and a dosage range for bilateral ECT between 50% and 150% above initial seizure threshold (i.e., 1.5–2.5 times initial threshold). Stimuli marginally above seizure threshold are likely to be less therapeutic than those delivered at a higher intensity, especially with right unilateral electrode placement. Grossly suprathreshold stimuli may be associated with greater cognitive side effects.

11.8. Physiologic Monitoring

11.8.1. Seizure Monitoring

11.8.1.1. General Considerations

a. Seizure duration should be monitored to ensure an adequate ictal response (see Sections 11.9.1 and 11.9.2), to detect prolonged seizure activity (see Section 11.9.3), and to enable appropriate decisions to be made regarding stimulus dosing strategy (see Section 11.7).

b. Seizure monitoring consists of observing the presence and duration of both ictal motor activity (see Section 11.8.1.2) and ictal EEG activity (see Section 11.8.1.3).

11.8.1.2. Ictal Motor Activity

a. Seizure duration should be documented at each treatment and should be monitored by timing the duration of convulsive movements.

b. The simplest and most reliable means of monitoring the ictal motor response is by visual observation. This measurement should be facilitated by preventing the flow of relaxant to the distal portion of an extremity by placing a blood pressure cuff at the wrist or ankle prior to relaxant infusion and inflating it substantially above the anticipated systolic pressure during the seizure.

c. If unilateral stimulus electrode placement is used, the occluded limb should be ipsilateral to the stimulated cerebral hemisphere to ensure contralateral spread of the seizure activity.

d. Because ictal movements may persist for a longer time in body regions other than the cuffed extremity, the longest duration of any seizure-related motor activity should be determined.

e. The duration of cuff inflation should be minimized to prevent prolonged tissue ischemia. Similarly, care should be taken when using this technique in patients at risk for skin or musculoskeletal complications or who have severe peripheral vascular disease, deep vein thrombosis, or sickle cell disease.

11.8.1.3. Ictal EEG Activity

a. Scalp electroencephalographic (EEG) monitoring should be carried out on at least a one-channel basis. This is because monitoring of the motor response alone may be associated with gross underestimation of true seizure duration and may lead to unnecessary restimulation or failure to detect prolonged seizures (nonconvulsive prolonged seizures or status epilepticus may be discernible only in the EEG).

b. EEG recording electrodes should be in good contact with the scalp. The location of EEG monitoring leads should maximize the detection of ictal EEG activity. The use of a frontal-mastoid montage is preferred.

c. EEG may be monitored either on a visual (i.e., chart recorder or video monitor) or an auditory basis.

d. Because excessive impedance at EEG sites is the most common cause of poor EEG recordings, careful attention should be paid to EEG site preparation.

e. The ECT psychiatrist should also be aware of the different manifestations of EEG seizure onset and termination as well as artifacts likely to occur during monitoring, such as ECG, pulse, EMG activity, and anesthesia effects.

11.8.2. EEG Seizure Adequacy Measures

Some ECT devices provide measures that convey quantitative information about EEG changes during and after the seizure. However, none of the present measures has been sufficiently validated, and changes in treatment technique should not be based on this information alone. Rather, this information could be used in concert with information on the rate and degree of clinical response and other aspects of treatment adequacy when considering changes in treatment technique.

11.8.3. Other Physiologic Monitoring

11.8.3.1. Cardiovascular Monitoring

a. ECG monitoring should begin prior to anesthesia induction and continue until spontaneous respiration resumes and any treatment-associated ECG abnormalities have resolved.

b. There should be capacity to provide a paper copy of ECG activity in the event that later consultation is necessary. If ECG paper copy is to be entered into the clinical record but was recorded at a nonstandard ECG recording speed, the actual chart speed or labeled timing marks should be included.

c. Systolic and diastolic blood pressure, as well as heart rate or pulse, should be measured before anesthetic induction and at intervals throughout the procedure, including during the patient's stay in the recovery area (see Section 11.10). Such monitoring should continue until any ECT-related changes have stabilized. Automatic noninvasive assessment of blood pressure is preferred.

11.8.3.2. Oximetry

a. Pulse oximetry should be used during ECT.
b. Oximetry is particularly valuable in patients at risk for hypoxia.

11.8.4. Electrical Safety Considerations Regarding Monitoring

a. External physiologic monitoring devices that are connected to the patient during the passage of stimulus current should be electrically isolated. If electrical isolation is uncertain, a biomedical engineer or other qualified person should be consulted prior to the use of monitoring devices.
b. Adequacy of the ground in the electrical circuit should be verified.

11.9. Management of Missed, Abortive, and Prolonged Seizures

11.9.1. Missed Seizures

a. If seizure activity is absent after the electrical stimulus, the patient should be restimulated at a higher intensity (e.g., 50%–100% increase).
b. In general, up to a total of four or five stimulations may be administered within a single treatment session, if necessary.
c. Each restimulation should be preceded by at least a 20-second delay to account for the possibility of delayed seizure onset.
d. The muscular contraction that usually accompanies the delivery of the electrical stimulus should not be mistaken for a brief seizure.
e. Although generally not required, additional doses of anesthetic or relaxant agents may occasionally need to be readministered.
f. Because missed seizures may be caused by premature termination of the stimulus, poor electrode contact, disconnection of the stimulus cable, or device malfunction, the electrical continuity of stimulus cables and electrodes should be checked prior to restimulation.
g. The following techniques, alone or in combination, should be considered as means of augmenting seizures (no specific order of importance is implied):

  • Diminish dose of anesthetic agent

- Diminish or omit doses of any concomitant medications with anticonvulsant action, especially benzodiazepines
- Use flumazenil to reverse the action of benzodiazepines
- Provide vigorous hyperventilation before and during the induced seizure
- Ensure adequate patient hydration
- Use an alternative anesthetic agent with less effect on seizure threshold and/or duration, such as ketamine or etomidate

11.9.2. Abortive or Brief Seizures

a. Although uncertainty exists about the minimal seizure duration necessary for an adequate treatment, many practitioners believe that it is unlikely that seizures lasting less than 15 seconds in motor and EEG manifestations are adequate.
b. The most common causes of abortive seizures (lasting less than 15 seconds) are excessive anesthetic dosage, concomitant anticonvulsant medications, inadequate ventilation, and insufficient electrical dosage. Abortive seizures may also be caused by premature termination of the stimulus, poor electrode contact, disconnection of the stimulus cable, and device malfunction.
c. It should be recognized that seizure duration may also be decreased if the electrical dosage is markedly in excess of seizure threshold. In such cases, the ictal EEG may show high-amplitude seizure expression.
d. Abortive seizures may be followed by restimulation at a higher intensity, as described in Section 11.9.1.
e. The electrical continuity of stimulus cables and electrodes should be checked prior to restimulation.
f. Because of the presence of a relative refractory period, a longer time interval (e.g., 45–90 seconds) should be used before restimulating than that used after a missed seizure. This longer waiting period before restimulating increases the likelihood that additional doses of anesthetic or relaxant agents will be necessary.
g. When an abortive seizure occurs at maximal stimulus intensity, the procedures outlined in Section 11.9.1 (g) should be considered.

11.9.3. Prolonged Seizures

a. Seizures persisting for more than 180 seconds by motor and/or EEG manifestations should be considered "prolonged."

b. The presence of prolonged seizures may be apparent only with EEG monitoring. The practitioner should determine whether seizure activity is ongoing as opposed to EEG artifact.

c. Prolonged seizures should be terminated pharmacologically with an anesthetic agent or benzodiazepine.

d. During and immediately after prolonged seizures, oxygenation should be maintained, with intubation performed as clinically indicated.

e. To detect adverse cardiovascular changes, cardiovascular monitoring should be continued throughout a prolonged seizure.

f. Appropriate medical consultation should be considered if difficulties are experienced in terminating a prolonged seizure, if spontaneous seizures occur, or if neurologic or other medical sequelae appear to be present. In such cases, ECT should be resumed only after correcting any treatable conditions known to increase the likelihood of prolonged seizures and assessing applicable risk/benefit considerations.

11.10. Postictal Recovery Period

11.10.1. Management in the Treatment Area

a. The patient should not be released from the treatment area until spontaneous respiration has resumed, with adequate tidal volume and return of pharyngeal reflexes; vital signs are sufficiently stable that the patient can return to a lower level of observation; and no adverse effects requiring immediate medical evaluation or intervention are present.

b. Physiologic monitoring should continue as specified in Section 11.8.

11.10.2. Management in the Recovery Area

a. Management of the patient while in the recovery area should be under the supervision of the anesthesia provider.

b. The recovery nurse(s) should provide continuous observation and supportive care (including reorientation), measure vital signs on at least 15-minute intervals beginning with the patient's arrival in the recovery area, and alert the anesthesia provider in a timely fashion of any situation potentially requiring medical intervention.

c. The patient should not leave the recovery area until he or she is awake with stable vital signs and is otherwise prepared to return to ward care, a step-down unit, or to the care of the responsible person accompanying the outpatient.

11.10.3. Postictal Delirium

a. Postictal delirium and agitation should be managed supportively using either an intravenous anesthetic agent or an intravenous or intramuscular benzodiazepine sedative/hypnotic agent. If this treatment is ineffective, intravenous haloperidol or droperidol may be used.
b. When recurrent or particularly severe, postictal delirium can often be prevented with the prophylactic use of the above agents. In such cases, administration of these medications should be delayed until after spontaneous respiration returns.

11.10.4. Postrecovery Care

a. It is advisable that space be provided in an adjacent area for outpatients to be observed after release from the recovery area but prior to release from the facility.
b. Observation should be provided either by facility nursing staff or by the individual accompanying the patient to the facility.
c. It is advisable that outpatients leave the facility in the care of a significant other or caregiver after each ECT treatment.

11.11. Frequency and Number of Treatments

11.11.1. Frequency of Treatments

a. Usually two or three treatments per week are administered on nonconsecutive days. Most facilities in the United States presently use three treatments per week.
b. Some practitioners believe that transient use of daily treatments may be useful early in the treatment course when a rapid onset of response is important, as in severe mania, catatonia, high suicidal risk, and severe inanition. Particularly with bilateral ECT, prolonged use of daily treatments increases cognitive impairment. Use of more frequent treatment regimens has not been justified.

c. A reduction in treatment frequency should be considered if delirium or severe cognitive dysfunction occurs.

d. The relative benefits and risks of MMECT (defined as the delivery of more than one adequate seizure per treatment session) compared with standard ECT have yet to be adequately defined. For this reason, MMECT should not be routinely used, and given concerns regarding safety, eliciting three or more adequate seizures in the same treatment session is not recommended. Under urgent clinical circumstances, the induction of two adequate seizures in the same session may be justified.

11.11.2. Number of Treatments

a. The total number of ECT treatments administered should be a function of the patient's response and the severity of adverse effects. Response should be determined by changes in target symptoms (see Section 12.1), with assessment made between each ECT treatment.

b. In major depression, an ECT course generally consists of 6–12 treatments, although a plateau in response may occur either earlier or later than this. Larger numbers of treatments are more likely to be required when a change in ECT technique has taken place because of lack of response and possibly also in some cases of schizophrenia.

c. For ECT responders, the treatment course should be ended or tapered as soon as it is clear that a maximum response has been reached.

d. In the absence of significant clinical improvement after 6–10 treatments, the indication for continued ECT should be reassessed with consideration given to modification of ECT technique—for example, an increase in stimulus dosage levels, a change from unilateral to bilateral electrode placement, or the use of medications to potentiate the clinical response.

e. Repeated courses of ECT are sometimes necessary. The decision to readminister a course of ECT should take into account the presence, severity, and persistence of cognitive deficits associated with prior ECT because cumulative effects may occur, particularly with bilateral electrode placement.

f. Each facility should develop a policy regarding the number of treatments after which a formal assessment of the need for continued ECT should be evaluated and discussed with the consentor, as outlined in Section 8.3.

CHAPTER 12

Evaluation of Outcome

12.1. Therapeutic Response

Before beginning an acute or index course of ECT, each patient should have a documented treatment plan indicating specific criteria for remission. The type and severity of prominent symptoms should be described. It is helpful if therapeutic goals take into account the aspects of symptomatology that are expected to improve. For example, some patients with schizoaffective disorder have relatively chronic forms of thought disturbance (e.g., delusions) with superimposed episodes of prominent affective symptomatology. In a number of these patients, ECT may ameliorate the affective component without influencing the chronic thought disturbance. Prolonging the ECT course because of persistent thought disturbance may result in unnecessary treatment. In contrast, many patients with mood disorder present with chronic dysthymia preceding a clear-cut episode of major depression. Some practitioners may be uncertain whether remission of a major depressive episode is associated with return to the chronic dysthymia or whether dysthymic symptoms also respond to ECT. Evidence has shown that the extent of residual symptoms shortly after ECT does not differ among patients with double depression (i.e., major depression superimposed on dysthymia) and patients with major depression without a history of dysthymia (Prudic et al. 1993). Thus, in patients with double depression, basing treatment termination only on resolution of the major depressive episode may result in incomplete treatment and possibly heighten the risk of relapse.

After the start of ECT, clinical assessments should be performed and documented by the attending physician or designee after every one or two treatments. To allow for clearing of acute cognitive side effects, it is preferable to conduct these assessments at least 24 hours after a treatment. For outpatients, this may involve evaluation prior to the subsequent treatment. Assessments should document changes in the disorder being treated with ECT, in terms of both improvement in the signs and symptoms that were present initially and the emergence of new symptoms. Although infrequent, switches from depression to mania may occur during the course of ECT. In this context, it is important to distinguish between mania and a delirium with euphoria (Devanand et al. 1988b) (see also Section 5.6). Serial assessments of cognitive function may help in making this differential diagnosis.

In patients treated for catatonia, the presence of mutism or negativism prior to ECT may have made other symptoms difficult to discern. After catatonic symptoms improve with ECT, other aspects of psychopathology may become evident and should be assessed and documented. Other patients may have experienced delusions or hallucinations before or during the ECT course, but these symptoms may have been difficult to verify because of patient guardedness or other factors. With clinical improvement, additional symptoms may become apparent that have an impact on future treatment.

Some practitioners find it useful to use a standardized rating instrument when assessing symptomatic change. Changes in rating scale scores over time are particularly helpful in determining whether the degree of improvement has accelerated, decelerated, or reached a plateau and in documenting the extent of residual symptoms at the completion of ECT. For patients with major depression, the Hamilton Rating Scale for Depression (HRSD; Hamilton 1967) is a commonly used instrument. The 24-item version of the HRSD contains items assessing symptoms of hopelessness, helplessness, and worthlessness, features that are particularly common in patients receiving ECT. An alternative instrument is the Montgomery-Åsberg Rating Scale for Depression (Montgomery and Åsberg 1979). For patients with psychotic disorder, clinician assessments of symptoms may be performed with the Brief Psychiatric Rating Scale (Overall and Gorham 1962). The Young Mania Scale (Young et al. 1978) may be used for patients with acute mania. Instruments such as the HRSD traditionally instruct the examiner to assess symptoms over the past week. Because symptomatic change with ECT is often rapid and requires more frequent assessment, it is useful to reduce the interval being examined to a few days.

Prior to ECT, clinician and self-report assessments of depression severity show only moderate correlation (Sayer et al. 1993). This discrepancy is largely attributable to a subgroup of patients who clinicians rate as moderately or severely depressed but who have low levels of symptoms by self-report. These patients most commonly present with psychotic depression (Sayer et al. 1993). After completion of ECT, the degree of agreement between self- and clinician-rated assessments is considerably greater. Some clinicians find that a formal self-report instrument is of supplemental value in documenting the effects of ECT on symptoms. The Beck Depression Inventory II (Beck et al. 1996; Dozois et al. 1998) may be used, with the period being assessed modified from 2 weeks to at most 1 week. An alternative self-rating instrument is the Inventory for Depressive Symptomatology (Rush et al. 1985), which has the advantage of having a complementary clinician-rated version. For elderly depressed patients, the Geriatric Depression Scale may be used (Yesavage et al. 1983). It should be noted, however, that self-ratings of depression severity are supplemental and should never substitute for clinician evaluations.

Before ECT is used as a continuation treatment, the type and severity of residual symptoms after acute phase treatment should be ascertained. As with acute phase treatment, the ECT physician should interview patients before each continuation treatment to determine changes in symptoms and cognition. Emergence of symptoms suggestive of potential relapse should trigger consideration of changes in treatment frequency and/or technique.

12.2. Adverse Effects

12.2.1. Cognitive Changes

The impact of ECT on cognition, particularly orientation and memory, should be assessed in terms of both objective findings and patient report during and after the ECT course (see Section 5.8). This assessment should be conducted before the start of ECT to establish a baseline level of functioning and should be repeated at least weekly throughout the ECT course. Like assessment of therapeutic change, it is suggested that cognitive assessment be conducted at least 24 hours after an ECT treatment to avoid contamination by acute postictal effects.

The evaluation of cognitive function may include bedside assessment and/or formal neuropsychologic measures. In either case, cognitive assessment should minimally include evaluations of orientation, anterograde amnesia, and retrograde amnesia. For bedside or informal assessment, orientation in the three spheres (person, place, and time) should be determined. Informal assessment of anterograde and retrograde amnesia can be conducted by discussion with the patient of events in the recent and distant past (e.g., events associated with the day of the interview, recent trips or special occasions, and memory for personal details, such as address or phone number).

Formal cognitive testing instruments provide quantitative measures for tracking change. To assess global cognitive functioning, including orientation, an instrument such as the Mini-Mental State Exam (MMSE, Folstein et al. 1975) may be used. Significantly diminished MMSE scores (e.g., reductions of 20% or more) may reflect or suggest the development of a sustained delirium and lead to consideration of modifications in ECT technique. Similarly, such reductions after the end of the ECT course may have implications for discharge planning and for the level of supervision required after ECT. It should be noted, however, that changes in global cognitive status as measured by the MMSE are not necessarily associated with the degree of anterograde or retrograde amnesia. Patients may show unchanged or improved MMSE scores and still manifest considerable amnesia (Sobin et al. 1995).

Various instruments are available to assess delayed recall of newly learned information, including subtests of the Wechsler Memory Scale III (WMS-III, Wechsler 1997), which provides age-adjusted norms for delayed memory components. Unfortunately, no alternative versions of the WMS-III exist, and repeated assessment may be confounded by practice effects. In contrast, the Randt Memory Test (Randt and Brown 1983; Randt et al. 1980) subscales that assess delayed memory for verbal and pictorial material have shown sensitivity to the anterograde amnesia associated with ECT (Zervas and Jandorf 1993), and this instrument has five alternative forms. When used with a delay recall procedure, the Buschke Selective Reminding Test (Hannay and Levin 1985) is also useful for repeated assessment (Sackeim et al. 1993, 2000). Tasks involving delayed copying of complex figures (Lezak 1995), delayed recognition memory for unfamiliar faces, and the Benton Visual Retention Test (Benton 1950; Sivan 1992) have shown sensitivity to ECT-associated anterograde amnesia for nonverbal information (Meyendorf et al. 1980; Sackeim et al. 1993, 2000; Steif et al. 1986; Weiner et al. 1986b).

Brief and valid assessment instruments to gauge the extent of retrograde amnesia are less readily available. Tests that formally assess recall and/or recognition of famous people or public events (e.g., Butters and

Albert 1982; Goldberg and Barnett 1985) have been used (Squire 1986; Weiner et al. 1986b). However, most of these instruments categorize events in relation to the decade of their prominence (e.g., 1990s, 1980s, 1970s). The retrograde amnesia resulting from ECT displays a temporal gradient, such that events closest in time to the treatment course are most vulnerable to memory loss and remote events are spared (Sackeim 1992; Squire 1986; Squire et al. 1975). Consequently, these instruments are unlikely to be sufficiently sensitive.

An alternative approach has been to assess amnesia for autobiographical or personal memories (Lisanby et al. 2000; McElhiney et al. 1995; Sackeim et al. 1993, 2000; Sobin et al. 1995; Weiner et al. 1986b). Memory loss for events in the patient's life is often the most distressing aspect of ECT's cognitive side effects. Unfortunately, the instruments shown to be sensitive in research are lengthy and generally not amenable to routine clinical use. Efforts are under way to validate a brief instrument that may be sensitive to ECT-induced retrograde amnesia for autobiographical information.

When cognitive status is assessed formally or informally, the patient's perception of cognitive changes should also be ascertained (Prudic et al. [in press]). This assessment may be done by informally inquiring whether the patient has noticed any changes in the ability to concentrate (e.g., to follow a television program or a magazine article), to remember visitors or events of the day, or to recall more remote events. Patient perception of memory functioning may also be examined using a quantitative instrument. The Squire Memory Complaint Questionnaire (Squire et al. 1979) has been used most commonly with patients receiving ECT.

As noted in Section 5.8, recent studies have repeatedly found that patients report fewer memory complaints shortly after the ECT course than at their pre-ECT baseline (Coleman et al. 1996). These changes in self-reported cognitive function are independent of changes in objective neuropsychologic measures but are substantially correlated with the degree of improvement in depressive symptoms (Calev et al. 1991a; Coleman et al. 1996; Cronholm and Ottosson 1963a; Frith et al 1983; Squire and Slater 1983; Squire and Zouzounis 1988; Weiner et al. 1986b). Some concerns have been raised about the reliability of the Squire Memory Complaint Questionnaire because it requires patients to compare their current cognitive functioning with their functioning before the psychiatric episode, a complex judgment (Coleman et al. 1996; Prudic et al. [in press]). The Cognitive Failures Questionnaire (Broadbent et al. 1982) is an alternative self-report instrument with a wider sampling of aspects of cognitive function.

If orientation or memory functioning showed substantial deterioration during the ECT course that is unresolved on hospital discharge, a plan should be made for follow-up of cognitive status and the assessment intervals should be specified. Most commonly, cognitive functioning recovers markedly within days of the end of the ECT course (Sackeim 1992; Sackeim et al. 1993; Steif et al. 1986; Weeks et al. 1980) and patients should be reassured that this will likely be the case.

It should be kept in mind that the suggested evaluation procedures provide only gross measures of cognitive status. Furthermore, interpretation of cognitive change may be subject to a number of difficulties. Patients frequently have cognitive impairments before receiving ECT (Sackeim and Steif 1988) and therapeutic response may be associated with improvement in many cognitive domains (Frith et al. 1983; Malloy et al. 1982; Sackeim et al. 1992a, 1993; Weeks et al. 1980). However, although some patients show improved scores relative to their pre-ECT baseline, they still may not have fully returned to their preepisode level of cognitive functioning (Sackeim 1992; Steif et al. 1986). This discrepancy may be a basis for complaints about lingering cognitive deficits. In addition, the procedures suggested here sample only limited aspects of cognitive functioning, for example, deliberate (conscious or intentional) learning and retention of information. Patients may also have deficits in incidental (unattended) learning. Furthermore, the suggested procedures concentrate on verbal memory, although both right unilateral and bilateral ECT produce deficits in memory for nonverbal material (Sackeim et al. 2000; Squire 1986).

12.2.2. Other Adverse Effects

During the ECT course, the onset of any new risk factors or significant worsening of those present prior to ECT should be evaluated before the next treatment. When such developments alter the risks of administering ECT, the consentor should be informed and the results of this discussion documented. Patient complaints about ECT should be considered carefully. The attending physician and/or a member of the ECT treatment team should discuss these complaints with the patient, attempt to determine their source, and ascertain whether corrective measures are indicated.

RECOMMENDATIONS

12.1. Therapeutic Response

a. Each treatment plan should indicate specific criteria for remission.
b. Clinical assessments should be performed by the attending physician or designee and documented prior to ECT and after every one or two ECT treatments, preferably at least 24 hours after the treatment.
c. Formal clinical rating instruments may be useful in documenting changes in symptoms over the ECT course.

12.2. Adverse Effects

12.2.1. Cognitive Changes

a. During a course of ECT, the presence and severity of disorientation, anterograde amnesia, and retrograde amnesia should be monitored in terms of both objective findings and self-report (see Section 5.8). This evaluation should consist of bedside assessment of orientation and memory (both retention of newly learned material and recall of recent and remote events) and/or administration of formal neuropsychologic measures.
b. Assessment should be carried out before ECT and at least weekly throughout an ECT course. When possible, cognitive assessment should be performed at least 24 hours after an ECT treatment.
c. If orientation and/or memory deteriorate substantially during an ECT course (see Section 5.8), modifications to the ECT procedure should be considered. If such effects persist after completion of the ECT course, a plan should be made for post-ECT follow-up assessment.

12.2.2. Other Adverse Effects

Any sudden onset of new risk factors or worsening of previously identified risk factors should be evaluated before the next ECT treatment (see Chapter 5). In this regard, patient complaints concerning ECT should be considered carefully.

CHAPTER 13

Treatment Following Completion of the Index Electroconvulsive Therapy Course

13.1. Lack of Response to an Index ECT Course

Most patients respond acutely to an index ECT course (see Chapter 2). However, the management of those who do not is complex (Sackeim et al. 1990b; Shapira et al. 1988; Zimmerman et al. 1990) and often frustrating for patients and clinicians. Although precise prediction is not possible, the likelihood of such an outcome is increased in some patient populations, such as those who are resistant to medication prior to ECT.

It should not be concluded that patients are ECT nonresponders unless reasonable attempts have been made to potentiate the ECT response. This may involve 1) switching to bilateral electrode placement and/or increasing stimulus intensity; 2) removing or diminishing the dose of medications with anticonvulsant properties (including barbiturate anesthetic agents and propofol) in patients with very high seizure thresholds; and 3) providing at least 10 treatments (unless the patient is intolerant or refuses; see Chapter 11). Continuing with additional high-intensity bilateral ECT has been reported to be successful in some otherwise ECT-resistant patients in a research setting (Sackeim et al. 1990b, 1993). Nonetheless, the risks of such an extended series should be weighed against those of a persisting episode.

Some practitioners choose to augment ECT with psychotropic agents, such as an antidepressant agent in patients with depression or an antipsychotic or mood stabilizing medication in patients with psychotic or manic symptoms. However, with the exception of patients with schizophrenia (see Chapter 7), the extent to which this strategy is helpful in the management of ECT nonresponders is unproven. Still, some recent findings suggest that antidepressant medication might potentiate the effects of ECT (Lauritzen et al. 1996; Nelson and Benjamin 1989), and the relative safety of combining many such agents with ECT (see Chapter 7) make the use of this strategy attractive to some practitioners.

Once it has been determined that the patient has not benefited from ECT, the patient should be reassessed with respect to primary diagnosis as well as the presence of comorbidity (Sackeim et al. 1990b). In ECT nonresponders, the choice of treatment is uncertain. Although no data exist to guide such practice, most practitioners attempt further medication trials, generally with a combination of agents from different classes, such as antidepressant plus mood stabilizer or two different types of antidepressants. The possibility has been posed that an ineffective ECT course may increase the medication responsivity of resistant patients. However, this has not been substantiated (Shapira et al. 1988).

13.2. Continuation Therapy

13.2.1. General Considerations

Continuation treatment has become the rule in contemporary psychiatric practice (American Psychiatric Association 1993, 1994b, 1997) and is traditionally defined as the provision of somatic treatment over the 6-month period after the onset of remission in an index episode of mental illness. Treatment past that time is defined as maintenance treatment (American Psychiatric Association 1990; Fava and Kaji 1994; National Institute of Mental Health Consensus Development Panel 1985; Prien and Kupfer 1986).

Because individuals referred for ECT are particularly likely to be resistant to medication and to display psychotic ideation during the index episode of illness, the risk of relapse after ECT is very high, particularly during the first few months (Aronson et al. 1987; Bourgon and Kellner 2000; Grunhaus et al. 1995; Sackeim et al. 1990a, 1990b, 1993; Spiker et al. 1985; Stoudemire et al. 1994). For this reason, the need for aggressive continuation therapy after completion of an index ECT course is compelling and it should be instituted as soon as possible, if not during the ECT course itself (see Section 7.4). Uncommon exceptions to this practice include patients who are intolerant to such treatment and possibly those with a history of extremely long periods of remission (although compelling evidence is lacking for the latter). Continuation therapy may consist of pharmacotherapy (see Section 13.2.2) and/or ECT (see Section 13.2.3). In addition, there is a role for adjunctive continuation psychotherapy in some patients (see Section 13.2.4). For purposes of clarity, the topic of maintenance treatment is dealt with separately (see Section 13.3).

13.2.2. Continuation Pharmacotherapy

A course of ECT is usually completed over a 2- to 4-week period. Based on earlier studies (Imlah et al. 1965; Kay et al. 1970; Seager and Bird 1962) and on clinical experience, traditional practice has suggested that continuation pharmacotherapy should vary with the patient's clinical diagnosis. For example, patients with unipolar depression generally receive continuation therapy with antidepressant agents (and possibly antipsychotic agents in the presence of psychotic symptoms), patients with bipolar depression receive antidepressant and/or mood stabilizer medications, patients with mania receive mood stabilizer and possibly antipsychotic agents, and patients with schizophrenia receive antipsychotic medications (Sackeim 1994).

However, some recent evidence suggests that a combination of antidepressant and mood stabilizer pharmacotherapy might improve the effectiveness of continuation therapy for patients with unipolar depression (Sackeim 1994). Also, for patients with bipolar depression, it may be beneficial to discontinue antidepressant medications during the continuation phase of treatment (Sachs 1996). For patients with major depressive episodes, medication dosages during continuation therapy are maintained at the clinically effective dose range for acute treatment, with adjustment up or down depending on response (American Psychiatric Association 1993). For patients with bipolar disorder or schizophrenia, a somewhat less aggressive approach is used (American Psychiatric Association 1994b, 1997). Still, the role of continuation therapy with psychotropic drugs after a course of ECT continues to undergo assessment (Sackeim 1994). In particular, disappointingly high relapse rates, especially in patients with psychotic depression and in those who are resistant to medication during the index episode (Flint and Rifat 1998; Meyers 1992; Sackeim et al. 1990a; Shapira et al. 1995), compel re-evaluation of present practice and suggest consideration of novel medication strategies or continuation ECT.

13.2.3. Continuation ECT

Although psychotropic continuation therapy is the prevailing practice, few studies document the efficacy of such treatment after a course of ECT. Even in patients complying with such regimens, some recent studies report high relapse rates (Aronson et al. 1987; Sackeim et al. 1990a, 1993; Spiker et al. 1985; Stoudemire et al. 1994). These high relapse rates have led some practitioners to recommend continuation ECT for selected individuals (Decina et al. 1987; Jaffe et al. 1990c; Kramer 1987b; Mc-Call et al. 1992b). Recent reviews have tended to report surprisingly low relapse rates among patients receiving such treatment (Abrams 1997a; Escande et al. 1992; Fava and Kaji 1994; Fox 1996; Jarvis et al. 1992; Monroe 1991; Rabheru and Persad 1997; Sackeim 1994; Stephens et al. 1993). Continuation ECT has also been described as a viable option in contemporary guidelines for long-term management of patients with major depression (American Psychiatric Association 1993), bipolar disorder (American Psychiatric Association 1994b), and schizophrenia (American Psychiatric Association 1997).

Recent data on continuation ECT have consisted primarily of retrospective series in patients with major depression (Beale et al. 1996; Clarke et al. 1989; Decina et al. 1987; Dubin et al. 1992; Ezion et al. 1990; Grunhaus et al. 1990; Kramer 1990, 1999; Lôo et al. 1990; Matzen et al. 1988; Petrides et al. 1994; Puri et al. 1992; Schwartz et al. 1995; Thienhaus et al. 1990; Thornton et al. 1990; Vanelle et al. 1994), mania (Abrams 1990; Godemann and Hellweg 1997; Husain et al. 1993; Jaffe et al. 1991; Kellner et al. 1990; Vanelle et al. 1994), schizophrenia (Chanpattana 1998; Chanpattana et al. 1999b; Höflich et al. 1995; Lohr et al. 1994; Sajatovik and Meltzer 1993; Üçok and Üçok 1996), and Parkinson's disease (Aarsland et al. 1997; Friedman and Gordon 1992; Höflich et al. 1995; Jeanneau 1993; Wengel et al. 1998; Zervas and Fink 1991). Although some of these investigations have included comparison groups not receiving continuation ECT or have compared use of mental health resources before and after implementation of continuation ECT, controlled studies involving random assignment are not yet available. Still, in spite of the cost per treatment, evidence suggesting that continuation ECT is cost effective is particularly promising (Bonds et al. 1998; Schwarz et al. 1995; Steffens et al. 1995; Vanelle et al. 1994). In addition, a prospective multisite study funded by the National Institute of Mental Health comparing a continuation ECT and continuation pharmacotherapy combination with the combination of nortriptyline and lithium is under way (Kellner, personal communication, 1999).

13.2.3.1. General

After a successful course of ECT, continuation ECT appears to be a viable form of continuation management of patients. Thus, facilities should offer continuation ECT as a treatment option.

Because continuation ECT is typically administered to patients who are in clinical remission, and because relatively long intertreatment intervals are used, it is typically administered on an ambulatory basis (see Section 11.1). The specific timing of continuation ECT treatments has been the subject of considerable discussion (Abrams 1997a; Fink et al. 1996; Kramer 1987b; Longcope and Fink 1990; Monroe 1991; Petrides 1998; Petrides et al. 1994; Rabheru and Persad 1997; Sackeim 1994; Scott et al. 1991), but evidence supporting any set regimen is lacking. In many cases, treatments are started on a weekly basis, with the interval between treatments gradually extended to a month, depending on the clinical response. Such a plan is designed to counteract the high likelihood of early relapse noted previously. In general, the greater the likelihood of early relapse, the more intensive the regimen should be. The use of psychotropic agents during a series of continuation ECT remains an unresolved issue (Fink et al. 1996; Jarvis et al. 1992; Petrides 1998; Thornton et al. 1990). Because many such patients have treatment-resistant illness, some practitioners supplement continuation ECT with medication, particularly in those individuals who have limited benefit from continuation ECT alone. In addition, some practitioners believe that, in ECT-responsive patients undergoing continuation pharmacotherapy alone, symptoms of impending relapse may represent an indication for a short series of ECT treatments for therapeutic as well as prophylactic purposes (Grunhaus et al. 1990). However, controlled studies are not yet available to substantiate this practice.

13.2.3.2. Indications for Continuation ECT

Patients referred for continuation ECT should meet the following indications: 1) a history of illness that is responsive to ECT, 2) either a patient preference for continuation ECT or resistance or intolerance to pharmacotherapy alone, and 3) the ability and willingness of the patient (or surrogate consentor) to receive continuation ECT, provide informed consent, and comply with the overall treatment plan, including any necessary behavioral restrictions.

13.2.3.3. Pre-ECT Evaluation for Continuation ECT

Before each continuation ECT treatment, the attending physician should 1) assess clinical status and current medications, 2) determine whether the treatment is indicated, and 3) decide the timing of the next treatment. A monthly assessment may be used if continuation treatments are occurring at least twice monthly and the patient has been clinically stable for at least 1 month. In any case, the overall treatment plan, including the role of ECT, should be updated at least every 6 months. Informed consent should also be renewed no less frequently than every 6 months (see Chapter 8). To provide an ongoing assessment of risk factors, an interval medical history focusing on specific systems at risk with ECT and vital signs should be done before each treatment, with further assessment as clinically indicated. In many settings, this brief evaluation is accomplished by the ECT psychiatrist or anesthesia provider on the day of the treatment. In patients receiving continuation ECT, the frequency of routine repeated anesthesia preoperative evaluations and laboratory testing varies (see Chapter 6). In the absence of applicable research data, intervals of 6 months for the former and 1 year for the latter are suggested. Although cognitive effects appear to be less severe with continuation ECT than with more frequent treatments administered during an ECT course (Barnes et al. 1997; Ezion et al. 1990; Grunhaus et al. 1990; Thienhaus et al. 1990; Thornton et al. 1990), cognitive function should be monitored at least every three treatments. As discussed in Chapter 12, this may consist of simple bedside assessment of memory function.

13.2.4. Continuation Psychotherapy

For some patients, individual, group, or family psychotherapy after ECT may be useful in helping to resolve residual symptoms, prevent relapse, facilitate better ways to cope with stressors, assist the patient in reorganizing his or her social and vocational activities, and encourage a return to normal life. However, no specific data are available indicating which patients might benefit from such intervention.

13.3. Maintenance Therapy

13.3.1. General Considerations

Maintenance therapy is defined as the prophylactic use of psychotropics or ECT longer than 6 months past the end of the index episode.

Conceptually, maintenance therapy aims to protect against recurrence, and thus is distinct from continuation therapy, which aims to prevent relapse. Depending on risk/benefit considerations, the type of maintenance treatment and the type of continuation treatment may differ.

Maintenance treatment is most strongly indicated when the patient has a strong history of recurrent illness or when present or past attempts to stop or taper continuation therapy have been associated with return of symptoms (Lôo et al. 1990; Stiebel 1995; Thienhaus et al. 1990; Thornton et al. 1990; Vanelle et al. 1994). However, after ECT, concern over recurrence of illness is so great (Sackeim 1994) that maintenance therapy should be initiated in virtually all patients receiving continuation therapy.

At present, no applicable data indicate how long maintenance therapy should be sustained after ECT. After an index episode of major depression responds to antidepressant pharmacotherapy (where some data exist), maintenance therapy can be expected to decrease recurrence rates out to at least 5 years after the index episode (Kupfer et al. 1992). Assuming that the treatment is well tolerated, the highly recurrent illness of many patients referred for ECT coupled with the severity of recurrent episodes makes a prolonged period of maintenance therapy attractive. In deciding when to begin to taper a patient off maintenance treatment, the precise timing should be guided by factors such as past history of treatment tapering; number, frequency, and intensity of prior episodes; family history; the ability of the patient to tolerate the maintenance treatment; patient preference; and the ability of the patient to comply with the treatment plan (including treatment accessibility, support of significant others, and patient reliability and cognitive functioning). Rapid discontinuation of maintenance treatment should be avoided because of potential risk of triggering a recurrence or, with some medications, a pharmacologically induced withdrawal or discontinuation syndrome.

13.3.2. Maintenance ECT

The specific criteria for maintenance ECT, as opposed to maintenance psychotropic therapy, are the same as those described above for continuation ECT. The frequency of maintenance ECT treatments should be kept to the minimum compatible with sustained remission. Reevaluation of the need for extension in the treatment series and repeated application of informed consent procedures should be performed at the intervals listed above for continuation ECT. Despite the absence of controlled studies of the efficacy or safety of long-term maintenance ECT, no evidence indicates that a lifetime "maximum" number of treatments is applicable (Barnes et al. 1997; Lippman et al. 1985).

RECOMMENDATIONS

13.1. Lack of Response to an Index ECT Course

The following strategies should be considered in patients who have not responded to an index ECT course:

- Ensure that ECT has been optimized with respect to electrode placement and stimulus intensity, that any concurrent medications with anticonvulsant properties have been decreased or discontinued, and that at least 10 treatments have been administered.
- Consider further ECT with pharmacologic augmentation (e.g., antidepressant medication in patients with major depression).
- Consider a switch to novel medication strategies.

13.2. Continuation Treatment

13.2.1. General Considerations

a. Continuation therapy, typically consisting of psychotropic medication or ECT, is indicated for virtually all patients. If continuation therapy is not recommended, the rationale behind this decision should be documented.
b. Continuation therapy should begin as soon as possible after termination of the ECT course, except when adverse ECT effects such as delirium necessitate a delay.
c. Unless contravened by adverse effects, continuation therapy should be maintained for at least 6 months and followed by longer-term maintenance therapy (see Section 13.3).

13.2.2. Continuation Pharmacotherapy

a. The choice of agent should be determined by the type of underlying illness, a consideration of adverse effects, and response history.
b. When clinically feasible, practitioners should consider a class of pharmacologic agents for which the patient did not manifest resis-

tance during the treatment of the acute episode.

13.2.3. Continuation ECT

13.2.3.1. General

a. Continuation ECT should be available in programs administering ECT.
b. Continuation ECT may be given on either an inpatient or an outpatient basis. In the latter case, the recommendations presented in Section 11.1 apply.
c. The timing of treatments should be individualized for each patient and should be adjusted as necessary, giving consideration to both beneficial and adverse effects.

13.2.3.2. Indications for Continuation ECT

Continuation of ECT is indicated if the patient has a history of illness that has been responsive to ECT, and one of the following has occurred:

• Pharmacotherapy alone has not been effective in treating index episodes or in preventing relapse or recurrence.
• Pharmacotherapy cannot be safely administered.
• The patient prefers treatment with ECT, and the patient or surrogate consentor agrees to receive continuation ECT. The patient must be capable, with the assistance of others, of complying with the treatment plan.

13.2.3.3. Pre-ECT Evaluation for Continuation ECT

Each facility using continuation ECT should delineate procedures for the pre-ECT evaluation. With both continuation and maintenance ECT (see Section 13.2.3 and 13.3.2), the following recommendations are suggested for use, with the understanding that additions to or increased frequency of evaluative procedures should be included whenever clinically indicated.

a. The following should be performed prior to each treatment:

• Interval psychiatric evaluation (may be done monthly if treatments are at an interval of 2 weeks or less *and* the patient has been clinically stable for at least 1 month)
• Interval medical history and vital signs (this examination may be

done by the ECT psychiatrist or anesthesia provider at the time of the treatment session)

b. The overall clinical treatment plan should be updated at least every 6 months.
c. Cognitive function should be assessed (see Section 12.2.1) at least every three treatments.
d. Repeated consent for ECT should be obtained at least every 6 months (see Chapter 8).
e. The frequency of routine repeated anesthesia preoperative evaluations and laboratory testing varies (see Chapter 6) in patients receiving continuation/maintenance ECT; in the absence of applicable research data, it is suggested that these evaluations be repeated at intervals of 6 months for the former and 1 year for the latter.

13.2.4. Continuation Psychotherapy

After an index ECT course, psychotherapy, whether on an individual, group, or family basis, represents a useful component of the clinical management plan for some patients.

13.3. Maintenance Therapy

13.3.1. General Considerations

a. Maintenance therapy, which is treatment continuing longer than 6 months after completion of the most recent ECT course, is indicated in most patients.
b. Depending on risk/benefit considerations, the type of maintenance treatment may differ from that used to provide continuation treatment.
c. The duration of maintenance therapy should be determined on the basis of risk/benefit considerations, taking into account factors such as past history involving episodes of illness as well as continuation/maintenance treatment, tolerance of maintenance treatment, patient preference, and ability of the patient to comply with the treatment plan.

13.3.2. Maintenance ECT

a. Maintenance ECT is generally indicated in patients receiving continuation ECT (Section 13.2.3.2).

b. The pre-ECT evaluation of patients receiving maintenance ECT should follow that described for continuation ECT (see Section 13.2.3.3.).

c. Maintenance ECT treatments should be administered at the minimum frequency compatible with sustained remission.

d. The continued need for maintenance ECT should be reassessed at least every 6 months. This assessment should include consideration of both beneficial and adverse effects.

CHAPTER 14

Documentation

14.1. Facility Responsibilities

The patient's medical record is a legal document that provides evidence of what did or did not take place during his or her contact with the health care facility. Information contained in the medical record also helps the clinical management team provide safe, effective, and efficient care. In addition, such information facilitates future evaluation and treatment decisions. Finally, documentation assists with quality improvement and utilization review activities. Because the medical record represents the primary source of clinical information, the facility's medical director should maintain overall responsibility for ensuring the adequacy of documentation.

Although adequate documentation is essential to modern medical practice, time spent writing in the medical record is no substitute for time spent providing direct patient care. For this reason, the level of documentation should facilitate rather than hamper quality of care. In this regard, notes in the clinical record should be concise and to the point, with detail limited to essential material.

14.2. Prior to an Index ECT Course

An index course of ECT should not begin until a pre-ECT evaluation has taken place, with relevant risks and benefits assessed, informed consent obtained, and a treatment plan adopted. Documentation of this process helps ensure that it has been completed appropriately and that potential problems have been considered. Although the attending physician usually records such information, it is the responsibility of the ECT psychiatrist to make sure that necessary documentation is in order prior to treatment with ECT. A checklist or summary format can be helpful.

More specifically, it is important to address the rationale for the ECT referral and to delineate relevant risk/benefit considerations. Because determination of treatment endpoint will be influenced by baseline symptoms, major target symptoms and their severity should be noted before treatment begins. Similarly, the ongoing assessment of adverse effects requires a baseline determination of orientation and memory function (see Section 12.2.1).

Before ECT, in addition to a signed formal consent document, the clinical record should contain a summary of major consent-related discussions (see Chapter 8). Such a summary should either note that the patient has provided consent or clarify the consent procedure used when a patient referred for ECT lacks capacity. When applicable, the summary should also note any factors having a major impact on risk/benefit considerations discussed with the individual providing consent.

14.3. Prior to a Continuation Series of ECT

For continuation/maintenance ECT, both the rationale for initiating such treatment and the relevant aspects of the informed consent process (see Chapter 8) should be documented.

The clinical record should demonstrate the treatment team's awareness of the presence or absence of both therapeutic change and adverse effects.

14.4. During an Index ECT Course or Continuation/ Maintenance Series of ECT

14.4.1. Between ECT Treatment Sessions

For index ECT treatments, therapeutic outcome should be documented at least every two treatments (See Section 12.1), whereas the presence or absence of cognitive effects should be documented at least weekly. For continuation/maintenance ECT, such notes can occur at less frequent intervals (see Section 13.2.3.3). When an index ECT course is extended past the number noted in the initial informed consent (see Section 8.4.2 and 11.11), or a series of continuation/maintenance treatments is extended for an additional 6-month period (see Section 13.2.3.3 and 13.3.2), the rationale should be noted in the clinical record.

14.4.2. At the Time of Each ECT Treatment Session

It is good clinical practice to document the essential parameters of the treatment procedure at the time of each ECT treatment, and a dedicated form for this purpose can be helpful. Such information helps the treatment team administer subsequent treatments safely and effectively, assists future caregivers in the determining treatment parameters, and is useful for ongoing quality improvement. In many facilities, members of the ECT treatment team rotate on a weekly or even daily basis, rendering such data particularly important.

Documentation of specific treatment information should include the ECT device used, the electrical parameters for each stimulation, the stimulus electrode placement, the seizure duration (or other indices of seizure adequacy), all medications given in the treatment and recovery room (including dosage), and the patient's vital signs (e.g., blood pressure and pulse). As with any procedure requiring general anesthesia, the anesthesia provider should provide a brief note describing the patient's condition during the perioperative period. Similarly, recovery area staff should document vital signs and orientation while the patient is under their care. Any substantial adverse effects occurring in the treatment or recovery areas, including any actions taken and recommendations for future management, should also be summarized in the clinical record.

In addition to information entered into the clinical record, it is useful to also keep a copy of such information within the treatment area. This is helpful not only in the event that data in the clinical record are lost but also because it provides a means to reconstruct how the ECT was administered months or even years later if the patient returns with recurrent illness. Material of this type also facilitates quality improvement and utilization review activities.

14.5. Following Completion of an Index ECT Course or a Continuation/Maintenance ECT Series

Just as it is important to document the rationale for beginning ECT, it is also helpful to provide a basis for the decision to end the course or series of treatments. Typical reasons for stopping an index course of ECT include achievement of maximal clinical benefit, failure to respond therapeutically to an adequate trial, adverse effects (type and severity should be noted), and patient refusal. A plan for continuation treatment should be documented because the risk of relapse is high after an index ECT course or, for that matter, after acute treatment with psychopharmacologic agents (see Chapter 13). If adverse effects are present at the time of completion of the ECT course these should be briefly noted, along with the follow-up plan. For continuation/maintenance ECT, documentation of the rationale for terminating the series should be provided as well as the plan for future treatment and monitoring of side effects, if applicable.

RECOMMENDATIONS

14.1. Facility Responsibilities

It is the responsibility of the facility's medical director (or medical staff, if no such individual is defined) to ensure adequate documentation regarding ECT.

14.2. Prior to an Index ECT Course

The ECT psychiatrist should confirm that the following documentation is included in the patient's clinical record (a checklist or summary format is encouraged):

- Reasons for ECT referral, including an assessment of anticipated benefits and risks
- Mental status, including baseline information pertinent to later determinations of therapeutic outcome, orientation, and memory function
- Signed consent document
- Statement covering other elements of the informed consent process as described in Chapter 8
- Pertinent laboratory results
- Consultation reports as indicated (see Chapters 4, 6, and 8)
- Discussion of any substantial alterations planned in the ECT procedure

14.3. Prior to a Continuation Series of ECT

Before beginning a continuation series of ECT, the ECT psychiatrist should confirm that the patient's clinical record includes documentation of the following material:

- Rationale for continuation ECT
- Signed consent document
- Statement covering other elements of the informed consent process as described in Chapter 8

14.4. During an Index ECT Course or Continuation/ Maintenance Series of ECT

14.4.1. Between ECT Treatment Sessions

a. Notes by the attending physician or designee should be entered in the patient's clinical record at least every two treatments during an index ECT course and should contain information about the presence or lack of a therapeutic response and any other substantive change (see Section 12.1). Notes describing the presence or absence of adverse cognitive effects should be entered into the record at least weekly (see Section 12.2.1).
b. Documented justification should be provided before exceeding a specified maximum number of treatments (set by each facility) in an index ECT course (see Sections 8.4 and 11.11.2).
c. With continuation or maintenance ECT, documentation of the presence or absence of beneficial response should occur either prior to each treatment or at least monthly if the patient is stable and treatments occur more than twice per month (see Section 13.2.3.3). The presence or absence of adverse cognitive effects should be noted at least every three treatments.
d. When a continuation or maintenance ECT series is extended by an initial or subsequent 6-month period, the rationale should be documented (see Section 13.2.3.3 and 13.3.2).

14.4.2. At the Time of Each ECT Treatment Session

a. For each treatment session, at least the following information should be documented in the patient's clinical record:

- Baseline vital signs
- Medication, including dosage, given before entering the treatment room
- Note from the anesthetist describing the patient's condition while in treatment/recovery area
- Where applicable, a note from the ECT psychiatrist or anesthetist covering any major alterations in risk factors or presence of adverse effects or complications, including actions taken and recommendations made

- Medication, including dosage, given in treatment and recovery areas
- Stimulus electrode placement
- Stimulus parameter settings for each stimulus
- Seizure duration and/or other indices of seizure adequacy (noting whether motor or electroencephalographic)
- Vital signs taken in treatment room and recovery area
- Note from the recovery nurse or the anesthesia provider documenting occurrence and management of any complications during recovery and patient's condition on leaving the recovery area

b. It is useful to keep a copy of treatment information in the treatment area, especially data regarding electrode placement, stimulus parameters, and seizure duration.

14.5. Following Completion of an Index ECT Course or a Continuation/Maintenance ECT Series

The attending physician or designee should enter the following information into the clinical record:

- Summary of overall therapeutic outcome and adverse effects experienced as a result of ECT course or series and rationale for specific choice of endpoint
- Plan for post-ECT clinical management and any plans for follow-up of adverse effects

CHAPTER 15

Education and Training in Electroconvulsive Therapy

15.1. General Considerations

Since the 1930s, ECT has evolved into a highly technical and complex treatment (Abrams 1997a; American Psychiatric Association 1990; Beyer et al. 1998; Fink 1986, 1987; Kellner 1991; Kellner et al. 1997; Royal College of Psychiatrists 1995). Major technical advances directed toward maximizing its efficacy and minimizing its risks have occurred in instrumentation, stimulus dosing, stimulus electrode placement, pharmacologic modification of induced seizures, and physiologic monitoring. These technical improvements necessitate greater practitioner training (Bolwig 1987; Hermann et al. 1998; Scott 1995). Thus, the traditional training paradigm of observation followed by trial (and error) is inappropriate in the present practice of ECT.

ECT training in residency programs in the United States ranges from excellent to totally absent. In many cases, the training is no more than minimal. Similar reports have come from other countries (Duffet and Lelliot 1998b; Goldbloom and Kussin 1991; Halliday and Johnson 1995; Henderson 1993). This situation must be corrected to ensure that future generations of practitioners are able to deliver ECT in a safe and effective fashion (Fink 1986, 1987; Jaffe et al. 1990a; Peterson 1988; Raskin 1986). Recent surveys of ECT practice outside the United States have emphasized the dangers of inadequate training (Anonymous 1981; Duffet and Lelliot 1998a, 1998b; Pippard 1992; Pippard and Ellam 1981). Conversely, other surveys of residents before and after training in ECT have supported the value of formal ECT education (Benbow 1986; Szuba et al. 1992). Department chairs, residency training directors, and departmental faculty should recognize that all psychiatric residents should meet certain minimal ECT training requirements (see below) for clinical competency in psychiatry. Those responsible for providing privileging in ECT (see Chapter 16) should set a high priority on assessing applicants' training background.

The practice of ECT is multidisciplinary and involves professionals trained in psychiatry, anesthesiology, and nursing. In addition, other physicians are often asked to consult on patients being evaluated for ECT or to care for patients who are either receiving or have recently received this treatment. In this regard, recent reports have indicated the need for increased exposure to ECT in anesthesiology (Haddad and Benbow 1993), nursing (Creed et al. 1995; Duffy and Conradt 1989; Froimson et al. 1995; Gass 1998; Jacobsma 1991), and social work (Katz 1992) training programs. As the leader of the ECT treatment team, the ECT psychiatrist must have comprehensive knowledge of ECT-related topics. Thus, within psychiatric residency programs, the training curriculum in ECT must require a substantial time commitment. Although anesthetic considerations for ECT are considerably more narrow in their focus and therefore less time consuming to cover, anesthesiology and nurse anesthetist training programs should not ignore this material. Finally, Continuing Medical Education (CME) programs in ECT are needed to ensure continued competence of practitioners. For those whose prior training in ECT was insufficient, CME programs may provide a means for attaining the level of expertise needed for clinical privileging in ECT.

15.2. Medical School

Brief but comprehensive didactic coverage of ECT should be included as part of psychiatric training in medical school (Andrade and Rao 1996; Benbow 1990; Szuba et al. 1992). Medical students should also be encouraged to observe ECT practice either directly or on videotape. On a national level, the National Board of Medical Examiners should incorporate a reasonable coverage of ECT-related topics into their examinations.

15.3. Psychiatry Residency Programs

15.3.1. General Issues

To accomplish ECT training goals for psychiatric residency programs, it is important that department chairs and residency training directors set a priority on developing adequate curricula for education and training in ECT (including designating qualified faculty). These individuals should also monitor the program's adequacy on an ongoing basis and correct any identified deficiencies. It is understood that not all departments have faculty with sufficient qualifications to teach courses on ECT. In such cases, arrangements should be made to bring in outside practitioners for this purpose.

15.3.2. Didactic Material to Be Covered

The type and amount of didactic instruction on ECT provided in psychiatry residency training programs varies considerably. Whereas some programs provide formal lecture or seminar presentations, others incorporate ECT-related material into curricula for other aspects of psychiatry, such as psychopharmacology or affective disorders. Still other programs appear to make the ill-founded assumption that practical experience in ECT will somehow provide the breadth of information that might be covered in a didactic format.

The didactic curriculum required for residents in a program should cover all major aspects of the ECT procedure, including mechanisms of action, selection of patients across the age spectrum, risks and adverse effects, pre-ECT evaluation, informed consent, methods of administration, evaluation of therapeutic outcome, management of patients after completion of an ECT course (including the potential roles of continuation/maintenance pharmacotherapy and ECT), and malpractice considerations. In areas marked by controversy, alternative viewpoints should be presented. The amount of time necessary to cover the above material will vary, but a minimum of 4 hours is necessary to give a good overview. Programs for training and preparing the psychiatrist to serve as an anesthesia provider with ECT must provide adequate didactic and practical training in anesthetic medications, airway management (including intubation), use of relevant monitoring equipment, and acute care of medical emergencies that might occur at the time of ECT or shortly after its administration.

The ECT didactic curriculum should also include sufficient opportunities for interchange between faculty and trainees so that questions can be answered and views clarified. Programs that are unable to provide at least 4 hours of ECT didactics should take explicit steps to ensure that remaining topics are covered within the context of practical experience in ECT (see below). Residents with a particular interest in

ECT should be encouraged to pursue advanced electives in ECT as well as membership at the training level in professional organizations such as the Association for Convulsive Therapy.

15.3.3. Practical Training

15.3.3.1. General Aspects

As noted earlier, the practice of ECT is a highly technical and sophisticated medical procedure. Although important, didactic teaching is clearly insufficient to provide the expertise necessary to administer ECT and must be supplemented by an intensive, well-supervised practical training experience. Efforts should be made to ensure the presence of direct supervision by the most highly qualified individuals available, even if such personnel must be secured from outside the department. Alternatively, the department may send residents for practical training in other educational institutions that provide such opportunities. Although videotaped material is often a useful supplement to didactic instruction (Benbow 1986; Duffet and Lelliot 1998b; Geaney 1993), it should not be relied on exclusively. In addition to videotapes, the use of teaching materials such as assigned readings can further the educational impact of practical training in ECT and should be encouraged.

15.3.3.2. Specific Recommendations

The amount of practical experience in ECT necessary to allow development of adequate skills will vary from resident to resident as well as from program to program. At a minimum, a resident should participate in the administration of at least 10 ECT treatments directly supervised by a psychiatrist privileged in ECT. To provide exposure to differing case material, at least three separate cases should be included in the series. These minimal requirements represent a trade-off between what is optimally desirable and what is feasible in many training programs.

A 1976 survey involving the American Association of Directors of Psychiatric Residency Programs (undertaken by the American Psychiatric Association Task Force on ECT [1978]) revealed that, on average, residents participated in approximately twice this number of treatments (i.e., 21.2). Similarly higher requirements were reported in Denmark (Bolwig 1987). However, a 1988 survey of the directors of 23 psychiatry residency training programs in the United States revealed that most respondents believe that residents should administer ECT to a minimum of two to five patients during their training (Yager et al. 1988). To an extent, these latter views may well be based on an appreciation of the variable number of patients receiving ECT in teaching institutions. For that matter, approximately 20% of respondents in a 1986 survey of medical schools indicated that ECT was not used at all in their primary teaching hospitals (Raskin 1986).

In addition to the actual administration of ECT, residents should gain experience in the clinical management of patients undergoing ECT. This experience should include the pre-ECT evaluation; informed consent; choice of type, number, and frequency of ECT treatments; and post-ECT management. At a minimum, each resident should actively participate in the care of at least three patients being treated with ECT. Practical experience in evaluation and case management of ECT patients is particularly important, because the number of psychiatrists providing such care is much larger than the number who directly administer ECT. A 1988 survey of psychiatric practitioners, department chairs, and training directors reiterated this view (Langsley and Yager 1988).

These recommendations for didactic and practical training in ECT constitute minimal requirements, and residency programs are encouraged to exceed these levels. Clinical case conferences, ECT rounds, and elective opportunities for advanced training in ECT represent particularly useful ways of improving the overall learning experience. Still, it is understood that some residency training programs may not have sufficient resources to meet these requirements, particularly in those settings in which the practice of ECT is minimal or absent. In such cases, attempts should be made to cover as much of the above curriculum as possible, making use of assigned readings, videotaped material, and outside speakers. Residents in such programs should explicitly be told that supplementation of their training experience will be required before they administer ECT on an unsupervised basis.

15.3.4. Advanced Training in ECT

Residency programs should offer elective training opportunities for those residents who wish to obtain a more intensive learning experience in ECT. Such electives should include both didactic and practical components and should be directed toward providing the knowledge base and experience necessary for eventual privileging in ECT (see Chapter 16).

15.3.5. Evaluation of Resident Performance

To ensure that ECT training in psychiatry residency programs is adequate, the specific educational and training experiences offered by the program should be documented. In addition, programs should evaluate residents' performance in the ECT-related components of the curriculum. Records of such evaluations should be kept for the purpose of ongoing program evaluation and for use as credentials in the ECT privileging process (see Chapter 16). Taking appropriate measures to ensure confidentiality, psychiatry residents should be encouraged to keep records of both the number of ECT treatments in which they participated and the number of patients who received ECT while under their care. Tracking such information is useful in helping to satisfy ECT privileging requirements and is in line with training policies already implemented for some medical and surgical procedures.

15.3.6. Record of Education and Training in ECT

Educational and training experiences in ECT as well as relevant performance evaluations of individual residents and faculty should be documented by the residency training committee on an ongoing basis. These records should include material needed to establish compliance with the practical training recommendations of Section 15.3.3.2.

15.4. Geriatric Psychiatry Training Programs

Because of the very strong role of ECT in the treatment of the elderly (see Section 4.2), formal training in ECT should be part of geriatric psychiatry training programs. Minimum didactic requirements should include all topics noted above for psychiatry residents as well as specific coverage of the use of ECT in the elderly (see Section 4.2). Likewise, practical training in ECT should include clinical exposure to the use of ECT with elderly patients. Programs are encouraged to devote a sufficient portion of the geriatric psychiatry training experience to ensure that graduates are clinically competent in this area.

15.5. Anesthesiology Residency Programs

Anesthesiology residency programs should incorporate specific training in ECT into their curricula. It should not be assumed that general education and training in anesthesia will suffice (Haddad and Benbow 1993). It is particularly important that differences between ECT anesthesia practices and standard anesthesia practices be covered in depth. The physiologic effects associated with seizure induction, for example, represent a routine part of the ECT procedure and not a cause for alarm or emergency corrective action. In addition, because of concerns about anticonvulsant effects, the dosages of anesthetic agents used for ECT are generally lower than those used with other procedures. Finally, because ECT treatments are delivered as a series, practitioners should not approach each successive treatment as a totally new anesthetic situation.

Training in ECT for anesthesiology residents should be provided by qualified individuals and should include faculty involved in the ECT training of psychiatric residents. As with psychiatry residents, training in ECT for anesthesiology residents should include both didactic and practical components. In terms of the didactic exposure, a concise but comprehensive perspective should be provided, including a discussion of ECT's role in contemporary psychiatric practice. Areas of specific anesthetic interest should be covered in depth, including pre-ECT evaluation, use of medications during the ECT procedure, pertinent drug interactions, provision of oxygenation (including the effects of hyperventilation upon the ictal response), use of physiologic monitoring, physiologic and behavioral effects of the postictal state, and electrical safety considerations. Again, areas in which ECT anesthesia differs from standard anesthetic practice should be given particular attention. Major adverse effects that may occur in the treatment and recovery areas should also be enumerated and their management discussed. Just as it is important that psychiatric residents receive adequate supervision in ECT, anesthesiology residents should also be supervised by qualified individuals during their practical training experience.

15.6. Nursing Schools

Because nursing personnel are important members of the ECT treatment team, education in ECT should be provided as part of the nursing school experience (Froimsin et al. 1995; Gass 1998; Poster et al. 1985). In terms of didactic instruction, a general overview of ECT should be provided, supplemented by an in-depth focus on areas in which nursing personnel are likely to play a major role (see Chapter 9). As with all aspects of ECT training, instruction should be provided by qualified individuals involved in actual clinical administration of ECT. Opportunity for observation of ECT administration is useful, either directly or through use of videotaped material. Postgraduate training for psychiatric nursing administrators should include additional instruction and training in ECT. For nurse anesthesia programs, the curricula should incorporate the material described earlier for anesthesiology residents.

15.7. Specialty Board Examinations

As one means of helping to ensure adequate training, specialty board examinations, regardless of professional discipline, can require exposure to education or training in ECT for board eligibility. Precedents for such a requirement have already been considered for other procedures by boards in medical and surgical specialties. At a minimum, specialty boards in psychiatry, anesthesiology, and nursing should incorporate a representative number of questions on ECT into their examinations.

15.8. Continuing Education Programs

As noted earlier, CME opportunities allow practitioners to keep their knowledge and skills up to date and provide a means to help those with educational and training deficiencies gain clinical privileges for ECT (Creed et al. 1995; Duffy and Conradt 1989; Fink 1986, 1987; Gass 1998; Jacobsma 1991; Katz 1992). Participation in such programs is particularly important for psychiatrists but is also useful for anesthesiologists and nurses. Attendance at CME programs can and should be an important factor in maintaining ECT privileges (see Chapter 16).

Although a number of excellent CME programs have been offered, there is clearly room for more, particularly with respect to practical education and training. Professional organizations should take the initiative in encouraging the development and implementation of such programs at annual meetings and elsewhere. Symposia, courses, seminars, and fellowship opportunities in ECT at the local, regional, and national levels should be publicized widely. Annual meetings of the American Psychiatric Association, American Association of Geriatric Psychiatrists, and the Society for Biological Psychiatry routinely include ECT topics, whereas the annual meeting of the Association for Convulsive Therapy (ACT) provides a program focused primarily on ECT.

Several practical courses and visiting fellowships, generally 1 week in duration, are offered at locations around the United States. Contact the American Psychiatric Association (APA) website at www.psych.org (click on "Medical Education" and then on "CME"), call the APA Office of CME at 202-682-6179, or write to the Office of CME at 1400 K Street NW, Washington, DC 20005 for a current list. These opportunities are primarily for psychiatrists, although some are oriented toward nurses. From time to time, other experienced clinicians offer individual preceptorships for various lengths of stay at their facilities.

RECOMMENDATIONS

15.1. General Considerations

A comprehensive educational and training experience is necessary to convey the knowledge and skills for providing ECT safely and effectively.

15.2. Medical School

a. Psychiatric instructional programs for medical students should include didactic exposure to the role of ECT in the treatment of severe mental disorders.
b. Didactic instruction should provide an overview of the history (including social contexts), indications, risks, mechanisms of action, and technique of ECT.
c. Didactic experience should be supplemented by observation of ECT delivery, either directly or through the use of videotapes.
d. The National Board of Medical Examiners should incorporate a representative number of questions concerning ECT into their examinations.

15.3. Psychiatry Residency Programs

15.3.1. General Issues

a. Psychiatric residency programs should provide comprehensive training in ECT to all residents.
b. Ideally, didactic instruction should take place before or during the inpatient residency experience.
c. Department chairs and psychiatric residency training directors and committees should assess the ECT training in their program on an ongoing basis and correct deficiencies in a timely manner.
d. ECT training should be provided by qualified and privileged individuals (see Chapter 16). Departments without such personnel

should use consultants or appropriate community practitioners.

15.3.2. Didactic Material to Be Covered

Formal didactic education should include at least 4 hours of lecture and discussion and should cover the following topics:

- Indications and potential risks
- Patient selection and evaluation
- Consent procedures, including applicable legal ramifications
- Technique of ECT administration, including anesthetic and relaxant agents, oxygenation and airway maintenance, stimulus electrode placement, stimulus parameters and dosing, monitoring (electroencephalogram, motor convulsion, electrocardiogram, blood pressure), management of missed and otherwise inadequate seizures, and the number and frequency of treatments; situations in which major options exist, such as electrode placement, should be discussed
- Instrumentation, including electrical safety considerations
- Management of adverse effects during ECT, including anticipated medical emergencies
- Evaluation of therapeutic outcome
- Evaluation of cognitive side effects
- Clinical management of patients after completion of the ECT course
- Mechanisms of action
- Documentation and risk management

15.3.3. Practical Training

15.3.3.1. General Aspects

a. Staff members who are privileged in ECT administration should supervise psychiatry residents involved in the delivery of ECT and management of patients receiving ECT.
b. The residency training committee, in conjunction with the individual(s) or committee overseeing the practice of ECT within the department, should provide specific guidelines for this experience.
c. The use of videotaped material may be a useful adjunct but should not substitute for in vivo clinical experience.
d. The practical training should also be enriched with materials such as assigned readings.

15.3.3.2. Specific Recommendations

a. Under the direct supervision of a privileged ECT psychiatrist, each resident should actively participate in at least 10 ECT treatments involving at least three separate patients.
b. Each resident should actively participate in the care of at least three patients during the ECT workup, course of treatments, and post-ECT management.
c. Use of clinical case conferences or regular ECT rounds is encouraged.

15.3.4. Advanced Training in ECT

Elective opportunities for advanced training in ECT should be available.

15.3.5. Evaluation of Resident Performance

Evaluation should be the responsibility of the training staff and should be performed using mechanisms approved by the residency training committee.

15.3.6. Record of Education and Training in ECT

a. The residency training committee should maintain a description of specific educational and training experiences related to ECT as well as relevant performance evaluations for both residents and faculty.
b. Records of practical training should include quantitative information needed to assess compliance with recommendations made in Section 15.3.3.2.

15.4. Geriatric Psychiatry Training Programs

a. Formal training in ECT should be part of geriatric psychiatry training programs.
b. Minimum didactic and practical training requirements for ECT training for geriatric psychiatry trainees are the same as those listed above for psychiatry residents (Section 15.3), with the addition of an emphasis on the use of ECT in the elderly (see Section 4.2).
c. Programs are encouraged to substantially exceed these minimal requirements.

15.5. Anesthesiology Residency Programs

a. Anesthesiology residency and nurse anesthesia programs should provide didactic as well as practical training in ECT.
b. This training should be carried out by appropriately qualified personnel.
c. Departments of anesthesiology are also encouraged to involve individuals responsible for the education of psychiatry residents in ECT in the planning and delivery of this training experience.
d. Didactic instruction should include material on:

- The history of ECT
- Indications for and potential risks of ECT
- Pre-ECT evaluation
- Type and dosing of medications commonly used before, during, and immediately after the procedure
- Oxygenation requirements
- Effects of hyperventilation
- Physiologic monitoring
- Electrical safety considerations
- Effects of the postictal state on recovery from anesthesia
- Potential adverse reactions and their management

e. A clinical training experience should be provided involving delivery of anesthesia to patients undergoing ECT under the supervision of individuals who are privileged to deliver anesthesia for ECT.

15.6. Nursing Schools

a. An appreciation of the role of ECT in contemporary psychiatric practice is an important aspect of general psychiatric training in nursing school, particularly given the widespread misinformation in this area.
b. Nursing schools are encouraged to provide formal didactic instruction on ECT, including

- The history of ECT
- Indications for and potential risks of ECT
- Pre-ECT evaluation
- Informed consent procedures

- ECT technique
- Nursing participation in ECT treatment and postanesthetic recovery (including management of emergency situations)
- Other responsibilities of nursing personnel

c. Nursing educators are encouraged to incorporate observation of ECT into their psychiatric nursing training experience, either directly or through the use of videotaped material.

d. Nurse anesthetist training programs should cover the material described above for anesthesiology residents (see Section 15.5).

15.7. Specialty Board Examinations

a. Specialty board examinations for psychiatry, anesthesiology, and nursing should include questions about ECT.

b. Training in ECT, as described above, should be considered among the requirements for specialty board eligibility.

15.8. Continuing Education Programs

a. Continuing education and training opportunities in ECT should be available for practitioners in all pertinent clinical disciplines to maintain their knowledge and practical expertise in ECT and to allow those with insufficient training to develop a more adequate background in this area.

b. Although most such training opportunities may be geared toward the psychiatrist, efforts should also be made to make these opportunities relevant to other disciplines involved in the practice of ECT.

c. Attendance at CME programs should be a factor in ECT privileging (see Chapter 16).

d. Relevant professional organizations and facilities offering ECT are encouraged to develop clinically oriented CME programs on ECT, including provision of CME credit.

e. The American Psychiatric Association should take a major role in CME efforts and include clinically relevant material on ECT in the scientific program of its annual meeting.

f. When feasible, CME programs on ECT should include hands-on experience in addition to didactic material.

g. Available courses and fellowship opportunities should be publicized, and course descriptions should indicate whether the course offers a comprehensive overview or covers a single issue, such as ECT in the medically ill.

h. Professional organizations, relevant academic departments, and facilities providing ECT should be encouraged to sponsor clinically and research oriented lectures and symposia at the local, national, and international levels that focus on ECT-related topics.

i. When educational programs discuss disorders for which ECT may be indicated, specific information relating to ECT treatment should also be provided.

j. Medical and nursing schools as well as hospitals and clinics that provide ECT are encouraged to have a variety of reference materials applicable to ECT available, including videotapes, books, professional journals (especially *Journal of ECT*), copies of relevant published reviews, and clinical and research reports.

CHAPTER 16

Privileging in Electroconvulsive Therapy

Throughout this report, it has been made clear that provision of safe and effective ECT requires the involvement of competent staff (see especially Chapter 9). The determination of clinical competency of practitioners is usually handled by certification or privileging. Although certificate-granting courses in ECT are now available for practitioners, no national accrediting body presently provides assurance of clinical competence in ECT (Fink and Kellner 1998). Accordingly, clinical competency of practitioners is presently ensured through local privileging. In practice, clinical privileges for a given specialty, subspecialty, or procedure are typically granted by a designated committee of the facility's medical staff, which, in turn, reports to the facility director. Specific educational, training, experience, and skill criteria for such privileging are set by the facility's organized medical staff. The materials provided by the applicant in this process constitute his or her credentials. To maintain privileges, staff members must usually reapply at regular intervals. Through such a peer review process, each facility ensures that its clinical services are provided in as safe and effective a fashion as possible. Often, privileging covers the practice of an entire discipline, such as psychiatry or anesthesiology. In recent years, however, because of the growing level of technical sophistication involved in clinical practice as well as a heightened sensitivity to quality of care, there has been a trend toward greater specificity in privileging. Because of the extent of knowledge and skill required to administer ECT, it is clear that general privileging in psychiatry will not suffice and that specific clinical privileges to administer ECT should be required.

Privileges to administer ECT should be granted only to psychiatrists who meet formal, documented criteria set by the organized medical staff. Before an applicant administers ECT on an unsupervised basis, the facility's medical director should establish that these criteria are met. The medical director should use qualified personnel to assist with this determination, including outside consultants as appropriate. The applicant's education, training, experience (including history of past ECT privileging), and demonstrated skill should be the specific determinants in the granting of ECT privileges. The extent of training and experience required should at least be sufficient to satisfy the educational and training recommendations described in Chapter 15. Medical licensure, satisfactory completion of residency training, and board certification or eligibility should be considered in addition to ECT-related material such as evidence of satisfactory completion of relevant residency and continuing medical education (CME) training experiences, holding of malpractice insurance covering the practice of ECT, and letters of recommendation. To help establish the presence of adequate skills in the administration of ECT, the applicant should be observed in the delivery of ECT and should demonstrate sufficient skill to satisfy the privileging authority. The individual evaluating the applicant's clinical skills should be a psychiatrist already privileged in ECT. If no such person is available in the facility, provisions should be made for the use of an outside consultant. The proceedings of all privileging actions should be documented.

In cases in which an applicant's education, training, or skill in ECT is deficient, further training should be required. This training experience should consist of didactic instruction and/or individualized reading as well as a formal or informal clinical practicum, if indicated (see Chapter 15). Decisions about the scope and depth of the training program should be guided by the type and degree of deficiencies present. Following satisfactory completion of the training program, the applicant should still be required to demonstrate proficient administration of ECT in the facility granting privileges. He or she should become familiar with the facility's policies and procedures for ECT as well as the layout of the ECT treatment suite and the use of applicable ECT devices, seizure monitoring equipment, and supplies.

Each facility granting privileges for ECT should also devise policies and procedures to maintain such privileges. This practice is required to ensure that a sustained level of clinical competence is achieved. The plan for maintaining privileging should make use of ongoing quality improvement programs as well as the monitoring of individual practice patterns, especially the number of treatments administered yearly. Any evidence of deficiencies in practice should be corrected. This plan should also include a requirement for CME in ECT-related areas. Reapplication for clinical privileges should be made at least every 2 years or as otherwise specified by regulation or by general local policies covering clinical privileging. The plan should include a provision for reassessment of clinical skills for individuals whose practice of ECT has been inactive for a considerable time, for example, 1 year.

Problems occur when a facility is so small that it does not have an organized medical staff or when the facility does not have sufficient expertise to adequately evaluate candidates for ECT privileges. In such situations, the existence of concurrent clinical privileges obtained from a separate facility may be an acceptable substitute, although an attempt should be made to institute policies and procedures for formal in-house privileging as soon as possible, involving the use of outside consultants as deemed necessary. Ongoing monitoring of compliance with these policies and procedures should be undertaken by means of a quality improvement program or equivalent process, with corrective action taken as indicated.

RECOMMENDATIONS

a. Each member of the ECT treatment team, as defined in Chapter 9, should be clinically privileged to practice his or her respective ECT-related duties or be otherwise authorized by law to do so. Such privileging should be carried out according to procedures established by the organized medical staff of the facility or its equivalent under whose auspices ECT is administered.

b. The medical director of each facility should ensure that privileges to administer ECT are granted only to psychiatrists with demonstrated proficiency to deliver ECT in a safe and effective manner.

c. The medical director, with the assistance of appropriate individuals, should develop a formal written plan for provision and maintenance of ECT privileges. This plan should designate those responsible for determining whether privileging criteria have been met. Proceedings of all privileging actions should be documented.

d. The applicant's education, training, experience, and history of privileging in ECT should be reviewed by the body designated for this purpose to determine whether the applicant is competent to practice ECT. If so, clinical ECT privileges may be granted following satisfactory administration of ECT as observed by a designated in-house evaluator or, if necessary, by an outside consultant.

e. An applicant with deficiencies in ECT procedure should undertake an appropriate training experience. Privileges may then be awarded after completion of 1) the prescribed training experience, 2) the local orientation process, and 3) demonstration of proficient administration of ECT in the local setting.

f. Reassessment of privileges should occur at least every 2 years or as specified by policies of the institution. Policies developed by the facility for this purpose should contain the following components:

- Use of a quality improvement program to monitor selected aspects of ECT treatment team performance, review of any apparent deficits, and institution of corrective action
- Ongoing monitoring of number of ECT treatments administered by treating psychiatrists, so that individuals whose practice becomes inactive can be given the opportunity to demonstrate use

of proficient technique on resuming an active clinical role
- Demonstration of CME experience in ECT-related areas

References

Aarsland D, Larsen JP, Waage O, et al: Maintenance electroconvulsive therapy for Parkinson's disease. Convuls Ther 13:274–277, 1997

Abboud T, Raya J, Sadri S: Fetal and maternal cardiovascular effects of atropine and glycopyrrolate. Anesth Analg 62:426–430, 1983

Abraham KR, Kulhara P: The efficacy of electroconvulsive therapy in the treatment of schizophrenia: a comparative study. Br J Psychiatry 151:152–155, 1987

Abramczuk JA, Rose NM: Pre-anaesthetic assessment and the prevention of post-ECT morbidity. Br J Psychiatry 134:582–587, 1979

Abrams R: Is unilateral electroconvulsive therapy really the treatment of choice in endogenous depression? Ann N Y Acad Sci 462:50–55, 1986

Abrams R: Lateralized hemispheric mechanisms and the antidepressant effects of right and left unilateral ECT. Convuls Ther 5:244–249, 1989

Abrams R: ECT as prophylactic treatment for bipolar disorder (letter). Am J Psychiatry 147:373–374, 1990

Abrams R: Electroconvulsive therapy in the medically compromised patient. Psychiatr Clin North Am 14:871–885, 1991

Abrams R: Electroconvulsive Therapy, 3rd Edition. New York, Oxford University Press, 1997a

Abrams R: The mortality rate with ECT. Convuls Ther 13:125–127, 1997b

Abrams R: Electroconvulsive therapy requires higher dosage levels: Food and Drug Administration action is required. Arch Gen Psychiatry 57:445–446, 2000

Abrams R, Fink M: The present status of unilateral ECT: some recommendations. J Affect Disord 7:245–247, 1984

Abrams R, Swartz CM: ECT Instruction Manual for the Thymatron DG. Chicago, IL, Somatics, 1989

Abrams R, Taylor MA: Anterior bifrontal ECT: a clinical trial. Br J Psychiatry 122:587–590, 1973

Abrams R, Taylor MA: Unipolar and bipolar depressive illness: phenomenology and response to electroconvulsive therapy. Arch Gen Psychiatry 30:320–321, 1974

Abrams R, Taylor MA: Catatonia: a prospective clinical study. Arch Gen Psychiatry 33:579–581, 1976

Abrams R, Fink M, Feldstein S: Prediction of clinical response to ECT. Br J Psychiatry 122:457–460, 1973

Abrams R, Swartz CM, Vedak C: Antidepressant effects of right versus left unilateral ECT and the lateralization theory of ECT action. Am J Psychiatry 146:1190–1192, 1989

Abrams R, Swartz CM, Vedak C: Antidepressant effects of high-dose right unilateral electroconvulsive therapy. Arch Gen Psychiatry 48:746–748, 1991

Acevedo AG, Smith JK: Adverse reaction to use of caffeine in ECT. Am J Psychiatry 145:529–530, 1988

Ackermann RF, Engel J Jr, Baxter L: Positron emission tomography and autoradiographic studies of glucose utilization following electroconvulsive seizures in humans and rats. Ann N Y Acad Sci 462:263–269, 1986

Addonizio G, Susman VL: ECT as a treatment alternative for patients with symptoms of neuroleptic malignant syndrome. J Clin Psychiatry 48:102–105, 1987

Adverse Drug Reactions Advisory Committee: Premature closure of the fetal ductus arteriosus after maternal use of non-steroidal anti-inflammatory drugs. Med J Aust 169: 270–271, 1998

Agarwal A, Winny G: Role of ECT-phenothiazine combination in schizophrenia. Ind J Psychiatry 27:233–236, 1985

Agnew WF, McCreery DB: Considerations for safety in the use of extracranial stimulation for motor evoked potentials. Neurosurgery 20:143–147, 1987

Ahmed SK, Stein GS: Negative interaction between lithium and ECT. Br J Psychiatry 151:419–420, 1987

Aldrich CJ, Wyatt JS, Spencer JA, et al: The effect of maternal oxygen administration on human fetal cerebral oxygenation measured during labour by near infrared spectroscopy. Br J Obstet Gynaecol 101:509–503, 1994

Aldrich CJ, D'Antona D, Spencer JA, et al: The effect of maternal posture on fetal cerebral oxygenation during labour. Br J Obstet Gynaecol 102:14–19, 1995

Alexander RC, Salomon M, Pioggia MI, et al: Convulsive therapy in the treatment of mania: McLean hospital. Convuls Ther 4:115–125, 1988

Alexopoulos GS: ECT and cardiac patients with pacemakers. Am J Psychiatry 137:1111–1112, 1980

Alexopoulos GS, Shamoian CJ, Lucas J, et al: Medical problems of geriatric psychiatric patients and younger controls during electroconvulsive therapy. J Am Geriatr Soc 32:651–654, 1984

Alexopoulos GS, Meyers B, Young R, et al: Recovery in geriatric depression. Arch Gen Psychiatry 53:305–312, 1996

Ali-Melkkila T, Kaila T, Kanto J, et al: Pharmacokinetics of glycopyrronium in parturients. Anaesthesia 45:634–637, 1990

Allen RE, Pitts FN Jr: ECT for depressed patients with lupus erythematosus. Am J Psychiatry 135:367–368, 1978

Allen RM: Pseudodementia and ECT. Biol Psychiatry 17:1435–1443, 1982

Allman P, Hawton K: ECT for post-stroke depression: beta blockade to modify rise in blood pressure. Convuls Ther 3:218–221, 1987

Altshuler LL, Cohen L, Szuba MP, et al: Pharmacologic management of psychiatric illness during pregnancy: dilemmas and guidelines. Am J Psychiatry 153:592–606, 1996

American Academy of Neurology: Consensus statements: medical management of epilepsy. Neurology 51(suppl 4):S39–S43, 1998

American Academy of Pediatrics Committee on Drugs: The transfer of drugs and other chemicals into human milk. Pediatrics 93:137–150, 1994

American Academy of Pediatrics Work Group on Breastfeeding: Breastfeeding and the use of human milk. Pediatrics 100:1035–1039, 1997

American Medical Association: Adjuncts to anesthesia, in Drug Evaluation, I/PAIN-5. Chicago, IL, American Medical Association, 1990

American Psychiatric Association: The Practice of ECT: Recommendations for Treatment, Training, and Privileging. Washington, DC, American Psychiatric Press, 1990

American Psychiatric Association: Practice guideline for major depressive disorder in adults. Am J Psychiatry 150(suppl):1–26, 1993

American Psychiatric Association: Diagnostic and Statistical Manual of Mental Disorders, 4th Edition. Washington, DC, American Psychiatric Association, 1994a

American Psychiatric Association: Practice guideline for the treatment of patients with bipolar disorder. Am J Psychiatry 151(suppl):1–36, 1994b

American Psychiatric Association: Practice guideline for the treatment of patients with schizophrenia. Am J Psychiatry 154(suppl):1–63, 1997

American Psychiatric Association Council on Psychiatry and Law: American Psychiatric Association resource document on principles of informed consent in psychiatry. J Am Acad Psychiatry Law 25:121–125, 1997

American Psychiatric Association Task Force on ECT: Electroconvulsive Therapy (Task Force Report #14). Washington, DC, American Psychiatric Association, 1978

American Society of Anesthesiologists: New classification of physical status. Anesthesiology 24:111, 1963

American Society of Anesthesiologists Task Force on Preoperative Fasting: Practice guidelines for preoperative fasting and the use of pharmacologic agents to reduce the risk of pulmonary aspiration: application to healthy patients undergoing elective procedures. Anesthesiology 90:896–905, 1999

Aminoff MJ: Management of status epilepticus. Can J Neurol Sci 25:S4–S6, 1998

Ananth J: Side effects on fetus and infant of psychotropic drug use during pregnancy. International Pharmacopsychiatry 11:246–260, 1976

Ananth J, Samra D, Kolivakis T: Amelioration of drug-induced parkinsonism by ECT. Am J Psychiatry 136:1094, 1979

Andersen K, Balldin J, Gottfries CG, et al: A double-blind evaluation of electroconvulsive therapy in Parkinson's disease with "on–off" phenomena. Acta Neurol Scand 76:191–199, 1987

Andrade C: Double stimulation to elicit an adequate treatment. Convuls Ther 7:300–302, 1991

Andrade C, Rao NS: Medical students' attitudes toward electroconvulsive therapy: an Indian perspective. Convuls Ther 12:86–90, 1996

Andrade C, Gangadhar BN, Subbakrishna DK, et al: A double-blind comparison of sinusoidal wave and brief-pulse electroconvulsive therapy in endogenous depression. Convuls Ther 4:297–305, 1988a

Andrade C, Gangadhar BN, Swaminath G, et al: Mania as a side effect of electroconvulsive therapy. Convuls Ther 4:81–83, 1988b

Andrade C, Gangadhar BN, Channabasavanna SM: Further characterization of mania as a side effect of ECT. Convuls Ther 6:318–319, 1990

Andrade C, Udaya HB, Chandra JS: BR-16A restricts development of electroconvulsive shock-induced retrograde amnesia. Biol Psychiatry 37:820–822, 1995

Ang MS, Thorp JA, Parisi VM: Maternal lithium therapy and polyhydramnios. Obstet Gynecol 76:517–519, 1990

Angst J, Angst K, Baruffol I, et al: ECT-induced and drug-induced hypomania. Convuls Ther 8:179–185, 1992

Anonymous: ECT in Britain: a shameful state of affairs (editorial). Lancet 2:1207–1208, 1981

Applebaum PS, Lidz CW, Meisel A: Informed Consent: Legal Theory and Clinical Practice. New York, Oxford University Press, 1987

Applegate RJ: Diagnosis and management of ischemic heart disease in the patient scheduled to undergo electroconvulsive therapy. Convuls Ther 13:128–144, 1997

Aronson TA, Shukla S, Hoff A: Continuation therapy after ECT for delusional depression: a naturalistic study of prophylactic treatments and relapse. Convuls Ther 3:251–259, 1987

Aronson TA, Shukla S, Hoff A, et al: Proposed delusional depression subtypes: preliminary evidence from a retrospective study of phenomenology and treatment course. J Affect Disord 14:69–74, 1988

Askew G, Pearson KW, Cryer D: Informed consent: can we educate patients? J R Coll Surg Edinb 35:308–310, 1990

Assael MI, Halperin B, Alpern S: Centrencephalic epilepsy induced by electrical convulsive treatment. Electroencephalogr Clin Neurophysiol 23:195, 1967

Atre-Vaidya N, Jampala VC: Electroconvulsive therapy in parkinsonism with affective disorder. Br J Psychiatry 152:55–58, 1988

Auerbach JG, Hans SL, Marcus J, et al: Maternal psychotropic medication and neonatal behavior. Neurotoxicol Teratol 14:399–406, 1992

Avery D, Winokur G: Mortality in depressed patients treated with electroconvulsive therapy and antidepressants. Arch Gen Psychiatry 33:1029–1037, 1976

Avery D, Lubrano A: Depression treated with imipramine and ECT: the De Carolis study reconsidered. Am J Psychiatry 136:549–562, 1979

Avramov MN, Husain MM, White PF: The comparative effects of methohexital, propofol, and etomidate for electroconvulsive therapy. Anesth Analg 81:596–602, 1995

Ayres C: The relative value of various somatic therapies in schizophrenia. Journal of Neuropsychiatry 1:154–162, 1960

Babigian HM, Guttmacher LB: Epidemiologic considerations in electroconvulsive therapy. Arch Gen Psychiatry 41:246–253, 1984

Bader GM, Silk KR, DeQuardo JR, et al: Electroconvulsive therapy and intracranial aneurysm. Convuls Ther 11:139–143, 1995

Badrinath SS, Bhaskaran S, Sundararaj I, et al: Mortality and morbidity associated with ophthalmic surgery. Ophthalmic Surg Lasers 26:535–541, 1995

Bagadia VN, Dave KP, Shah LP: A comparative study of physical treatments in schizophrenia. Ind J Psychiatry 12:190–204, 1970

Bagadia VN, Abhyankar RR, Doshi J, et al: Report from a WHO collaborative center for psychopharmacology in India, 1: reevaluation of ECT in schizophrenia. Psychopharmacol Bull 19:550–555, 1983

Bagadia VN, Abhyankar R, Pradhan PV, et al: Reevaluation of ECT in schizophrenia: right temporoparietal versus bitemporal electrode placement. Convuls Ther 4:215–220, 1988

Bailine SH, Safferman A, Vital-Herne J, et al: Flumazenil reversal of benzodiazepine-induced sedation for a patient with severe pre-ECT anxiety. Convuls Ther 10:65–68, 1994

Bailine SH, Rifkin A, Kayne E, et al: Comparison of bifrontal and bitemporal ECT for major depression. Am J Psychiatry 157:121–123, 2000

Baker AA, Game JA, Thorpe JG: Physical treatment for schizophrenia. Journal of Mental Science 104:860–864, 1958

Baker AA, Bird G, Lavin NI, et al: ECT in schizophrenia. Journal of Mental Science 106:1506–1511, 1960a

Baker AA, Game JA, Thorpe JG: Some research into the treatment of schizophrenia in the mental hospital. Journal of Mental Science 106:203–213, 1960b

Bali IM: The effect of modified electroconvulsive therapy on plasma potassium concentration. Br J Anaesth 47:398–401, 1975

Balldin J, Edén S, Granérus AK, et al: Electroconvulsive therapy in Parkinson's syndrome with "on–off" phenomenon. J Neural Transm 47:11–21, 1980

Balldin J, Granérus AK, Lindstedt G, et al: Predictors for improvement after electroconvulsive therapy in parkinsonian patients with on–off symptoms. J Neural Transm 52:199–211, 1981

Barnes RC, Hussein A, Anderson DN, et al: Maintenance electroconvulsive therapy and cognitive function. Br J Psychiatry 170:285–287, 1997

Barton JL, Mehta S, Snaith RP: The prophylactic value of extra ECT in depressive illness. Acta Psychiatr Scand 49:386–392, 1973

Battersby M, Ben-Tovim D, Eden J: Electroconvulsive therapy: a study of attitudes and attitude change after seeing an educational video. Aust N Z J Psychiatry 27:613–619, 1993

Baxter LRJ, Roy-Byrne P, Liston EH, et al: Informing patients about electroconvulsive therapy: effects of a videotape presentation. Convuls Ther 2:25–29, 1986

Beale MD, Kellner CH, Lemert R, et al: Skeletal muscle relaxation in patients undergoing electroconvulsive therapy (letter). Anesthesiology 80:957, 1994a

Beale MD, Kellner CH, Pritchett JT, et al: Stimulus dose-titration in ECT: a 2-year clinical experience. Convuls Ther 10:171–176, 1994b

Beale MD, Pritchett JT, Kellner CH: Supraventricular tachycardia in a patient receiving ECT, clozapine, and caffeine. Convuls Ther 10:228–231, 1994c

Beale MD, Bernstein HJ, Kellner CH: Maintenance electroconvulsive therapy for geriatric depression: a one year follow-up. Clinical Gerontologist 16:86–90, 1996

Beale MD, Kellner CH, Gurecki P, et al: ECT for the treatment of Huntington's disease: a case study. Convuls Ther 13:108–112, 1997a

Beale MD, Kellner CH, Parsons PJ: ECT for the treatment of mood disorders in cancer patients. Convuls Ther 13:222–226, 1997b

Bean G, Nishisato S, Rector NA, et al: The assessment of competence to make a treatment decision: an empirical approach. Can J Psychiatry 41:85–92, 1996

Beck AT, Steer RA, Brown GK: Beck Depression Inventory Manual, 2nd Edition. San Antonio, TX, Psychological Corporation, 1996

Benatov R, Sirota P, Megged S: Neuroleptic-resistant schizophrenia treated with clozapine and ECT. Convuls Ther 12:117–121, 1996

Benbow SM: Effect of training on administration of electroconvulsive therapy by junior doctors. Convuls Ther 2:19–24, 1986

Benbow SM: The role of electroconvulsive therapy in the treatment of depressive illness in old age. Br J Psychiatry 155:147–152, 1989

Benbow SM: Medical students and electroconvulsive therapy: their knowledge and attitudes. Convuls Ther 6:32–37, 1990

Bennett-Levy J, Powell GE: The subjective memory questionnaire (SMQ): an investigation into the self-reporting of "real-life" memory skills. British Journal of Social and Clinical Psychology 19:177–188, 1980

Benton AL: A multiple choice type of visual retention test. Arch Neurol Psychiatry 64:699–707, 1950

Bergsholm P, Gran L, Bleie H: Seizure duration in unilateral electroconvulsive therapy: the effect of hypocapnia induced by hyperventilation and the effect of ventilation with oxygen. Acta Psychiatr Scand 69:121–128, 1984

Berigan TR, Harazin J, Williams HL II: Use of flumazenil in conjunction with electroconvulsive therapy (letter). Am J Psychiatry 152:957, 1995

Berman E, Wolpert EA: Intractable manic-depressive psychosis with rapid cycling in an 18-year-old woman successfully treated with electroconvulsive therapy. J Nerv Ment Dis 175:236–239, 1987

Berry M, Whittaker M: Incidence of suxamethonium apnea in patients undergoing ECT. Br J Anaesth 47:1195–1197, 1975

Bertagnoli MW, Borchardt CM: A review of ECT for children and adolescents. J Am Acad Child Adolesc Psychiatry 29:302–307, 1990

Beyer JL, Weiner RD, Glenn MD: Electroconvulsive Therapy: A Programmed Text, 2nd Edition. Washington, DC, American Psychiatric Press, 1998

Bhatia SC, Bhatia SK, Gupta S: Concurrent administration of clozapine and ECT: a successful therapeutic strategy for a patient with treatment-resistant schizophrenia. J ECT 14:280–283, 1998

Bhatia SC, Baldwin SA, Bhatia SK: Electroconvulsive therapy during the third trimester of pregnancy. J ECT 15:270–274, 1999

Bibb RC, Guze SB: Hysteria (Briquet's syndrome) in a psychiatric hospital: the significance of secondary depression. Am J Psychiatry 129:224–228, 1972

Bidder TG, Strain JJ, Brunschwig L: Bilateral and unilateral ECT: follow-up study and critique. Am J Psychiatry 127:737–745, 1970

Black DW, Winokur G, Nasrallah A: ECT in unipolar and bipolar disorders: a naturalistic evaluation of 460 patients. Convuls Ther 2:231–237, 1986

Black DW, Winokur G, Nasrallah A: Treatment and outcome in secondary depression: a naturalistic study of 1,087 patients. J Clin Psychiatry 48:438–441, 1987a

Black DW, Winokur G, Nasrallah A: The treatment of depression: electroconvulsive therapy vs antidepressants. A naturalistic evaluation of 1,495 patients. Compr Psychiatry 28:169–182, 1987b

Black DW, Winokur G, Nasrallah A: Treatment of mania: a naturalistic study of electroconvulsive therapy versus lithium in 438 patients. J Clin Psychiatry 48:132–139, 1987c

Black DW, Bell S, Hulbert J, et al: The importance of Axis II in patients with major depression: a controlled study. J Affect Disord 14:115–122, 1988

Black DW, Hulbert J, Nasrallah A: The effect of somatic treatment and comorbidity on immediate outcome in manic patients. Compr Psychiatry 30:74–79, 1989a

Black DW, Winokur G, Mohandoss E, et al: Does treatment influence mortality in depressives? A follow-up of 1076 patients with major affective disorders. Ann Clin Psychiatry 1:165–173, 1989b

Black DW, Winokur G, Nasrallah A: Illness duration and acute response in major depression. Convuls Ther 5:338–343, 1989c

Black DW, Winokur G, Nasrallah A: A multivariate analysis of the experience of 423 depressed inpatients treated with electroconvulsive therapy. Convuls Ther 9:112–120, 1993

Blackwood DH, Cull RE, Freeman CP, et al: A study of the incidence of epilepsy following ECT. J Neurol Neurosurg Psychiatry 43:1098–1102, 1980

Bloch M, Admon D, Bonne O, et al: Electroconvulsive therapy in a depressed heart transplant patient. Convuls Ther 8:290–293, 1992

Bloch Y, Pollack M, Mor I: Should the administration of ECT during clozapine therapy be contraindicated? Br J Psychiatry 169:253–254, 1996

Bloomstein JR, Rummans TA, Maruta T, et al: The use of electroconvulsive therapy in pain patients. Psychosomatics 37:374–379, 1996

Boey WK, Lai FO: Comparison of propofol and thiopentone as anaesthetic agents for electroconvulsive therapy. Anaesthesia 45:623–628, 1990

Bolwig TG: Training in convulsive therapy in Denmark (letter). Convuls Ther 3:156–157, 1987

Bond ED: Results of treatment in psychoses with a control series, IV: general data and summary. Am J Psychiatry 110:885–887, 1954

Bonds C, Frye MA, Coudreaut MF, et al: Cost reduction with maintenance ECT in refractory bipolar disorder. J ECT 14:36–41, 1998

Bone ME, Wilkins CJ, Lew JK: A comparison of propofol and methohexitone as anaesthetic agents for electroconvulsive therapy. Eur J Anaesthesiol 5:279–286, 1988

Book WJ, Abel M, Eisenkraft JB: Adverse effects of depolarizing neuromuscular blocking agents: incidence, prevention, and management. Drug Safety 10:331–349, 1994

Borgatta L, Jenny RW, Gruss L, et al: Clinical significance of methohexital, meperidine, and diazepam in breast milk. J Clin Pharmacol 37:186–192, 1997

Boronow J, Stoline A, Sharfstein SS: Refusal of ECT by a patient with recurent depression, psychosis, and catatonia. Am J Psychiatry 154:1285–1291, 1997

Borowitz AH: An investigation into combined electroconvulsive and chlorpromazine therapy in the treatment of schizophrenia. S Afr Med J 33:836–840, 1959

Bouckoms AJ, Welch CA, Drop LJ, et al: Atropine in electroconvulsive therapy. Convuls Ther 5:48–55, 1989

Bourgon LN, Kellner CH: Relapse of depression after ECT: a review. J ECT 16:19–31, 2000

Boylan LS, Haskett RF, Mulsant BF, et al: Determinants of seizure threshold in ECT: benzodiazepine use, anesthetic dosage, and other factors. J ECT 16:3–18, 2000

Brand N, Clarke Q, Eather L, et al: Surgical morbidity in the North Coast Health Region. J Qual Clin Pract 14:103–110, 1994

Brandon S, Cowley P, McDonald C, et al: Electroconvulsive therapy: results in depressive illness from the Leicestershire trial. BMJ 288:22–25, 1984

Brandon S, Cowley P, McDonald C, et al: Leicester ECT trial: results in schizophrenia. Br J Psychiatry 146:177–183, 1985

Breakey WR, Kala AK: Typhoid catatonia responsive to ECT. BMJ 2:357–359, 1977

Brill NQ, Crumpton E, Eiduson S, et al: Investigation of the therapeutic components and various factors associated with improvement with electroconvulsive treatment: a preliminary report. Am J Psychiatry 113:997–1008, 1957

Brill NQ, Crumpton E, Eiduson S, et al: An experimental study of the relative effectiveness of various components of electroconvulsive therapy. Am J Psychiatry 115:734–735, 1959a

Brill NQ, Crumpton E, Eiduson S, et al: Predictive and concomitant variables related to improvement with actual and simulated ECT. Arch Gen Psychiatry 1:263–272, 1959b

Brill NQ, Crumpton E, Eiduson S, et al: Relative effectiveness of various components of electroconvulsive therapy. Arch Neurol Psychiatry 81:627–635, 1959c

Brimacombe JR, Berry AM: Cricoid pressure. Can J Anaesth 44:414–425, 1997

Broadbent DE, Cooper PF, Fitzgerald P, et al: The cognitive failures questionnaire (CFQ) and its correlates. Br J Clin Psychol 21:1–16, 1982

Bross R: Near fatality with combined ECT and reserpine. Am J Psychiatry 113:933, 1957

Broussard CN, Richter JE: Nausea and vomiting of pregnancy. Gastroenterol Clin North Am 27:123–151, 1998

Bruce EM, Crone N, Fitzpatrick G, et al: A comparative trial of ECT and Tofranil. Am J Psychiatry 117:76–80, 1960

Bryden M: Laterality: Functional Asymmetry in the Intact Brain. New York, Academic Press, 1982

Bryden MP, Steenhuis RE: Issues in the assessment of handedness, in Cerebral Laterality: Theory and Research. Edited by Kitterle FL. Hillsdale, NJ, Erlbaum, 1991, pp 35–51

Buchan H, Johnstone E, McPherson K, et al: Who benefits from electroconvulsive therapy? Combined results of the Leicester and Northwick Park trials. Br J Psychiatry 160:355–359, 1992

Bulbena A, Berrios GE: Pseudodementia: facts and figures. Br J Psychiatry 148:87–94, 1986

Burnstein RM, Denny N: Mivacurium in electroconvulsive therapy (letter). Anesthesia 48:1116, 1993

Burke WJ, Rutherford JL, Zorumski CF, et al: Electroconvulsive therapy and the elderly. Compr Psychiatry 26:480–486, 1985

Burke WJ, Rubin EH, Zorumski CF, et al: The safety of ECT in geriatric psychiatry. J Am Geriatr Soc 35:516–521, 1987

Burns CM, Stuart GW: Nursing care in electroconvulsive therapy. Psychiatr Clin North Am 14:971–988, 1991

Burt DB, Zembar MJ, Niederehe G: Depression and memory impairment: a meta-analysis of the association, its pattern, and specificity. Psychol Bull 117:285–305, 1995

Bush G, Fink M, Petrides G, et al: Catatonia, II: treatment with lorazepam and electroconvulsive therapy. Acta Psychiatr Scand 93:137–143, 1996

Butters N, Albert M: Processes underlying failures to recall remote events, in Human Memory and Amnesia. Edited by Cermak L. Hillsdale, NJ, Erlbaum, 1982, pp 257–274

Byrne D: Affect and vigilance performance in depressive illness. J Psychiatr Res 13:185–191, 1977

Caine ED: Pseudodementia: current concepts and future directions. Arch Gen Psychiatry 38:1359–1364, 1981

Calev A, Ben-Tzvi E, Shapira B, et al: Distinct memory impairments following electroconvulsive therapy and imipramine. Psychol Med 19:111–119, 1989

Calev A, Kochavlev E, Tubi N, et al: Change in attitude toward electroconvulsive therapy: effects of treatment, time since treatment, and severity of depression. Convuls Ther 7:184–189, 1991a

Calev A, Nigal D, Shapira B, et al: Early and long-term effects of electroconvulsive therapy and depression on memory and other cognitive functions. J Nerv Ment Dis 179:526–533, 1991b

Calev A, Fink M, Petrides G, et al: Caffeine pretreatment enhances clinical efficacy and reduces cognitive effects of electroconvulsive therapy. Convuls Ther 9:95–100, 1993

Calev A, Gaudino EA, Squires NK, et al: ECT and non-memory cognition: a review. Br J Clin Psychol 34:505–515, 1995

Cameron D, Lohrenz J, Handcock K: The depatterning treatment of schizophrenia. Compr Psychiatry 3:65–76, 1962

Caplan G: Treatment of epilepsy by electrically induced convulsions. BMJ 1:511–513, 1945

Caplan G: Electrical convulsion therapy in treatment of epilepsy. Journal of Mental Science 92:784–793, 1946

Caplan RA, Benumof JL, Berry FA, et al: Practice guidelines for management of the difficult airway: a report by the American Society of Anesthesiologists Task Force on Management of the Difficult Airway. Anesthesiology 78:597–602, 1993

Caracci G, Decina P: Fluoxetine and prolonged seizure. Convuls Ther 7:145–147, 1991

Cardno AG, Simpson CJ: Electroconvulsive therapy in Paget's disease and hydrocephalus. Convuls Ther 7:48–51, 1991

Cardwell BA, Nakai B: Seizure activity in combined clozapine and ECT: a retrospective view. Convuls Ther 11:110–113, 1995

Carney MWP, Roth M, Garside RF: The diagnosis of depressive syndromes and the prediction of ECT response. Br J Psychiatry 111:659–674, 1965

Carney MW, Rogan PA, Sebastian J, et al: A controlled comparative trial of unilateral and bilateral sinusoidal and pulse ECT in endogenous depression. Physicians Drug Manual 7:77–79, 1976

Carr ME Jr, Woods JW: Electroconvulsive therapy in a patient with unsuspected pheochromocytoma. South Med J 78:613–615, 1985

Carrasco Gonzalez MD, Palomar M, Rovira R: Electroconvulsive therapy for status epilepticus. Ann Intern Med 127:247–248, 1997

Casey DA: Electroconvulsive therapy in the neuroleptic malignant syndrome. Convuls Ther 3:278–283, 1987

Castelli I, Steiner LA, Kaufmann MA, et al: Comparative effects of esmolol and labetalol to attenuate hyperdynamic states after electroconvulsive therapy. Anesth Analg 80:557–561, 1995

Centers for Disease Control: Recommendations for prevention of HIV transmission in health care settings. MMWR Morb Mortal Wkly Rep 36(suppl):1S–18S, 1987

Centers for Disease Control and Prevention: Recommended infection-control practices for dentistry. MMWR Morb Mortal Wkly Rep 42:1–12, 1993

Chafetz ME: An active treatment for chronically ill patients. J Nerv Ment Dis 98:464–473, 1943

Chambers CD, Johnson KA, Dick LM, et al: Birth outcomes in pregnant women taking fluoxetine. N Engl J Med 335:1010–1015, 1996

Chan CH, Janicak PG, Davis JM, et al: Response of psychotic and nonpsychotic depressed patients to tricyclic antidepressants. J Clin Psychiatry 48:197–200, 1987

Chanpattana W: Maintenance ECT in schizophrenia: a pilot study. J Med Assoc Thai 81:17–24, 1998

Chanpattana W, Chakrabhand ML, Kongsakon R, et al: Short-term effect of combined ECT and neuroleptic therapy in treatment-resistant schizophrenia. J ECT 15:129–139, 1999a

Chanpattana W, Chakrabhand ML, Sackeim HA, et al: Continuation ECT in treatment-resistant schizophrenia: a controlled study. J ECT 15:178–192, 1999b

Chater SN, Simpson KH: Effect of passive hyperventilation on seizure duration in patients undergoing electroconvulsive therapy. Br J Anaesth 60:70–73, 1988

Chen P, Ganguli M, Mulsant BH, et al: The temporal relationship between depressive symptoms and dementia: a community-based prospective study. Arch Gen Psychiatry 56:261–266, 1999

Cheney CO, Drewry PH: Results of nonspecific treatment in dementia praecox. Am J Psychiatry 95:203–217, 1938

Childers RT: Comparison of four regimens in newly admitted female schizophrenics. Am J Psychiatry 120:1010–1011, 1964

Childers RT, Therrien R: A comparison of trifluoperazine and chlorpromazine in schizophrenia. Am J Psychiatry 118:552–554, 1961

Christensen P, Kragh-Sorensen P, Sorensen C, et al: EEG-monitored ECT: a comparison of seizure duration under anesthesia with etomidate and thiopentone. Convuls Ther 2:145–150, 1986

Ciraulo D, Lind L, Salzman C, et al: Sodium nitroprusside treatment of ECT-induced blood pressure elevations. Am J Psychiatry 135:1105–1106, 1978

Clarke TB, Coffey CE, Hoffman GW, et al: Continuation therapy for depression using outpatient electroconvulsive therapy. Convuls Ther 5:330–337, 1989

Cleophas TJ, Niemeyer MC, van der Wall EE, et al: Nitrate-induced headache in patients with stable angina pectoris: beneficial effect of starting on a low dosage. 5-ISMN headache study group. Angiology 47:679–685, 1996

Clinical Research Centre, Division of Psychiatry: The Northwick Park ECT trial: predictors of response to real and simulated ECT. Br J Psychiatry 144:227–237, 1984

Coffey CE: The Clinical Science of Electroconvulsive Therapy. Washington, DC, American Psychiatric Press, 1993

Coffey CE: Brain morphology in primary mood disorders: implications for electroconvulsive therapy. Psychiatric Annals 26:713–716, 1996

Coffey CE: The pre-ECT evaluation. Psychiatric Annals 28:506–508, 1998

Coffey CE, Kellner CH: Electroconvulsive therapy, in Textbook of Geriatric Neuropsychiatry, 2nd Edition. Edited by Coffey CE, Cummings JL. Washington, DC, American Psychiatric Press, 2000, pp 829–860

Coffey CE, Weiner RD, Kalayjian R, et al: Electroconvulsive therapy in osteogenesis imperfecta: issues of muscular relaxation. Convuls Ther 2:207–211, 1986

Coffey CE, Hinkle PE, Weiner RD, et al: Electroconvulsive therapy of depression in patients with white matter hyperintensity. Biol Psychiatry 22:629–636, 1987a

Coffey CE, Hoffman G, Weiner RD, et al: Electroconvulsive therapy in a depressed patient with a functioning ventriculoatrial shunt. Convuls Ther 4:302–306, 1987b

Coffey CE, Weiner RD, Hinkle PE, et al: Augmentation of ECT seizures with caffeine. Biol Psychiatry 22:637–649, 1987c

Coffey CE, Weiner RD, McCall WV, et al: Electroconvulsive therapy in multiple sclerosis: a magnetic resonance imaging study of the brain. Convuls Ther 3:137–144, 1987d

Coffey CE, Figiel GS, Weiner RD, et al: Caffeine augmentation of ECT. Am J Psychiatry 147:579–585, 1990

Coffey CE, Lucke J, Weiner RD, et al: Seizure threshold in electroconvulsive therapy, I: initial seizure threshold. Biol Psychiatry 37:713–720, 1995a

Coffey CE, Lucke J, Weiner RD, et al: Seizure threshold in electroconvulsive therapy, II: the anticonvulsant effect of ECT. Biol Psychiatry 37:777–788, 1995b

Cohen D, Paillere-Martinot ML, Basquin M: Use of electroconvulsive therapy in adolescents. Convuls Ther 13:25–31, 1997

Cohen D, Taieb O, Flament M, et al: Absence of cognitive impairment at long-term follow-up in adolescents treated with ECT for severe mood disorder. Am J Psychiatry 157:460–462, 2000

Cohen LS, Friedman JM, Jefferson JW, et al: A reevaluation of risk of in utero exposure to lithium. JAMA 271:146–150, 1994

Cohen LS, Rosenbaum JF: Psychotropic drug use during pregnancy: weighing the risks. J Clin Psychiatry 59:18–28, 1998

Coleman EA, Sackeim HA, Prudic J, et al: Subjective memory complaints before and after electroconvulsive therapy. Biol Psychiatry 39:346–356, 1996

Colenda CC, McCall WV: A statistical model predicting the seizure threshold for right unilateral ECT in 106 patients. Convuls Ther 12:3–12, 1996

Consensus Conference: Electroconvulsive therapy. JAMA 254:2103–2108, 1985

Constant J: Treatment of delirious episodes. Rev Prat 22:4465–4473, 1972

Coryell W, Zimmerman M: Outcome following ECT for primary unipolar depression: a test of newly proposed response predictors. Am J Psychiatry 141:862–867, 1984

Coryell W, Pfohl B, Zimmerman M: Outcome following electroconvulsive therapy: a comparison of primary and secondary depression. Convuls Ther 1:10–14, 1985

Cousins L: Fetal oxygenation, assessment of fetal well-being, and obstetric management of the pregnant patient with asthma. J Allergy Clin Immunol 103:S343–S349, 1999

Coverdale JH, Chervenak FA, McCullough LB, et al: Ethically justified clinically comprehensive guidelines for the management of the depressed pregnant patient. Am J Obstet Gynecol 174:169–173, 1996

Creed P, Froimson L, Mathew L: Survey of the practice of electroconvulsive therapy in North Carolina. Convuls Ther 11:182–187, 1995

Crimson ML, Trivedi M, Pigott TA, et al: The Texas Medication Algorithm Project: report of the Texas Consensus Conference Panel on Medication Treatment of Major Depressive Disorder. J Clin Psychiatry 60:142–156, 1999

Cronholm B, Molander L: Memory disturbances after electroconvulsive therapy, IV: influence of interpolated electroconvulsive shock on retention of memory material. Acta Psychiatrica et Neurologica Scandinavica 36:83–90, 1961

Cronholm B, Molander L: Memory disturbances after electroconvulsive therapy. Acta Psychiatr Scand 40:212–216, 1964

Cronholm B, Ottosson J-O: Memory functions in endogenous depression: before and after electroconvulsive therapy. Arch Gen Psychiatry 5:193–199, 1961

Cronholm B, Ottosson J-O: The experience of memory function after electroconvulsive therapy. Br J Psychiatry 109:251–258, 1963a

Cronholm B, Ottosson J-O: Ultrabrief stimulus technique in electroconvulsive therapy, II: comparative studies of therapeutic effects and memory disturbances in treatment of endogenous depression with the Elther ES electroshock apparatus and Siemens Konvulsator III. J Nerv Ment Dis 137:268–276, 1963b

Crosby ET, Cooper RM, Douglas MJ, et al: The unanticipated difficult airway with recommendations for management. Can J Anaesth 45:757–776, 1998

Crow S, Meller W, Christenson G, et al: Use of ECT after brain injury. Convuls Ther 12:113–116, 1996

Crowe RR: Current concepts. Electroconvulsive therapy: a current perspective. N Engl J Med 311:163–167, 1984

Culver CM, Ferrell RB, Green RM: ECT and special problems of informed consent. Am J Psychiatry 137:586–591, 1980

Cumming J, Kort K: Apparent reversal by cortisone of an electroconvulsive refractory state in a psychotic patient with Addison's disease. CMAJ 74:291–292, 1956

Cummins RO: Textbook of Advanced Cardiac Life Support. Dallas, TX, American Heart Association, 1994

Cunningham SJ, Anderson DN: Delusional depression, hyperparathyroidism, and ECT. Convuls Ther 11:129–133, 1995

Currier GE, Cullinan C, Rothschild D: Results of treatment of schizophrenia in a state hospital: changing trends since advent of electroshock therapy. Arch Neurol Psychiatry 67:80–82, 1952

Daniel WF, Crovitz HF: Recovery of orientation after electroconvulsive therapy. Acta Psychiatr Scand 66:421–428, 1982

Daniel WF, Crovitz HF: Acute memory impairment following electroconvulsive therapy, 1: effects of electrical stimulus waveform and number of treatments. Acta Psychiatr Scand 67:1–7, 1983a

Daniel WF, Crovitz HF: Acute memory impairment following electroconvulsive therapy, 2: effects of electrode placement. Acta Psychiatr Scand 67:57–68, 1983b

Daniel WF, Crovitz HF: Disorientation during electroconvulsive therapy: technical, theoretical, and neuropsychological issues. Ann N Y Acad Sci 462:293–306, 1986

Danziger L, Kendwall JA: Prediction of immediate outcome of shock therapy in dementia. Diseases of the Nervous System 7:299–303, 1946

Das PS, Saxena S, Mohan D, et al: Adjunctive electroconvulsive therapy for schizophrenia. Natl Med J India 4:183–184, 1991

Davidson J: Seizures and bupropion: a review. J Clin Psychiatry 50:256–261, 1989

Davidson J, McLeod M, Law-Yone B, et al: A comparison of electroconvulsive therapy and combined phenelzine-amitriptyline in refractory depression. Arch Gen Psychiatry 35:639–642, 1978

Davidson RJ: Cerebral asymmetry, emotion, and affective style, in Brain Asymmetry. Edited by Davidson RJ, Hugdahl K. Cambridge, MA, MIT Press, 1995, pp 361–387

Davis EW, McCulloch WS, Roseman E: Rapid changes in the O2 tension of cerebral cortex during induced convulsions. Am J Psychiatry 100:825–829, 1944

Davis JM, Janicak PG, Sakkas P, et al: Electroconvulsive therapy in the treatment of the neuroleptic malignant syndrome. Convuls Ther 7:111–120, 1991

DeBattista C, Mueller K: Sumatriptan prophylaxis for post electroconvulsive therapy headaches. Headache 35:502–503, 1995

Decina P, Malitz S, Sackeim HA, et al: Cardiac arrest during ECT modified by beta-adrenergic blockade. Am J Psychiatry 141:298–300, 1984

Decina P, Guthrie EB, Sackeim HA, et al: Continuation ECT in the management of relapses of major affective episodes. Acta Psychiatr Scand 75:559–562, 1987

Delgado-Escueta AV, Janz D: Consensus guidelines: preconception counseling, management, and care of the pregnant woman with epilepsy. Neurology 42:149–160, 1992

d'Elia G: Unilateral electroconvulsive therapy. Acta Psychiatr Scand Suppl 215:1–98, 1970

d'Elia G: Memory changes after unilateral electroconvulsive therapy with different electrode positions. Cortex 12:280–289, 1976

d'Elia G: Electrode placement and antidepressant efficacy. Convuls Ther 8:294–296, 1992

Dempsey GM, Tsuang MT, Struss A, et al: Treatment of schizo-affective disorder. Compr Psychiatry 16:55–59, 1975

DeQuardo JR, Tandon R: ECT in post-stroke major depression. Convuls Ther 4:221–224, 1988

Devanand DP, Sackeim HA: Seizure elicitation blocked by pretreatment with lidocaine. Convuls Ther 4:225–229, 1988

Devanand DP, Sackeim HA: Use of increased anesthetic dose prior to electroconvulsive therapy to prevent postictal excitement. Gen Hosp Psychiatry 14:345–349, 1992

Devanand DP, Decina P, Sackeim HA, et al: Status epilepticus during ECT in a patient receiving theophylline. J Clin Psychopharm 8:153, 1988a

Devanand DP, Sackeim HA, Decina P, et al: The development of mania and organic euphoria during ECT. J Clin Psychiatry 49:69–71, 1988b

Devanand DP, Briscoe KM, Sackeim HA: Clinical features and predictors of postictal excitement. Convuls Ther 5:140–146, 1989

Devanand DP, Malitz S, Sackeim HA: ECT in a patient with aortic aneurysm. J Clin Psychiatry 51:255–256, 1990

Devanand DP, Verma AK, Tirumalasetti F, et al: Absence of cognitive impairment after more than 100 lifetime ECT treatments. Am J Psychiatry 148:929–932, 1991

Devanand DP, Prudic J, Sackeim HA: Electroconvulsive therapy–induced hypomania is uncommon. Convuls Ther 8:296–298, 1992

Devanand DP, Dwork AJ, Hutchinson ER, et al: Does ECT alter brain structure? Am J Psychiatry 151:957–970, 1994

Devanand DP, Fitzsimons L, Prudic J, et al: Subjective side effects during electroconvulsive therapy. Convuls Ther 11:232–240, 1995

Devanand DP, Sano M, Tang MX, et al: Depressed mood and the incidence of Alzheimer's disease in the elderly living in the community. Arch Gen Psychiatry 53:175–182, 1996

Devanand DP, Lisanby SH, Nobler MS, et al: The relative efficiency of altering pulse frequency or train duration when determining seizure threshold. J ECT 14:227–235, 1998

Devinsky O, Duchowny MS: Seizures after convulsive therapy: a retrospective case survey. Neurology 33:921–925, 1983

DeWet JST: Evaluation of a common method of convulsion therapy in Bantu schizophrenics. Journal of Mental Science 103:739–757, 1957

Diaz-Cabal R, Pearlman C, Kawecki A: Hyperthyroidism in a patient with agitated depression: resolution after electroconvulsive therapy. J Clin Psychiatry 47:322–323, 1986

Dighe-Deo D, Shah A: Electroconvulsive therapy in patients with long bone fractures. J ECT 14:115–119, 1998

Dillon AE, Wagner CL, Wiest D, et al: Drug therapy in the nursing mother. Obstet Gynecol Clin North Am 24:675–696, 1997

Dillon P: Electroconvulsive therapy patient/family education. Convuls Ther 11:188–191, 1995

Dinan TG, Barry S: A comparison of electroconvulsive therapy with a combined lithium and tricyclic combination among depressed tricyclic nonresponders. Acta Psychiatr Scand 80:97–100, 1989

Dinwiddie SH, Drevets WC, Smith DR: Treatment of phencyclidine-associated psychosis with ECT. Convuls Ther 4:230–235, 1988

Dodwell D, Goldberg D: A study of factors associated with response to electroconvulsive therapy in patients with schizophrenic symptoms. Br J Psychiatry 154:635–639, 1989

Doering EB, Ball WA: Flumazenil before electroconvulsive therapy: outstanding issues (letter). Anesthesiology 83:642–643, 1995

Dolinski SY, Zvara DA: Anesthetic considerations of cardiovascular risk during electroconvulsive therapy. Convuls Ther 13:157–164, 1997

Donahue JC: Electroconvulsive therapy and memory loss: anatomy of a debate. J ECT 16:133–143, 2000

Doongaji DR, Jeste DV, Saoji NJ, et al: Unilateral versus bilateral ECT in schizophrenia. Br J Psychiatry 123:73–79, 1973

Douglas CJ, Schwartz HI: ECT for depression caused by lupus cerebritis: a case report. Am J Psychiatry 139:1631–1632, 1982

Douyon R, Serby M, Klutchko B, et al: ECT and Parkinson's disease revisited: a "naturalistic" study. Am J Psychiatry 146:1451–1455, 1989

Dozois DJA, Dobson KS, Ahnberg JL: A psychometric evaluation of the Beck Depression Inventory, II. Psychological Assessment 10:83–89, 1998

Drop LJ, Welch CA: Anesthesia for electroconvulsive therapy in patients with major cardiovascular risk factors. Convuls Ther 5:88–101, 1989

Dubin WR, Jaffe R, Roemer R, et al: The efficacy and safety of maintenance ECT in geriatric patients. J Am Geriatr Soc 40:706–709, 1992

DuBois JC: Obsessions and mood: apropos of 43 cases of obsessive neurosis treated with antidepressive chemotherapy and electroshock. Ann Med Psychol (Paris) 142:141–151, 1984

Dubovsky SL: Using electroconvulsive therapy for patients with neurological disease. Hospital and Community Psychiatry 37:819–825, 1986

Dudley WH Jr, Williams JG: Electroconvulsive therapy in delirium tremens. Compr Psychiatry 13:357–360, 1972

Duffett R, Lelliott P: Auditing electroconvulsive therapy: the third cycle. Br J Psychiatry 172:401–405, 1998a

Duffett R, Lelliott P: Junior doctors' training in the theory and the practice of electroconvulsive therapy. J ECT 14:127–130, 1998b

Duffy WJ Jr, Conradt H: Electroconvulsive therapy: the perioperative process. AORN J 50:806–812, 1989

Dunlop E: Combination of antidepressants with electroshock therapy. Diseases of the Nervous System 21:513–514, 1960a

Dunlop E: Electroshock and monoamine oxidase inhibitors in the treatment of depressed reactions. Diseases of the Nervous System 21:130–131, 1960b

Dunn CG, Quinlan D: Indicators of ECT response and non-response in the treatment of depression. J Clin Psychiatry 39:620–622, 1978

Dwersteg JF, Avery DH: Atracurium as a muscle relaxant for electroconvulsive therapy in a burned patient (letter). Convuls Ther 3:49–53, 1987

Dwyer R, McCaughey W, Lavery J, et al: Comparison of propofol and methohexitone as anaesthetic agents for electroconvulsive therapy. Anaesthesia 43:459–462, 1988

Dysken M, Evans HM, Chan CH, et al: Improvement of depression and parkinsonism during ECT: a case study. Neuropsychobiology 2:81–86, 1976

Eagle KA, Brundage BH, Chaitman BR, et al: Guidelines for perioperative cardiovascular evaluation for noncardiac surgery: report of the American College of Cardiology/American Heart Association Task Force on Practice Guidelines (Committee on Perioperative Cardiovascular Evaluation for Noncardiac Surgery). Circulation 93:1278–1317, 1996

Echevarria Moreno M, Martin Munoz J, Sanchez Valderrabanos J, et al: Electroconvulsive therapy in the first trimester of pregnancy. J ECT 14:251–254, 1998

Edlund MJ, Craig TJ: Antipsychotic drug use and birth defects: an epidemiologic reassessment. Compr Psychiatry 25:32–37, 1984

Edwards RM, Stoudemire A, Vela MA, et al: Intraocular pressure changes in nonglaucomatous patients undergoing elecrtoconvulsive therapy. Convuls Ther 6:209–213, 1990

Eisenkraft JB, Book WJ, Mann SM, et al: Resistance to succinylcholine in myasthenia gravis: a dose–response study. Anesthesiology 69:760–763, 1988

El-Ganzouri A, Ivankovich AD, Braveman B, et al: Monoamine oxidase inhibitors: should they be discontinued preoperatively? Anesth Analg 64:592–596, 1985 el-Islam MF, Ahmed SA, Erfan ME: The effect of unilateral ECT on schizophrenic delusions and hallucinations. Br J Psychiatry 117:447–448, 1970

Elliot DL, Linz DH, Kane JA: Electroconvulsive therapy: pretreatment medical evaluation. Arch Intern Med 142:979–981, 1982

Ellison FA, Hamilton DM: The hospital treatment of dementia praecox: part II. Am J Psychiatry 106:454–461, 1949

El-Mallakh RS: Complications of concurrent lithium and electroconvulsive therapy: a review of clinical material and theoretical considerations. Biol Psychiatry 23:595–601, 1988

Endler NS: The origins of electroconvulsive therapy (ECT). Convuls Ther 4:5–23, 1988

Endler NS: Holiday of Darkness: A Psychologist's Journey Out of His Depression, Revised Edition. Toronto, Canada, Wall & Thompson, 1990

Endler NS, Persad E: Electroconvulsive therapy: the myths and the realities. Toronto, Canada, Hans Huber, 1988

Engel J Jr: Seizures and epilepsy. Philadelphia, PA, FA Davis, 1989

Enns M, Karvelas L: Electrical dose titration for electroconvulsive therapy: a comparison with dose prediction methods. Convuls Ther 11:86–93, 1995

Enns M, Peeling J, Sutherland GR: Hippocampal neurons are damaged by caffeine-augmented electroshock seizures. Biol Psychiatry 40:642–647, 1996

Erman MK, Welch CA, Mandel MR: A comparison of two unilateral ECT electrode placements: efficacy and electrical energy considerations. Am J Psychiatry 136:1317–1319, 1979

Escande M, Nordman S, Loustalan JM, et al: Value of electroconvulsive therapy as maintenance treatment for recurrent depression unresponsive to pharmacologic therapy. Annales de Psychiatrie 7:161–164, 1992

Everman PD, Kellner CH, Beale MD, et al: Modified electrode placement in patients with neurosurgical skull defects. J ECT 15:237–239, 1999

Exner JE Jr, Murillo LG: Effectiveness of regressive ECT with process schizophrenia. Diseases of the Nervous System 34:44–48, 1973

Exner JE Jr, Murillo LG: A long term follow-up of schizophrenics treated with regressive ECT. Diseases of the Nervous System 38:162–168, 1977

Ezion T, Levy A, Levin Y, et al: Should electroconvulsive therapy be used as an ambulatory preventative treatment? Isr J Psychiatry Relat Sci 27:168–174, 1990

Faber R, Trimble MR: Electroconvulsive therapy in Parkinson's disease and other movement disorders. Mov Disord 6:293–303, 1991

Fahy P, Imlah N, Harrington J: A controlled comparison of electroconvulsive therapy, imipramine, and thiopentone sleep in depression. Journal of Neuropsychiatry 4:310–314, 1963

Fantz RM, Markowitz JS, Kellner CH: Sumatriptan for post-ECT headache. J ECT 14:272–274, 1998

Farah A, McCall WV: Electroconvulsive therapy stimulus dosing: a survey of contemporary practices. Convuls Ther 9:90–94, 1993

Farah A, McCall WV: ECT administration to a hyperthyroid patient. Convuls Ther 11:126–128, 1995

Farah A, Beale MD, Kellner CH: Risperidone and ECT combination therapy: a case series. Convuls Ther 11:280–282, 1995

Farah A, McCall WV, Amundson RH: ECT after cerebral aneurysm repair. Convuls Ther 12:165–170, 1996

Fava M, Davidson RG: Definition and epidemiology of treatment-resistant depression. Psychiatr Clin North Am 19:179–200, 1996

Fava M, Kaji J: Continuation and maintenance treatments of major depressive disorder. Psychiatric Annals 24:281–290, 1994

Fawver J, Milstein V: Asthma/emphysema complication of electroconvulsive therapy: a case study. Convuls Ther 1:61–64, 1985

Fear CF, Littlejohns CS, Rouse E, et al: Propofol anaesthesia in electroconvulsive therapy: reduced seizure duration may not be relevant. Br J Psychiatry 165:506–509, 1994

Ferrill MJ, Kehoe WA, Jacisin JJ: ECT during pregnancy: physiologic and pharmacologic considerations. Convuls Ther 8:186–200, 1992

Figiel GS, Jarvis MR: ECT in a depressed patient receiving bupropion. J Clin Psychopharmacol 10:376, 1990

Figiel GS, Coffey CE, Djang WT, et al: Brain magnetic resonance imaging findings in ECT-induced delirium. J Neuropsychiatry Clin Neurosci 2:53–58, 1990

Figiel GS, Hassen MA, Zorumski C, et al: ECT-induced delirium in depressed patients with Parkinson's disease. J Neuropsychiatry Clin Neurosci 3:405–411, 1991

Figiel GS, DeLeo B, Zorumski CF, et al: Combined use of labetalol and nifedipine in controlling the cardiovascular response from ECT. J Geriatr Psychiatry Neurol 6:20–24, 1993

Figiel GS, McDonald L, LaPlante R: Cardiovascular complications of ECT. Am J Psychiatry 151:790–791, 1994

Finestone DH, Weiner RD: Effects of ECT on diabetes mellitus: an attempt to account for conflicting data. Acta Psychiatr Scand 70:321–326, 1984

Fink M: Convulsive therapy: theory and practice. New York, Raven Press, 1979

Fink M: Meduna and the origins of convulsive therapy. Am J Psychiatry 141:1034–1041, 1984

Fink M: Training in convulsive therapy (editorial). Convuls Ther 2:227–229, 1986

Fink M: New technology in convulsive therapy: a challenge in training. Am J Psychiatry 144:1195–1198, 1987

Fink M: Is catatonia a primary indication for ECT? Convuls Ther 5:1–4, 1989

Fink M: Electroconvulsive therapy in children and adolescents (editorial). Convuls Ther 9:155–157, 1993

Fink M: Electroshock: Restoring the Mind. New York, Oxford University, 1999

Fink M, Coffey CE: ECT in pediatric neuropsychiatry, in Textbook of Pediatric Neuropsychiatry. Edited by Coffey CE, Brumback R. Washington, DC, American Psychiatric Press, 1998, pp 1389–1408

Fink M, Kellner CH: Certification in ECT (editorial). J ECT 14:1–4, 1998

Fink M, Sackeim HA: Convulsive therapy in schizophrenia? Schizophr Bull 22:27–39, 1996

Fink M, Sackeim HA: Theophylline and the risk of status epilepticus in ECT. J ECT 14:286–290, 1998

Fink M, Abrams R, Bailine S, et al: Ambulatory electroconvulsive therapy: report of a task force of the Association for Convulsive Therapy. Convuls Ther 12:42–55, 1996

Fink M, Kellner CH, Sackeim HA: Intractable seizures, status epilepticus, and ECT J ECT 15:282–284, 1999

Finlayson AJ, Vieweg WV, Wilkey WD, et al: Hyponatremic seizure following ECT. Can J Psychiatry 34:463–464, 1989

Fisher DM, Kahwaji R, Bevan D, et al: Factors affecting the pharmacokinetic characteristics of rapacuronium. Anesthesiology 90:993–1000, 1999

Fleminger JJ, Horne DJ, Nair NPV, et al: Differential effect of unilateral and bilateral ECT. Am J Psychiatry 127:430–436, 1970

Flint AJ, Rifat SL: The effect of sequential antidepressant treatment on geriatric depression. J Affect Disord 36:95–105, 1996

Flint AJ, Rifat SL: Two-year outcome of psychotic depression in late life. Am J Psychiatry 155:178–183, 1998

Flor-Henry P: Electroconvulsive therapy and lateralized affective systems. Ann N Y Acad Sci 462:389–397, 1986

Fochtmann LJ: Animal studies of electroconvulsive therapy: foundations for future research. Psychopharmacol Bull 30:321–444, 1994

Folkerts H: Electroconvulsive therapy in neurologic diseases. Nervenarzt 66:241–251, 1995

Folkerts H: The ictal electroencephalogram as a marker for the efficacy of electroconvulsive therapy. Eur Arch Psychiatry Clin Neurosci 246:155–164, 1996

Folkerts HW, Michael N, Tolle R, et al: Electroconvulsive therapy vs. paroxetine in treatment-resistant depression: a radnomized study. Acta Psychiatr Scand 96:334–342, 1997

Folstein M, Folstein S, McHugh PR: Clinical predictors of improvement after electroconvulsive therapy of patients with schizophrenia, neurotic reactions, and affective disorders. Biol Psychiatry 7:147–152, 1973

Folstein M, Folstein S, McHugh P: "Mini-Mental State." J Psychiatric Res 12:189–198, 1975

Fox HA: Patients' fear of and objection to electroconvulsive therapy. Hospital and Community Psychiatry 44:357–360, 1993

Fox HA: Continuation and maintenance ECT. Journal of Practical Psychiatry and Behavioral Health 6:357–363, 1996

Francis A, Fochtmann L: Caffeine augmentation of electroconvulsive seizures. Psychopharmacology (Berl) 115:320–324, 1994

Frankenburg FR, Suppes T, McLean PE: Combined clozapine and electroconvulsive therapy. Convuls Ther 9:176–180, 1993

Fraser RM, Glass IB: Recovery from ECT in elderly patients. Br J Psychiatry 133:524–528, 1978

Fraser RM, Glass IB: Unilateral and bilateral ECT in elderly patients: a comparative study. Acta Psychiatr Scand 62:13–31, 1980

Frasure-Smith N, L'Esperance F, Talajic M: Depression following myocardial infarction: impact on 6-month survival. JAMA 270:1819–1825, 1993

Fredman B, d'Etienne J, Smith I, et al: Anesthesia for electroconvulsive therapy: effects of propofol and methohexital on seizure activity and recovery. Anesth Analg 79:75–79, 1994

Freeman CP, Cheshire KE: Attitude studies on electroconvulsive therapy. Convuls Ther 2:31–42, 1986

Freeman CP, Kendell RE: ECT, I: patients' experiences and attitudes. Br J Psychiatry 137:8–16, 1980

Freeman CP, Kendell RE: Patients' experiences of and attitudes to electroconvulsive therapy. Ann N Y Acad Sci 462:341–352, 1986

Freeman CP, Basson JV, Crighton A: Double-blind controlled trial of electroconvulsive therapy (ECT) and simulated ECT in depressive illness. Lancet 1:738–740, 1978

Freeman CP, Weeks D, Kendell RE: ECT, II: patients who complain. Br J Psychiatry 137:17–25, 1980

Freese KJ: Can patients safely undergo electroconvulsive therapy while receiving monoamine oxidase inhibitors? Convuls Ther 1:190–194, 1985

Fricchione GL, Kaufman LD, Gruber BL, et al: Electroconvulsive therapy and cyclophosphamide in combination for severe neuropsychiatric lupus with catatonia. Am J Med 88:442–443, 1990

Fried D, Mann JJ: Electroconvulsive treatment of a patient with known intracranial tumor. Biol Psychiatry 23:176–180, 1988

Friedel RO: The combined use of neuroleptics and ECT in drug resistant schizophrenic patients. Psychopharmacol Bull 22:928–930, 1986

Friedman J: Teratogen update: anesthetic agents. Teratology 37:69–77, 1988

Friedman J, Gordon N: Electroconvulsive therapy in Parkinson's disease: a report on five cases. Convuls Ther 8:204–210, 1992

Frith CD, Stevens M, Johnstone EC, et al: Effects of ECT and depression on various aspects of memory. Br J Psychiatry 142:610–617, 1983

Frith CD, Stevens M, Johnstone EC, et al: A comparison of some retrograde and anterograde effects of electroconvulsive shock in patients with severe depression. Br J Psychol 78:53–63, 1987

Froimson L, Creed P, Mathew L: State of the art: nursing knowledge and electroconvulsive therapy. Convuls Ther 11:205–211, 1995

Fromholt P, Christensen AL, Strömgren LS: The effects of unilateral and bilateral electroconvulsive therapy on memory. Acta Psychiatr Scand 49:466–478, 1973

Fu W, Stool LA, White PF, et al: Is oral clonidine effective in modifying the acute hemodynamic response during electroconvulsive therapy? Anesth Analg 86:1127–1130, 1998

Fuenmayor AJ, el Fakih Y, Moreno J, et al: Effects of electroconvulsive therapy on cardiac function in patients without heart disease. Cardiology 88:254–257, 1997

Gaines GY III, Rees DI: Electroconvulsive therapy and anesthetic considerations. Anesth Analg 65:1345–1356, 1986

Gaitz CM, Pokorny AD, Mills MJ: Death following electroconvulsive therapy. AMA Archives of Neurology and Psychiatry (Chicago) 75:493–499, 1956

Gangadhar BN (ed): Proceedings of the National Workshop on ECT: Priorities for Research and Practice in India. Bangalore, India, National Institute of Mental Health and Neurologic Sciences, 1992

Gangadhar BN, Kapur RL, Kalyanasundaram S: Comparison of electroconvulsive therapy with imipramine in endogenous depression: a double blind study. Br J Psychiatry 141:367–371, 1982

Gangadhar BN, Janakiramaiah N, Subbakrishna DK, et al: Twice versus thrice weekly ECT in melancholia: a double-blind prospective comparison. J Affect Disord 27:273–278, 1993

Gangadhar BN, Girish K, Janakiramaiah N, et al: Formula method for stimulus setting in bilateral electroconvulsive therapy: relevance of age. J ECT 14:259–265, 1998

Garrett MD: Use of ECT in a depressed hypothyroid patient. J Clin Psychiatry 46:64–66, 1985

Gaspar D, Samarasinghe LA: ECT in psychogeriatric practice: a study of risk factors, indications and outcome. Compr Psychiatry 23:170–175, 1982

Gass JP: The knowledge and attitudes of mental health nurses to electro-convulsive therapy. J Adv Nurs 27:83–90, 1998

Geaney D: Electroconvulsive therapy: the official video of the Royal College of Psychiatrists Special Committee on ECT. Psychiatric Bulletin 17:702–703, 1993

Geretsegger C, Rochowanski E: Electroconvulsive therapy in acute life-threatening catatonia with associated cardiac and respiratory decompensation. Convuls Ther 3:291–295, 1987

Gerson SC, Plotkin DA, Jarvik LF: Antidepressant drug studies, 1964 to 1986: empirical evidence for aging patients. J Clin Psychopharmacol 8:311–322, 1988

Ghaziuddin N, King CA, Naylor MW, et al: Electroconvulsive treatment in adolescents with pharmacotherapy-refractory depression. J Child Adolesc Psychopharmacol 6:259–271, 1996

Girish K, Jayaprakash MS, Gangadhar BN, et al: Etophylline as a proconvulsant. Convuls Ther 12:196–198, 1996

Gitlin MC, Jahr JS, Margolis MA, et al: Is mivacurium chloride effective in electroconvulsive therapy? A report of four cases, including a patient with myasthenia gravis. Anesth Analg 77:392–394, 1993

Glassman AH, Shapiro PA: Depression and the course of coronary artery disease. Am J Psychiatry 155:4–11, 1998

Godemann F, Hellweg R: 20 years' unsuccessful prevention of bipolar affective psychosis recurrence. Nervenarzt 68:582–585, 1997

Goetz KL, Price TRP: Electroconvulsive therapy in Creutzfeldt-Jakob disease. Convuls Ther 9:58–62, 1993

Gold L, Chiarello CJ: Prognostic value of clinical findings in cases treated with electroshock. J Nerv Ment Dis 100:577–583, 1944

Gold MI, Duarte I, Muravchick S: Arterial oxygenation in conscious patients after 5 minutes and after 30 seconds of oxygen breathing. Anesth Analg 60:313–315, 1981

Goldberg E, Barnett J: The Goldberg-Barnett Remote Memory Questionnaire. New York, Albert Einstein Medical College, 1985

Goldberg RJ, Badger JM: Major depressive disorder in patients with the implantable cardioverter defibrillator: two cases treated with ECT. Psychosomatics 34:273–277, 1993

Goldbloom DS, Kussin DJ: Electroconvulsive therapy training in Canada: a survey of senior residents in psychiatry. Can J Psychiatry 36:126–128, 1991

Goldfarb W, Kieve H: The treatment of psychotic like regressions of combat soldiers. Psychiatr Q 19:555–565, 1945

Goldman D: Brief stimulus electric shock therapy. J Nerv Ment Dis 110:36–45, 1949

Goldstein DJ, Corbin LA, Sundell KL: Effects of first-trimester fluoxetine exposure on the newborn. Obstet Gynecol 89:713–718, 1997

Gomez J: Subjective side-effects of ECT. Br J Psychiatry 127:609–611, 1975

Goodwin FK: New directions for ECT research. Psychopharmacol Bull 30:265–268, 1994

Goodwin FK, Jamison KR: Manic-Depressive Illness. New York, Oxford University, 1990

Goswami U, Dutta S, Kuruvilla K, et al: Electroconvulsive therapy in neuroleptic-induced parkinsonism. Biol Psychiatry 26:234–238, 1989

Gottlieb JS, Huston PE: Treatment of schizophrenia. J Nerv Ment Dis 113:237–246, 1951

Green A, Nutt D, Cowen P: Increased seizure threshold following convulsion, in Psychopharmacology of Anticonvulsants. Edited by Sandler M. Oxford, England, Oxford University Press, 1982, pp 16–26

Greenan J, Dewar M, Jones C: Intravenous glycopyrrolate and atropine at the induction of anaethesia: a comparison. J R Soc Med 76:369–371, 1985

Greenberg LB, Mofson R, Fink M: Prospective electroconvulsive therapy in a delusional depressed patient with a frontal meningioma: a case report. Br J Psychiatry 153:105–107, 1988

Greenberg LB, Boccio RV, Fink M: A comparison of etomidate and methohexital anesthesia forelectroconvulsive therapy. Ann Clin Psychiatry 1:39–42, 1989

Greenberg RM, Pettinati HM: Benzodiazepines and electroconvulsive therapy. Convuls Ther 9:262–273, 1993

Greenblatt M, Grosser GH, Wechsler HA: A comparative study of selected anti-depressant medications and ECT. Am J Psychiatry 119:144–153, 1962

Greenblatt M, Grooser GH, Wechsler HA: Differential response of hospitalized depressed patients in somatic therapy. Am J Psychiatry 120:935–943, 1964

Greer RA, Stewart RB: Hyponatremia and ECT. Am J Psychiatry 150:1272, 1993

Gregory S, Shawcross CR, Gill D: The Nottingham ECT Study: a double-blind comparison of bilateral, unilateral, and simulated ECT in depressive ill-ness. Br J Psychiatry 146:520–524, 1985

Griesemer DA, Kellner CH, Beale MD, et al: Electroconvulsive therapy for treat-ment of intractable seizures: initial findings in two children. Neurology 49:1389–1392, 1997

Grisso T, Appelbaum PS: Comparison of standards for assessing patients' capacities to make treatment decisions. Am J Psychiatry 152:1033–1037, 1995

Grogan R, Wagner DR, Sullivan T, et al: Generalized nonconvulsive status epi-lepticus after electroconvulsive therapy. Convuls Ther 11:51–56, 1995

Grossman J: Electroconvulsive therapy for patient with cardiac pacemaker. JAMA 255:1501, 1986

Gruber RP: ECT for obsessive-compulsive symptoms (possible mechanisms of action). Diseases of the Nervous System 32:180–182, 1971

Grunhaus L, Dilsaver S, Greden JF, et al: Depressive pseudodementia: a sug-gested diagnostic profile. Biol Psychiatry 18:215–225, 1983

Grunhaus L, Pande AC, Haskett RF: Full and abbreviated courses of mainte-nance electroconvulsive therapy. Convuls Ther 6:130–138, 1990

Grunhaus L, Dolberg O, Lustig M: Relapse and recurrence following a course of ECT: reasons for concern and strategies for further investigation. J Psychi-atr Res 29:165–172, 1995

Guay J, Grenier Y, Varin F: Clinical pharmacokinetics of neuromuscular relax-ants in pregnancy. Clin Pharmacokinet 34:483–496, 1998

Gujavarty K, Greenberg LB, Fink M: Electroconvulsive therapy and neuroleptic medication in therapy-resistant positive-symptom psychosis. Convuls Ther 3:185–195, 1987

Gunderson-Falcone G: Developing an outpatient electroconvulsive therapy program: a nursing perspective. Convuls Ther 11:202–204, 1995

Gustafson Y, Nilsson I, Mattsson M, et al: Epidemiology and treatment of post-stroke depression. Drugs Aging 7:298–309, 1995

Gutheil TG, Bursztajn H: Clinician's guidelines for assessing and presenting subtle forms of patient incompetence in legal settings. Am J Psychiatry 137:586–591, 1986

Gutierrez Esteinou R, Pope HG: Does fluoxetine prolong electrically induced seizures? Convuls Ther 5:344–348, 1989

Guttmacher LB, Cretella H: Electroconvulsive therapy in one child and three adolescents. J Clin Psychiatry 49:20–23, 1988

Guttmann E, Mayer-Gross W, Slater ETO: Short-distance prognosis of schizophrenia. Journal of Neurology and Psychiatry 2:25–34, 1939

Guze BH, Baxter LR Jr, Liston EH, et al: Attorneys' perceptions of electroconvulsive therapy: impact of instruction with an ECT videotape demonstration. Compr Psychiatr 29:520–522, 1988

Guze SB: The occurrence of psychiatric illness in systemic lupus erythematosus. Am J Psychiatry 123:1562–1570, 1967

Haddad PM, Benbow SM: Electroconvulsive therapy–related psychiatric knowledge among British anesthetists. Convuls Ther 9:101–107, 1993

Hafeiz HB: Psychiatric manifestations of enteric fever. Acta Psychiatr Scand 75:69–73, 1987

Hagemann TM: Gastrointestinal medications and breastfeeding. Journal of Human Lactation 14:259–262, 1998

Hall MJ, Kozak LJ, Gillum BS: National survey of ambulatory surgery 1994. Statistical Bulletin of the Metropolitan Insurance Company 78:18–27, 1997

Halliday G, Johnson G: Training to administer electroconvulsive therapy: a survey of attitudes and experiences. Aust N Z J Psychiatr 29:133–138, 1995

Halsall SM, Lock T, Atkinson A: Nursing guidelines for ECT, in Royal College of Psychiatrists, The ECT Handbook: The Second Report of the Royal College of Psychiatrists' Special Committee on ECT. London, England, Royal College of Psychiatrists, 1995, pp 114–121

Hamilton DM, Wall JH: The hospital treatment of dementia praecox. Am J Psychiatry 105:346–352, 1948

Hamilton M: Development of a rating scale for primary depressive illness. Br J Soc Clin Psychol 6:278–296, 1967

Hamilton M: Electroconvulsive therapy. Indications and contraindications. Ann N Y Acad Sci 462:5–11, 1986

Hamilton M, White J: Factors related to the outcome of depression treated with ECT. Journal of Mental Science 106:1031–1041, 1960

Hamilton RW, Walter-Ryan WG: ECT and thrombocythemia (letter). Am J Psychiatry 143:258, 1986

Hanin B, Lerner Y, Srour N: An unusual effect of ECT on drug-induced parkinsonism and tardive dystonia. Convuls Ther 11:271–274, 1995

Hannay HJ, Levin HS: Selective reminding test: an examination of the equivalence of four forms. J Clin Exp Neuropsychol 7:251–263, 1985

Hanretta AT, Malek-Ahmadi P: Use of ECT in a patient with a Harrington rod implant. Convuls Ther 11:266–270, 1995

Harsch HH: Atrial fibrillation, cardioversion, and electroconvulsive therapy. Convuls Ther 7:139–142, 1991

Harsch HH, Haddox JD: Electroconvulsive therapy and fluoxetine (letter). Convuls Ther 6:250–251, 1990

Hartmann SJ, Saldivia A: ECT in an elderly patient with skull defects and shrapnel. Convuls Ther 6:165–171, 1990

Heath ES, Adams A, Wakeling PL: Short courses of ECT and simulated ECT in chronic schizophrenia. Br J Psychiatry 110:800–807, 1964

Heinonen OP, Slone D, Shapiro S: Birth Defects and Drugs in Pregnancy. Littleton, MA, Publishing Sciences Group, 1977

Henderson T: Administration of electroconvulsive therapy: training, practice, and attitudes. Psychiatric Bulletin 17:154–155, 1993

Hermann RC, Ettner SL, Dorwart RA, et al: Characteristics of psychiatrists who perform ECT. Am J Psychiatry 155:889–894, 1998

Hermesh H, Aizenberg D, Weizman A: A successful electroconvulsive treatment of neuroleptic malignant syndrome. Acta Psychiatr Scand 75:237–239, 1987

Hermesh H, Aizenberg D, Friedberg G, et al: Electroconvulsive therapy for persistent neuroleptic-induced akathisia and parkinsonism: a case report. Biol Psychiatry 31:407–411, 1992

Hermle L, Oepen G: Differential diagnosis of acute life threatening catatonia and malignant neuroleptic syndrome: a case report. Fortschr Neurol Psychiatr 54:189–195, 1986

Herz DA, Looman JE, Lewis SK: Informed consent: is it a myth? Neurosurgery 31:380–381, 1992

Herzberg F: Prognostic variables for electro-shock therapy. J Gen Psychol 50:79–86, 1954

Herzog A, Detre T: Psychotic reactions associated with childbirth. Diseases of the Nervous System 37:229–235, 1976

Heshe J, Röder E: Electroconvulsive therapy in Denmark: review of the technique, employment, indications, and complications. Ugeskr Laeger 137:939–944, 1975

Heshe J, Röder E: Electroconvulsive therapy in Denmark. Br J Psychiatry 128:241–245, 1976

Heshe J, Röder E, Theilgaard A: Unilateral and bilateral ECT: a psychiatric and psychological study of therapeutic effect and side effects. Acta Psychiatr Scand Suppl 275:1–180, 1978

Hickey DR, O'Connor JP, Donati F: Comparison of atracurium and succinylcholine for electroconvulsive therapy in a patient with atypical plasma cholinesterase. Can J Anaesth 34:280–283, 1987

Hickie I, Parsonage B, Parker G: Prediction of response to electroconvulsive therapy: preliminary validation of a sign-based typology of depression. Br J Psychiatry 157:65–71, 1990

Hickie I, Mason C, Parker G, et al: Prediction of ECT response: validation of a refined sign-based (CORE) system for defining melancholia (see comments). Br J Psychiatry 169:68–74, 1996

Hicks FG: ECT modified by atracurium. Convuls Ther 3:54–59, 1987

Hill MA, Courvoisie H, Dawkins K, et al: ECT for the treatment of intractable mania in two prepubertal male children. Convuls Ther 13:74–82, 1997

Himmelhoch JM, Neil JF, May SJ, et al: Age, dementia, dyskineisa, and lithium response. Am J Psychiatry 137:941–945, 1980

Hinkle PE, Coffey CE, Weiner RD, et al: Use of caffeine to lengthen seizures in ECT. Am J Psychiatry 144:1143–1148, 1987

Hobson RF: Prognostic factors in ECT. J Neurol Neurosurg Psychiatry 16:275–281, 1953

Höflich G, Kasper S, Burghof KW, et al: Maintenance ECT for treatment of therapy-resistant paranoid schizophrenia and Parkinson's disease. Biol Psychiatry 37:892–894, 1995

Holmberg G: The influence of oxygen administration on electrically induced convulsions in man. Acta Psychiatrica et Neurologica Scandinavica 28:365–386, 1953

Hood DD, Mecca RS: Failure to initiate electroconvulsive seizures in a patient pretreated with lidocaine. Anesthesiology 58:379–381, 1983

House A: Depression after stroke. BMJ 294:76–78, 1987

Hovorka EJ, Schumsky DA, Work MS: Electroconvulsive thresholds as related to stimulus parameters of unidirectional ECS. Journal of Comparative and Physiological Psychology 53:412–414, 1960

Howie MB, Black HA, Zvara D, et al: Esmolol reduces autonomic hypersensitivity and length of seizures induced by electroconvulsive therapy. Anesth Analg 71:384–388, 1990

Hsiao JK, Evans DL: ECT in a depressed patient after craniotomy. Am J Psychiatry 141:442–444, 1984

Hsiao JK, Messenheimer JA, Evans DL: ECT and neurological disorders. Convuls Ther 3:121–136, 1987

Husain MM, Meyer DE, Muttakin MH, et al: Maintenance ECT for treatment of recurrent mania (letter). Am J Psychiatry 150:985, 1993

Huston PE, Strother CR: The effect of electric shock on mental efficiency. Am J Psychiatry 104:707–712, 1948

Hutchinson JT, Smedberg D: Treatment of depression: a comparative study of ECT and six drugs. Br J Psychiatry 109:536–538, 1963

Hutson MM, Blaha JD: Patients' recall of preoperative instruction for informed consent for an operation. J Bone Joint Surg 73:160–162, 1991

Hyman SE, Nestler EJ: Initiation and adaptation: a paradigm for understanding psychotropic drug action. Am J Psychiatry 153:151–162, 1996

Hyrman V, Palmer LH, Cernik J, et al: ECT: the search for the perfect stimulus. Biol Psychiatry 20:634–645, 1985

Ilivicky H, Caroff SN, Simone AF: Etomidate during ECT for elderly seizure-resistant patients. Am J Psychiatry 152:957–958, 1995

Imlah NW, Ryan E, Harrington JA: The influence of antidepressant drugs on the response to electroconvulsive therapy and on subsequent relapse rates. Neuropsychopharmacology 4:438–442, 1965

Impastato D, Almansi N: A study of over 2000 cases of electrofit treated patients. N Z Med J 43:2057–2065, 1943

Ingvar M: Cerebral blood flow and metabolic rate during seizures: relationship to epileptic brain damage. Ann N Y Acad Sci 462:194–206, 1986

Irving AD, Drayson AM: Bladder rupture during ECT. Br J Psychiatry 144:670, 1984

Jackson B: The effects of unilateral and bilateral ECT on verbal and visual spatial memory. J Clin Psychol 34:4–13, 1978

Jacobsma B: A balancing act: continuing education for staff nurses. J Psychosoc Nurs Ment Health Serv 29:15–21, 1991

Jaffe R, Shoyer B, Siegel L, et al: An assessment of psychiatric residents' knowledge and attitudes regarding ECT. Academic Psychiatry 14:204–210, 1990a

Jaffe R, Brubaker G, Dubin WR, et al: Caffeine-associated cardiac dysrhythmia during ECT: report of three cases. Convuls Ther 6:308–313, 1990b

Jaffe R, Dubin W, Shoyer B, et al: Outpatient electroconvulsive therapy: efficacy and safety. Convuls Ther 6:231–238, 1990c

Jaffe RL, Rives W, Dubin WR, et al: Problems in maintenance ECT in bipolar disorder: replacement by lithium and anticonvulsants. Convuls Ther 7:288–294, 1991

Janakiramaiah N, Channabasavanna SM, Murthy NS: ECT/chlorpromazine combination versus chlorpromazine alone in acutely schizophrenic patients. Acta Psychiatr Scand 66:464–470, 1982

Janakiramaiah N, Motreja S, Gangadhar BN, et al: Once vs. three times weekly ECT in melancholia: a randomized controlled trial. Acta Psychiatr Scand 98:316–320, 1998

Janicak PG, Davis JM, Gibbons RD, et al: Efficacy of ECT: a meta-analysis. Am J Psychiatry 142:297–302, 1985

Janike MA, Baer L, Minichiello WE: Somatic treatments for obsessive-compulsive disorders. Compr Psychiatry 28:250–263, 1987

Janis IL: Psychologic effects of electric convulsive treatments (I: post-treatment amnesias). J Nerv Ment Dis 111:359–382, 1950

Janis K, Hess J, Fabian JA, et al: Substitution of mivacurium for succinylcholine for ECT in elderly patients. Can J Anaesth 42:612–613, 1995

Jarvis MR, Goewert AJ, Zorumski CF: Novel antidepressants and maintenance electroconvulsive therapy: a review. Ann Clin Psychiatry 4:275–284, 1992

Jeanneau A: Electroconvulsive therapy in the treatment of Parkinson disease. Encephale 19:573–578, 1993

Jha AK, Stein GS, Fenwick P: Negative interaction between lithium and electroconvulsive therapy: a case-control study. Br J Psychiatry 168:241–243, 1996

Johnson SY: Regulatory pressures hamper the effectiveness of electroconvulsive therapy. Law and Psychology Review 17:155–170, 1993

Johnstone EC, Deakin JF, Lawler P, et al: The Northwick Park electroconvulsive therapy trial. Lancet 2:1317–1320, 1980

Jones BP, Henderson M, Welch CA: Executive functions in unipolar depression before and after electroconvulsive therapy. Int J Neurosci 38:287–297, 1988

Kales H, Raz J, Tandon R, et al: Relationship of seizure duration to antidepressant efficacy in electroconvulsive therapy. Psychol Med 27:1373–1380, 1997

Kalinowsky LB: Electric convulsion therapy with emphasis on importance of adequate treatment. AMA Archives of Neurology and Psychiatry (Chicago) 50:652–660, 1943

Kalinowsky LB, Hoch PH: Shock Treatments and Other Somatic Procedures in Psychiatry. New York, Grune & Stratton, 1946

Kalinowsky LB, Hoch PH: Somatic Treatments in Psychiatry. New York, Grune & Stratton, 1961

Kalinowsky LB, Kennedy F: Observation in electroschock therapy applied to problems in epilepsy. J Nerv Ment Dis 98:56–67, 1943

Kalinowsky LB, Worthing H: Results with electric convulsive therapy in 200 cases of schizophrenia. Psychiatr Q 17:144–153, 1943

Kant R, Bogyi AM, Carosella NW, et al: ECT as a therapeutic option in severe brain injury. Convuls Ther 11:45–50, 1995

Kant R, Coffey CE, Bogyi AM: Safety and efficacy of ECT in patients with head injury. J Neuropsychiatry Clin Neurosci 11:32–37, 1999

Kanto JH: Use of benzodiazepines during pregnancy, labour and lactation, with particular reference to pharmacokinetic considerations. Drugs 23:354–380, 1982

Kardener SH: EST in a patient with idiopathic thrombocytopenic purpura. Diseases of the Nervous System 29:465–466, 1968

Karliner W: Electroshock therapy in the presence of retinal detachment. Diseases of the Nervous System 19:401, 1958

Katona CL: Puerperal mental illness: comparisons with non-puerperal controls. Br J Psychiatry 141:447–452, 1982

Katz G: Electroconvulsive therapy from a social work perspective. Social Work Health Care 16:55–68, 1992

Katz PO, Castell DO: Gastroesophageal reflux disease during pregnancy. Gastroenterol Clin North Am 27:153–167, 1998

Kaufman KR: Asystole with electroconvulsive therapy. J Intern Med 235:275–277, 1994

Kay DW, Fahy T, Garside RF: A seven-month double-blind trial of amitriptyline and diazepam in ECT-treated depressed patients. Br J Psychiatry 117:667–671, 1970

Kellam AMP: The neuroleptic malignant syndrome. Br J Psychiatry 150:752–759, 1987

Keller MB, Lavori PW, Klerman GL, et al: Low levels and lack of predictors of somatotherapy and psychotherapy received by depressed patients. Arch Gen Psychiatry 43:458–466, 1986

Kellner C (ed): Electroconvulsive therapy. Psychiatr Clin North Am Dec:793–1035, 1991

Kellner CH: The cognitive effects of ECT: bridging the gap between research and clinical practice (editorial). Convuls Ther 12:133–135, 1996a

Kellner CH: The CT scan (or MRI) before ECT: a wonderful test has been overused (editorial). Convuls Ther 12:79–80, 1996b

Kellner CH, Bernstein HJ: ECT as a treatment for neurologic illness, in The Clinical Science of Electroconvulsive Therapy. Edited by Coffey CE. Washington, DC, American Psychiatric Press, 1993, pp 183–210

Kellner CH, Bruno RM: Fluoxetine and ECT (letter). Convuls Ther 5:367–368, 1989

Kellner CH, Rames L: Dexamethasone pretreatment for ECT in a patient with meningioma. Clinical Gerontologist 10:67–72, 1990

Kellner C, Batterson JR, Monroe R: ECT as an alternative to lithium for preventive treatment of bipolar disorder. Am J Psychiatry 147:953, 1990

Kellner CH, Monroe RR, Burns CM, et al: Electroconvulsive therapy in a patient with a heart transplant. N Engl J Med 325:663, 1991a

Kellner CH, Tolhurst JE, Burns CM: ECT in the presence of severe cervical spine disease (case report). Convuls Ther 7:52–55, 1991b

Kellner CH, Rubey RN, Burns C, et al: Safe administration of ECT in a patient taking selegiline. Convuls Ther 8:144–145, 1992

Kellner CH, Beale MD, Pritchett JT, et al: Electroconvulsive therapy and Parkinson's disease: the case for further study. Psychopharmacol Bull 30:495–500, 1994a

Kellner CH, Pritchett JT, Jackson CW: Bupropion coadministration with electroconvulsive therapy: two case reports. J Clin Psychopharmacology 14:215–216, 1994b

Kellner CH, Pritchett JT, Beale MD, et al: Handbook of ECT. Washington, DC, American Psychiatric Press, 1997

Kellner CH, Beale MD, Bernstein HJ: Electroconvulsive therapy, in Handbook of Child and Adolescent Psychiatry, Vol 6. Edited by Noshpitz JD. New York, Wiley, 1998, pp 269–272

Kelly D, Brull SJ: Neuroleptic malignant syndrome and mivacurium: a safe alternative to succinylcholine? Can J Anaesth 41:845–849, 1994

Kelway B, Simpson KH, Smith RJ, et al: Effects of atropine and glycopyrrolate on cognitive function following anaesthesia and electroconvulsive therapy (ECT). Int Clin Psychopharmacol 1:296–302, 1986

Kendell RE: Psychiatric diagnosis in Britain and the United States. Br J Psychiatry 9:453–461, 1975

Kennedy CJ, Anchel D: Regressive electric shock in schizophrenics refractory to other shock therapies. Psychiatr Q 22:317–320, 1948

Kessing L, LaBianca JH, Bolwig TG: HIV-induced stupor treated with ECT. Convuls Ther 10:232–235, 1994

Khanna S, Gangadhar BN, Sinha V, et al: Electroconvulsive therapy in obsessive-compulsive disorder. Convuls Ther 4:314–320, 1988

Kiloh LG: Pseudo-dementia. Acta Psychiatr Scand 37:336–351, 1961

Kiloh LG, Child JP, Latner G: A controlled trial of iproniazid in the treatment of endogenous depression. Journal of Mental Science 106:1139–1144, 1960

Kiloh LG, Smith JS, Johnson GF: Physical Treatments in Psychiatry. Melbourne, Australia, Blackwell Scientific, 1988

Kindler S, Shapira B, Hadjez J, et al: Factors influencing response to bilateral electroconvulsive therapy in major depression. Convuls Ther 7:245–254, 1991

King PD: Phenelzine and ECT in the treatment of depression. Am J Psychiatry 116:64–68, 1959

King PD: Chlorpromazine and electroconvulsive therapy in the treatment of newly hospitalized schizophrenics. J Clin Exp Psychopathol 21:101–105, 1960

Kino FF, Thorpe TF: Electrical convulsion therapy in 500 selected psychotics. Journal of Mental Science 92:138–145, 1946

Kirkby KC, Beckett WG, Matters RM, et al: Comparison of propofol and methohexitone in anaesthesia for ECT: effect on seizure duration and outcome. Aust N Z J Psychiatry 29:299–303, 1995

Klapheke MM: Clozapine, ECT, and schizoaffective disorder, bipolar type. Convuls Ther 7:36–39, 1991

Klapheke MM: Combining ECT and antipsychotic agents: benefits and risks. Convuls Ther 9:241–255, 1993

Klapheke MM: Electroconvulsive therapy consultation: an update. Convuls Ther 13:227–241, 1997

Koenig HG, Kuchibhatla M: Use of health services by hospitalized medically ill depressed elderly patients. Am J Psychiatry 155:871–877, 1998

Koester J: Voltage-gated channels and the generatioin of the action potential, in Principles of Neural Science. Edited by Kandel ER, Schwartz JH. New York, Elsevier, 1985, pp 75–86

Kolano JE, Chibber A, Calalang CC: Use of esmolol to control bleeding and heart rate during electroconvulsive therapy in a patient with an intracranial aneurysm. J Clin Anesth 9:493–495, 1997

König P, Glatter-Götz U: Combined electroconvulsive and neuroleptic therapy in schizophrenia refractory to neuroleptics. Schizophr Res 3:351–354, 1990

Koren G, Zemlickis DM: Outcome of pregnancy after first trimester exposure to H2 receptor antagonists. Am J Perinatol 8:37–38, 1991

Koren G, Pastuszak A, Ito S: Drugs in pregnancy. N Engl J Med 338:1128–1137, 1998

Korin H, Fink M, Kwalwasser S: Relation of changes in memory and learning to improvement in electroshock. Confinia Neurologica 16:83–96, 1956

Kovac AL, Goto H, Pardo MP, et al: Comparison of two esmolol bolus doses on the haemodynamic response and seizure duration during electroconvulsive therapy (comments). Can J Anaesth 38:204–209, 1991

Krahn LE, Rummans TA, Peterson GC, et al: Electroconvulsive therapy for depression after temporal lobectomy for epilepsy. Convuls Ther 9:217–219, 1993

Kramer BA: Use of ECT in California, 1977–1983. Am J Psychiatry 142:1190–1192, 1985

Kramer BA: Electroconvulsive therapy use in geriatric depression. J Nerv Ment Dis 175:233–235, 1987a

Kramer BA: Maintenance ECT: a survey of practice (1986). Convuls Ther 3:260–268, 1987b

Kramer BA: Maintenance electroconvulsive therapy in clinical practice. Convuls Ther 6:279–286, 1990

Kramer BA: Anticholinergics and ECT. Convuls Ther 9:293–300, 1993

Kramer BA: A naturalistic view of maintenance ECT at a university setting. J ECT 15:226–231, 1999

Kramer BA, Afrasiabi A: Atypical cholinesterase and prolonged apnea during electroconvulsive therapy. Convuls Ther 7:129–132, 1991

Kramer BA, Allen RE, Friedman B: Atropine and glycopyrrolate as ECT preanesthesia. J Clin Psychiatry 47:199–200, 1986

Kramer BA, Afrasiabi A, Pollock VE: Intravenous versus intramuscular atropine in ECT. Am J Psychiatry 149:1258–1260, 1992

Kramp P, Bolwig TG: Electroconvulsive therapy in acute delirious states. Compr Psychiatry 22:368–371, 1981

Kraus RP, Remick RA: Diazoxide in the management of severe hypertension after electroconvulsive therapy. Am J Psychiatry 139:504–505, 1982

Kreisman NR, Sick TJ, Rosenthal M: Importance of vascular responses in determining cortical oxygenation during recurrent paroxysmal events of varying duration and frequency of repetition. J Cereb Blood Flow Metab 3:330–339, 1983

Kristiansen ES: A comparison of treatment of endogenous depression with electroshock and with imipramine (Tofranil). Acta Psychiatr Scand 37:179–188, 1961

Kroessler D: Relative efficacy rates for therapies of delusional depression. Convuls Ther 1:173–182, 1985

Krueger RB, Sackeim HA: Electroconvulsive therapy and schizophrenia, in Schizophrenia. Edited by Hirsch SR, Weinberger D. Oxford, England, Blackwell Scientific, 1995, pp 503–545

Krueger RB, Sackeim HA, Gamzu ER: Pharmacological treatment of the cognitive side effects of ECT: a review. Psychopharmacol Bull 28:409–424, 1992

Krueger RB, Fama JM, Devanand DP, et al: Does ECT permanently alter seizure threshold? Biol Psychiatry 33:272–276, 1993

Krystal AD, Coffey CE: Neuropsychiatric considerations in the use of electro-convulsive therapy. J Neuropsychiatry Clin Neurosci 9:283–292, 1997

Krystal AD, Weiner RD, McCall WV, et al: The effects of ECT stimulus dose and electrode placement on the ictal electroencephalogram: an intraindividual crossover study. Biol Psychiatry 34:759–767, 1993

Krystal AD, Weiner RD, Coffey CE: The ictal EEG as a marker of adequate stimulus intensity with unilateral ECT. J Neuropsychiatry Clin Neurosci 7:295–303, 1995

Krystal AD, Weiner RD, Coffey CE, et al: Effect of ECT treatment number on the ictal EEG. Psychiatry Res 62:179–189, 1996

Krystal AD, Watts BV, Weiner RD, et al: The use of flumazenil in the anxious and benzodiazepine-dependent ECT patient. J ECT 14:5–14, 1998

Krystal AD, Dean MD, Weiner RD, et al: ECT stimulus intensity: are present ECT devices too limited? Am J Psychiatry 157:963–967, 2000

Kukopulos A, Reginaldi D, Tondo L, et al: Spontaneous length of depression and response to ECT. Psychol Med 7:625–629, 1977

Kulin NA, Pastuszak A, Sage SR, et al: Pregnancy outcome following maternal use of the new selective serotonin reuptake inhibitors: a prospective controlled multicenter study. JAMA 279:609–610, 1998

Kuller JA, Katz VL, McMahon MJ, et al: Pharmacologic treatment of psychiatric disease in pregnancy and lactation: fetal and neonatal effects. Obstet Gynecol 87:789–794, 1996

Kupfer DJ, Frank E, Perel JM, et al: Five-year outcomes for maintenance therapies in recurrent depression. Arch Gen Psychiatry 49:769–773, 1992

LaGrone D: ECT in secondary mania, pregnancy, and sickle cell anemia. Convuls Ther 6:176–180, 1990

Lambourn J, Gill D: A controlled comparison of simulated and real ECT. Br J Psychiatry 133:514–519, 1978

Landmark J, Joseph L, Merskey H: Characteristics of schizophrenic patients and the outcome of fluphenazine and of electroconvulsive treatments. Can J Psychiatry 32:425–428, 1987

Landy DA: Combined use of clozapine and electroconvulsive therapy. Convuls Ther 7:218–221, 1991

Langsley DG, Yager J: The definition of a psychiatrist: eight years later. Am J Psychiatry 145:469–475, 1988

Langsley DG, Enterline JD, Hickerson GXJ: A comparison of chlorpromazine and ECT in treatment of acute schizophrenic and manic reactions. Arch Neurol Psychiatry 81:384–391, 1959

Larrabee GJ, Levin HS: Memory self-ratings and objective test performance in a normal elderly sample. J Clin Exp Neuropsychol 8:275–284, 1986

Lauritzen L, Odgaard K, Clemmesen L, et al: Relapse prevention by means of paroxetine in ECT-treated patients with major depression: a comparison with imipramine and placebo in medium-term continuation therapy. Acta Psychiatr Scand 94:241–251, 1996

Lawson JS, Inglis J, Delva NJ, et al: Electrode placement in ECT: cognitive effects. Psychol Med 20:335–344, 1990

Lazarus A: Treatment of neuroleptic malignant syndrome with electroconvulsive therapy. J Nerv Ment Dis 174:47–49, 1986

Lebensohn ZM, Jenkins RB: Improvement of Parkinsonism in depressed patients treated with ECT. Am J Psychiatry 132:283–285, 1975

Lee JJ, Rubin AP: Breast feeding and anesthesia. Anesthesia 48:616–625, 1993

Leentjens AF, van den Broek WW, Kusuma A, et al: Facilitation of ECT by intravenous administration of theophylline. Convuls Ther 12:232–237, 1996

Leff JP, Wing JK: Trial of maintenance therapy in schizophrenia. BMJ 3:599–604, 1971

Lerer B, Shapira B, Calev A, et al: Antidepressant and cognitive effects of twice- versus three-times-weekly ECT. Am J Psychiatry 152:564–570, 1995

Letemendia FJ, Delva NJ, Rodenburg M, et al: Therapeutic advantage of bifrontal electrode placement in ECT. Psychol Med 23:349–360, 1993

Levin Y, Elizur A, Korczyn AD: Physostigmine improves ECT-induced memory disturbances. Neurology 37:871–875, 1987

Levine SB, Blank K, Schwartz HI, et al: Informed consent in the electroconvulsive treatment of geriatric patients. Bull Am Acad Psychiatry Law 19:395–403, 1991

Levy SD: "Cuff" monitoring, osteoporosis, and fracture. Convuls Ther 4:248–249, 1988

Lew JK, Eastley RJ, Hanning CD: Oxygenation during electroconvulsive therapy: a comparison of two anaesthetic techniques. Anaesthesia 41:1092–1097, 1986

Lewis AB: ECT in drug-refractory schizophrenics. Hillside Journal of Clinical Psychiatry 4:141–154, 1982

Lewis BS, Rabinowitz B, Schlesinger Z, et al: Effect of isosorbide-5-mononitrate on exercise performance and clinical status in patients with congestive heart failure: results of the Nitrates in Congestive Heart Failure (NICE) study. Cardiology 91:1–7, 1999

Lezak MD: Neuropsychological Assessment, 3rd Edition. New York, Oxford University Press, 1995

Liberson WT: Time factors in electric convulsive therapy. Yale J Biol Med 17:571–578, 1945

Liberson WT: Some technical observations concerning brief stimulus therapy. Digest of Neurology and Psychiatry 15:72–78, 1947

Liberson WT: Brief stimulus therapy: physiological and clinical observations. Am J Psychiatry 105:28–29, 1948

Lim SK, Lim WL, Elegbe EO: Comparison of propofol and methohexitone as an induction agent in anaesthesia for electroconvulsive therapy. West Afr J Med 15:186–189, 1996

Lippman SB, El-Mallakh R: Can electroconvulsive therapy be given during lithium treatment. Lithium 5:205–209, 1994

Lippman SB, Tao CA: Electroconvulsive therapy and lithium: safe and effective treatment. Convuls Ther 9:54–57, 1993

Lippman S, Manshadi M, Wehry M, et al: 1,250 electroconvulsive treatments without evidence of brain injury. Br J Psychiatry 147:203–204, 1985

Lisanby SH, Devanand DP, Nobler MS, et al: Exceptionally high seizure threshold: ECT device limitations. Convuls Ther 12:156–164, 1996

Lisanby S, Luber B, Osman M, et al: The effect of pulse width on seizure threshold during electroconvulsive shock (ECS). Convul Ther 13:56, 1997

Lisanby SH, Sackeim HA: Therapeutic brain interventions and the nature of emotion, in The Neuropsychology of Emotion. Edited by Borod J. New York, Oxford University Press, 2000, pp 456–491

Lisanby SH, Maddox JH, Prudic J, et al: The effects of electroconvulsive therapy on memory of autobiographical and public events. Arch Gen Psychiatry 57:581–590, 2000

Livingston JC, Johnstone WM Jr, Hadi HA: Electroconvulsive therapy in a twin pregnancy: a case report. Am J Perinatol 11:116–118, 1994

Llewellyn A, Stowe ZN: Psychotropic medications in lactation. J Clin Psychiatry 59(suppl 2):41–52, 1998

Lohr WD, Figiel GS, Hudziak JJ, et al: Maintenance electroconvulsive therapy in schizophrenia (letter). J Clin Psychiatr 55:217–218, 1994

Longcope JC, Fink M: Guidelines for long-term use of electroconvulsive therapy. JAMA 264:1174, 1990

Lôo H, de Carvalho W, Galinowski A: Towards the rehabilitation of maintenance electroconvulsive therapy? Ann Med Psychol (Paris) 148:1–15, 1990

Lowenstein DH, Alldredge BK: Status epilepticus. N Engl J Med 338:970–976, 1998

Lowinger L, Huddleson JH: Outcome on dementia praecox under electric shock therapy as related to mode of onset and to number of convulsions induced. J Nerv Ment Dis 102:243–246, 1945

Luber B, Nobler MS, Moeller JR, et al: Quantitative EEG during seizures induced by electroconvulsive therapy: relations to treatment modality and clinical features, II. Topographic analyses. J ECT, in press

Lui PW, Ma JY, Chan KK: Modification of tonic-clonic convulsions by atracurium in multiple-monitored electroconvulsive therapy. J Clin Anesth 5:16–21, 1993

Lunn RJ, Savageau MM, Beatty WW, et al: Anesthics and electroconvulsive therapy seizure duration: implications for therapy from a rat model. Biol Psychiatry 16:1163–1175, 1981

Lykouras E, Malliaras D, Christodoulou GN, et al: Delusional depression: phenomenology and response to treatment. A prospective study. Acta Psychiatr Scand 73:324–329, 1986

Mac DS, Pardo MP: Systemic lupus erythematosus and catatonia: a case report. J Clin Psychiatry 44:155–156, 1983

MacKenzie TB, Thurston J, Rogers L, et al: Placement of an implantable venous access device for use in maintenance ECT. Convuls Ther 12:122–124, 1996

Magee LA, Inocencion G, Kamboj L, et al: Safety of first trimester exposure to histamine H2 blockers: a prospective cohort study. Dig Dis Sci 41:1145–1149, 1996

Magen JG, D'Mello D: Acute lymphocytic leukemia and psychosis: treatment with electroconvulsive therapy. Ann Clin Psychiatry 7:133–137, 1995

Magni G, Fisman M, Helmes E: Clinical correlates of ECT-resistant depression in the elderly. J Clin Psychiatry 49:405–407, 1988

Mahler H, Co BT Jr, Dinwiddie S: Studies in involuntary civil commitment and involuntary electroconvulsive therapy. J Nerv Ment Dis 174:97–106, 1986

Malek-Ahmadi P, Sedler RR: Electroconvulsive therapy and asymptomatic meningioma. Convuls Ther 5:168–170, 1989

Malek-Ahmadi P, Beceiro JR, McNeil BW, et al: Electroconvulsive therapy and chronic subdural hematoma. Convuls Ther 6:38–41, 1990

Maletzky BM: Multiple-Monitored Electroconvulsive Therapy. Boca Raton, FL, CRC Press, 1981

Maletzky BM: Conventional and multiple-monitored electroconvulsive therapy: a comparison in major depressive episodes. J Nerv Ment Dis 174:257–264, 1986

Maletzky B, McFarland B, Burt A: Refractory obsessive compulsive disorder and ECT. Convuls Ther 10:34–42, 1994

Malloy FW, Small IF, Miller MJ, et al: Changes in neuropsychological test performance after electroconvulsive therapy. Biol Psychiatry 17:61–67, 1982

Malone FD, D'Alton ME: Drugs in pregnancy: anticonvulsants. Semin Perinatol 21:114–123, 1997

Malsch E, Gratz I, Mani S, et al: Efficacy of electroconvulsive therapy after propofol and methohexital anesthesia. Convuls Ther 10:212–219, 1994

Maltbie AA, Wingfield MS, Volow MR, et al: Electroconvulsive therapy in the presence of brain tumor: case reports and an evaluation of risk. J Nerv Ment Dis 168:400–405, 1980

Mandel MR, Welch CA, Mieske M, et al: Prediction of response to ECT in tricyclic-intolerant or tricyclic-resistant depressed patients. McLean Hosp J 4:203–209, 1977

Maneksha FR: Hypertension and tachycardia during electroconvulsive therapy: to treat or not to treat? Convuls Ther 7:28–35, 1991

Mann SC, Caroff SN, Bleier HR, et al: Lethal catatonia. Am J Psychiatry 143:1374–1381, 1986

Mann SC, Caroff SN, Bleier HR, et al: Electroconvulsive therapy of the lethal catatonia syndrome. Convuls Ther 6:239–247, 1990

Manning M: Undercurrents: A Life Beneath the Surface. San Francisco, CA, Harper, 1994

Marco LA, Randels PM: Succinylcholine drug interactions during electroconvulsive therapy. Biol Psychiatry 14:433–445, 1979

Martensson B, Bartfai A, Hallen B, et al: A comparison of propofol and methohexital as anesthetic agents for ECT: effects on seizure duration, therapeutic outcome, and memory. Biol Psychiatry 35:179–189, 1994

Martin BA, Bean GJ: Competence to consent to electroconvulsive therapy. Convuls Ther 8:92–102, 1992

Martin BA, Glancy GD: Consent to electroconvulsive therapy: investigation of the validity of a competency questionnaire. Convuls Ther 10:279–286, 1994

Martin BA, Cooper RM, Parikh SV: Propofol anesthesia, seizure duration, and ECT: a case report and literature review. J ECT 14:99–108, 1998

Martin M, Figiel G, Mattingly G, et al: ECT-induced interictal delirium in patients with a history of a CVA. J Geriatr Psychiatry Neurol 5:149–155, 1992

Mashimo K, Kanaya M, Yamauchi T: Electroconvulsive therapy for a schizophrenic patient in catatonic stupor with joint contracture. Convuls Ther 11:216–219, 1995

Mashimo K, Sato Y, Yamauchi T: Effective electroconvulsive therapy for stupor in the high risk patient: a report of two cases. Psychiatry Clin Neurosci 50:129–131, 1996

Mashimo K, Yamauchi T, Harada T: Electroconvulsive therapy for a schizophrenic patient with burns in the critical care centre. Burns 23:85–86, 1997

Masiar SJ, Johns CA: ECT following clozapine. Br J Psychiatry 158:135–136, 1991

Matters RM, Beckett WG, Kirkby KC, et al: Recovery after electroconvulsive therapy: comparison of propofol with methohexitone anaesthesia. Br J Anaesth 75:297–300, 1995

Mattes JA, Pettinati HM, Stephens S, et al: A placebo-controlled evaluation of vasopressin for ECT-induced memory impairment. Biol Psychiatry 27:289–303, 1990

Mattingly G, Baker K, Zorumski CF, et al: Multiple sclerosis and ECT: possible value of gadolinium-enhanced magnetic resonance scans for identifying high-risk patients. J Neuropsychiatry Clin Neurosci 4:145–151, 1992

Matzen TA, Martin RL, Watt TJ, et al: The use of maintainence electroconvulsive therapy for relapsing depression. Jefferson Journal of Psychiatry 6:52–58, 1988

May PR: Treatment of Schizophrenia: A Comparative Study of Five Treatment Methods. New York, Science House, 1968

May PR, Tuma AH: Treatment of schizophrenia: an experimental study of five treatment methods. Br J Psychiatry 111:503–510, 1965

May PR, Tuma AH, Yale C, et al: Schizophrenia: a follow-up study of results of treatment, II: hospital stay over two to five years. Arch Gen Psychiatry 33:481–486, 1976

May PR, Tuma AH, Dixon WJ, et al: Schizophrenia: a follow-up study of the results of five forms of treatment. Arch Gen Psychiatry 38:776–784, 1981

Mayur PM, Shree RS, Gangadhar BN, et al: Atropine premedication and the cardiovascular response to electroconvulsive therapy. Br J Anaesth 81:466–467, 1998

Mayur P, Gangadhar BN, Janakiramaiah N, et al: Motor monitoring during electroconvulsive therapy. Br J Psychiatry 174:270–273, 1999

McAllister DA, Perri MG, Jordan RC, et al: Effects of ECT given two vs. three times weekly. Psychiatry Res 21:63–69, 1987

McAllister TW, Price TR: Severe depressive pseudodementia with and without dementia. Am J Psychiatry 139:626–629, 1982

McCabe M: ECT in the treatment of mania: a controlled study. Am J Psychiatry 133:688–691, 1976

McCabe M, Norris B: ECT versus chlorpromazine in mania. Biol Psychiatry 12:245–254, 1977

McCabe P: Morbidity and mortality rates for peripheral vascular surgery. Infect Control 6:94–95, 1985

McCall WV: Asystole in electroconvulsive therapy: report of four cases. J Clin Psychiatry 57:199–203, 1996

McCall WV: Cardiovascular risk during ECT: managing the managers. Convuls Ther 13:123–124, 1997

McCall WV, Coffey CE, Maltbie AA: Successful electroconvulsive therapy in a depressed patient with pseudohypoparathyroidism. Convuls Ther 5:114–117, 1989

McCall WV, Sheip FE, Weiner RD, et al: Effects of labetalol on hemodynamics and seizure duration during ECT. Convuls Ther 7:5–14, 1991

McCall WV, Minneman SA, Weiner RD, et al: Dental pathology in ECT patients prior to treatment. Convuls Ther 8:19–24, 1992a

McCall WV, Weiner RD, Shelp FE, et al: ECT in a state hospital setting. Convuls Ther 8:12–18, 1992b

McCall WV, Reid S, Rosenquist P, et al: A reappraisal of the role of caffeine in ECT. Am J Psychiatry 150:1543–1545, 1993

McCall WV, Reid S, Ford M: Electrocardiographic and cardiovascular effects of subconvulsive stimulation during titrated right unilateral ECT. Convuls Ther 10:25–33, 1994

McCall W, Farah B, Reboussin D, et al: Comparison of the efficacy of titrated, moderate dose and fixed, high-dose right unilateral ECT in elderly patients. Am J Geriatr Psychiatry 3:317–324, 1995

McCall WV, Colenda CC, Farah BA: Ictal EEG regularity declines during a course of RUL ECT. Convuls Ther 12:213–216, 1996a

McCall WV, Robinette GD, Hardesty D: Relationship of seizure morphology to the convulsive threshold. Convuls Ther 12:147–51, 1996b

McCall WV, Reboussin DM, Weiner RD, et al: Titrated, moderately suprathreshold versus fixed, high dose RUL ECT: acute antidepressant and cognitive effects. Arch Gen Psychiatry 57:438–444, 2000

McCormick AS, Saunders DA: Oxygen saturation of patients recovering from electroconvulsive therapy. Anaesthesia 51:702–704, 1996

McDonald IM, Perkins M, Marjerrison G, et al: A controlled comparison of amitriptyline and electroconvulsive therapy in the treatment of depression. Am J Psychiatry 122:1427–1431, 1966

McElhatton PR: The use of phenothiazines during pregnancy and lactation. Reprod Toxicol 6:475–490, 1992

McElhatton PR: The effects of benzodiazepine use during pregnancy and lactation. Reprod Toxicol 8:461–475, 1994

McElhiney MC, Moody BJ, Steif BL, et al: Autobiographical memory and mood: effects of electroconvulsive therapy. Neuropsychology 9:501–517, 1995

McElroy SL, Keck PE Jr, Friedman LM: Minimizing and managing antidepressant side effects. J Clin Psychiatry 56(suppl 2):49–55, 1995

McGarvey KA, Zis AP, Brown EE, et al: ECS-induced dopamine release: effects of electrode placement, anticonvulsant treatment, and stimulus intensity. Biol Psychiatry 34:152–157, 1993

McKinney PA, Kellner CH: Multiple ECT late in the course of neuroleptic malignant syndrome. Convuls Ther 13:269–273, 1997

McKinney PA, Beale MD, Kellner CH: Electroconvulsive therapy in a patient with a cerebellar meningioma. J ECT 14:49–52, 1998

McKinnon AL: Electric shock therapy in a private psychiatric hospital. CMAJ 58:478–483, 1948

Medical Research Council: Clinical trial of the treatment of depressive illness: report to the Medical Research Council by its Clinical Psychiatry Committee. BMJ 1:881–886, 1965

Meisel A, Roth LH: Toward an informed discussion of informed consent. Arizona Law Review 25:265–346, 1983

Meldrum BS: Neuropathological consequences of chemically and electrically induced seizures. Ann N Y Acad Sci 462:186–193, 1986

Meldrum BS, Horton RW, Brierley JB: Epileptic brain damage in adolescent baboons following seizures induced by allyglycine. Brain 97:417–428, 1974

Mellman LA, Gorman JM: Successful treatment of obsessive-compulsive disorder with ECT. Am J Psychiatry 141:596–597, 1984

Mendels J: Electroconvulsive therapy and depression, I: the prognostic significance of clinical factors. Br J Psychiatry 111:675–681, 1965a

Mendels J: Electroconvulsive therapy and depression, III: a method for prognosis. Br J Psychiatry 111:687–690, 1965b

Mendels J: The prediction of response to electroconvulsive therapy. Am J Psychiatry 124:153–159, 1967

Messer GJ, Stoudemire A, Knos G, et al: Electroconvulsive therapy and the chronic use of pseudocholinesterase-inhibitor (echothiophate iodide) eye drops for glaucoma: a case report. Gen Hosp Psychiatry 14:56–60, 1992

Messina AG, Paranicas M, Katz B, et al: Effect of electroconvulsive therapy on the electrocardiogram and echocardiogram. Anesth Analg 75:511–514, 1992

Meyendorf R, Bender W, Baumann E, et al: Comparison of nondominant unilateral and bilateral electroconvulsive therapy: clinical efficiency and side effects. Arch Psychiatr Nervenkr 229:89–112, 1980

Meyers BS: Geriatric delusional depression. Clin Geriatr Med 8:299–308, 1992

Middaugh LD: Phenobarbital during pregnancy in mouse and man. Neurotoxicology 7:287–301, 1986

Miller AL, Faber RA, Hatch JP, et al: Factors affecting amnesia, seizure duration, and efficacy in ECT. Am J Psychiatry 142:692–696, 1985

Miller AR, Isenberg KE: Reversible ischemic neurologic deficit after ECT. J ECT 14:42–48, 1998

Miller DH, Clancy J, Cumming E: A comparison between unidirectional current nonconvulsive electrical stimulation given with Reiters machine, standard alternating current electroshock (Cerletti method), and pentothal in chronic schizophrenia. Am J Psychiatry 109:617–620, 1953

Miller LJ: Use of electroconvulsive therapy during pregnancy. Hospital and Community Psychiatry 45:444–450, 1994

Miller LJ: Pharmacotherapy during the perinatal period. Directions in Psychiatry 18:49–64, 1998

Miller ME, Siris SG, Gabriel AN: Treatment delays in the course of electroconvulsive therapy. Hospital and Community Psychiatry 37:825–827, 1986

Miller ME, Gabriel A, Herman G, et al: Atropine sulfate premedication and cardiac arrhythmia in electroconvulsive therapy (ECT). Convuls Ther 3:10–17, 1987

Miller WH Jr, Bloom JD, Resnick MP: Chronic mental illness and perinatal outcome. Gen Hosp Psychiatry 14:171–176, 1992

Mills MJ, Avery D: The legal regulation of electroconvulsive therapy, in Mood Disorders: The World's Major Public Health Problem. Edited by Ayd FJ. Baltimore, MD, Frank Ayd Communications, 1978, pp 154–183

Milstein V, Small JG, Klapper MH, et al: Uni- versus bilateral ECT in the treatment of mania. Convuls Ther 3:1–9, 1987

Milstein V, Small JG, Miller MJ, et al: Mechanisms of action of ECT: schizophrenia and schizoaffective disorder. Biol Psychiatry 27:1282–1292, 1990

Milstein V, Small IF, French RN: ECT in a patient with Harrington Rods. Convuls Ther 8:137–140, 1992

Minneman SA: A history of oral protection for the ECT patient: past, present, and future. Convuls Ther 11:94–103, 1995

Mitchell P, Torda T, Hickie I, et al: Propofol as an anaesthetic agent for ECT: effect on outcome and length of course. Aust N Z J Psychiatry 25:255–261, 1991

Moellentine C, Rummans T, Ahlskog JE, et al: Effectiveness of ECT in patients with parkinsonism. J Neuropsychiatry Clin Neurosci 10:187–193, 1998

Moise FN, Petrides G: Case study: electroconvulsive therapy in adolescents. J Am Acad Child Adolesc Psychiatry 35:312–318, 1996

Monaco JT, Delaplaine RP: Tranycypromine with ECT. Am J Psychiatry 120:1003, 1964

Monroe RR, Jr: Maintenance electroconvulsive therapy. Psychiatr Clin North Am 14:947–960, 1991

Montgomery SA, Åsberg M: A new depression scale designed to be sensitive to change. Br J Psychiatry 134:382–389, 1979

Morgan DH: ECT given to people with pacemakers. Bulletin of the Royal College of Psychiatrists 11:135–135, 1987

Moscarillo FM: Cardiologist as alternative to anesthesiologist for ECT? (letter). Convuls Ther 5:194–196, 1989

Mosolov SN, Moshchevitin SI: Use of electroconvulsive therapy for breaking the continual course of drug-resistant affective and schizoaffective psychoses. Zh Nevropatol Psikhiatr Im S S Korsakova 90:121–125, 1990

Motamed C, Choquette R, Donati F: Rocuronium prevents succinylcholine-induced fasciculations. Can J Anaesth 44:1262–1268, 1997

Motoyama EK, Rivard G, Acheson F, et al: The effect of changes in maternal pH and PCO_2 on the PO_2 of fetal lambs. Anesthesiology 28:891–903, 1967

Moya F, Kvisselgaard N: Investigation of placental thresholds to succinylcholine. Anesthesiology 22:1–6, 1961

Mukherjee S: Mechanisms of the antimanic effect of electroconvulsive therapy. Convuls Ther 5:227–243, 1989

Mukherjee S: Combined ECT and lithium therapy. Convuls Ther 9:274–284, 1993

Mukherjee S, Debsikdar V: Unmodified electroconvulsive therapy of acute mania: a retrospective naturalistic study. Convuls Ther 8:5–11, 1992

Mukherjee S, Debsikdar V: Absence of neuroleptic-induced Parkinsonism in psychotic patients receiving adjunctive electroconvulsive therapy. Convuls Ther 10:53–58, 1994

Mukherjee S, Sackeim HA, Lee C: Unilateral ECT in the treatment of manic episodes. Convuls Ther 4:74–80, 1988

Mukherjee S, Sackeim HA, Schnur DB: Electroconvulsive therapy of acute manic episodes: a review of 50 years' experience. Am J Psychiatry 151:169–176, 1994

Muller D: 1. Nardil (phenelzine) as a potentiator of electroconvulsive therapy (ECT). 2. A survey of outpatient ECT. Journal of Mental Science 107:994–996, 1961

Mulsant BH, Rosen J, Thornton JE, et al: A prospective naturalistic study of electroconvulsive therapy in late-life depression. J Geriatr Psychiatry Neurol 4:3–13, 1991

Mulsant BH, Haskett RF, Prudic J, et al: Low use of neuroleptic drugs in the treatment of psychotic major depression. Am J Psychiatry 154:559–561, 1997

Murray GB, Shea V, Conn DK: Electroconvulsive therapy for poststroke depression. J Clin Psychiatry 47:258–260, 1986

National Institute of Mental Health Consensus Development Panel: Mood disorders: pharmacologic prevention of recurrences. Am J Psychiatry 142:469–476, 1985

Najjar F, Guttmacher LB: ECT in the presence of intracranial aneurysm. J ECT 14:266–271, 1998

Nelson JC, Price LH, Jatlow PI: Neuroleptic dose and desipramine concentrations during combined treatment of unipolar delusional depression. Am J Psychiatry 143:1151–1154, 1986

Nelson JP, Benjamin L: Efficacy and safety of combined ECT and tricyclic antidepressant therapy in the treatment of depressed geriatric patients. Convuls Ther 5:321–329, 1989

Nelson JP, Rosenberg DR: ECT treatment of demented elderly patients with major depression: a retrospective study of efficacy and safety. Convuls Ther 7:157–165, 1991

Nettlebladt P: Factors influencing number of treatments and seizure duration in ECT: drug treatment, social class. Convuls Ther 4:160–168, 1988

Nisijima K, Ishiguro T: Electroconvulsive therapy for the treatment of neuroleptic malignant syndrome with psychotic symptoms: a report of five cases. J ECT 15:158–166, 1999

Nobler MS, Sackeim HA: Augmentation strategies in electroconvulsive therapy: a synthesis. Convuls Ther 9:331–351, 1993

Nobler MS, Sackeim HA: Electroconvulsive therapy: clinical and biological aspects, in Predictors of Response in Mood Disorders. Edited by Goodnick PJ. Washington, DC, American Psychiatric Press, 1996, pp 177–198

Nobler MS, Sackeim HA, Solomou M, et al: EEG manifestations during ECT: effects of electrode placement and stimulus intensity. Biol Psychiatry 34:321–330, 1993

Nobler MS, Sackeim HA, Moeller JR, et al: Quantifying the speed of symptomatic improvement with electroconvulsive therapy: comparison of alternative statistical methods. Convuls Ther 13:208–221, 1997

Nobler MS, Luber B, Moeller JR, et al: Quantitative EEG during seizures induced by electroconvulsive therapy: relations to treatment modality and clinical features, I: global analyses. J ECT, VOL: in press

Nonacs R, Cohen LS: Postpartum mood disorders: diagnosis and treatment guidelines. J Clin Psychiatry 59:34–40, 1998

Norris AS, Clancy J: Hospitalized depressions: drugs or electrotherapy. Arch Gen Psychiatry 5:276–279, 1961

Nurmohamed MT, Rosendaal FR, Buller HR, et al:Low-molecular-weight heparin versus standard heparin in general and orthopaedic surgery: a meta-analysis. Lancet 340:152–156, 1992

Nurnberg HG: An overview of somatic treatment of psychosis during pregnancy and postpartum. Gen Hosp Psychiatry 11:328–338, 1989

Nymeyer L, Grossberg GT: Delirium in a 75-year-old woman receiving ECT and levodopa. Convuls Ther 13:114–116, 1997

Nystrom S: On relation between clinical factors and efficacy of ECT in depression. Acta Psychiatrica et Neurologica Scandinavica Supplement 181:11–135, 1964

Oates MR: The treatment of psychiatric disorders in pregnancy and the puerperium. Clin Obstet Gynecol 13:385–395, 1986

O'Brien PD, Morgan DH: Bladder rupture during ECT. Convuls Ther 7:56–59, 1991

O'Connell BK, Towfighi J, Kofke WA, et al: Neuronal lesions in mercaptopropionic acid-induced status epilepticus. Acta Neuropathol (Berl) 77:47–54, 1988

O'Connor CJ, Rothenberg DM, Soble JS, et al: The effect of esmolol pretreatment on the incidence of regional wall motion abnormalities during electroconvulsive therapy. Anesth Analg 82:143–147, 1996

Offner F: Electrical properties of tissues in shock therapy. Proc Soc Exp Biol Med 49:571–574, 1942

Offner FS: Stimulation with minimum power. Neurophysiology 9:387–390, 1946

O'Flaherty D, Husain MM, Moore M, et al: Circulatory responses during electroconvulsive therapy: the comparative effects of placebo, esmolol, and nitroglycerin. Anaesthesia 47:563–567, 1992

Oldfield RC: The assessment and analysis of handedness: the Edinburgh Inventory. Neuropsychologia 9:97–113, 1971

Olfson M, Marcus S, Sackeim HA, et al: Use of ECT for the inpatient treatment of recurrent major depression. Am J Psychiatry 155:22–29, 1998

O'Shea B, Lynch T, Falvey J, et al: Electroconvulsive therapy and cognitive improvement in a very elderly depressed patient. Br J Psychiatry 150:255–257, 1987

Ostensen M: Nonsteroidal anti-inflammatory drugs during pregnancy. Scand J Rheumatol Suppl 107:128–132, 1998

O'Toole JK, Dyck G: Report of psychogenic fever in catatonia responding to electroconvulsive therapy. Diseases of the Nervous System 38:852–853, 1977

Ottosson J-O: Experimental studies of the mode of action of electroconvulsive therapy. Acta Psychiatr Scand Suppl 145:1–141, 1960

Ottosson J-O: Ethics of electroconvulsive therapy. Convuls Ther 8:233–236, 1992

Overall JE, Gorham DR: The Brief Psychiatric Rating Scale. Psychol Rep 10:799–812, 1962

Packman PM, Meyer DA, Verdun RM: Hazards of succinylcholine administration during electrotherapy. Arch Gen Psychiatry 35:1137–1141, 1978

Palmer DM, Sprang HE, Hans CL: Electroshock therapy in schizophrenia: a statistical survey of 455 cases. J Nerv Ment Dis 114:162–171, 1951

Pande AC, Grunhaus LJ: ECT for depression in the presence of myasthenia gravis. Convuls Ther 6:172–175, 1990

Pande AC, Grunhaus LJ, Haskett RF, et al: Electroconvulsive therapy in delusional and non-delusional depressive disorder. J Affect Disord 19:215–219, 1990

Pargger H, Kaufmann MA, Schouten R, et al: Hemodynamic responses to electroconvulsive therapy in a patient 5 years after cardiac transplantation. Anesthesiology 83:625–627, 1995

Parker G, Roy K, Hadzi-Pavlovic D, et al: Psychotic (delusional) depression: a meta-analysis of physical treatments. J Affect Disord 24:17–24, 1992

Parker V, Nobler MS, Pedley TA, et al: A unilateral, prolonged, nonconvulsive seizure in a patient treated with bilateral ECT. J ECT 16:121–132, 2000

Parry J: Legal parameters of informed consent for ECT administered to mentally disabled persons. Psychopharmacol Bull 22:490–494, 1986

Pastuszak A, Schick-Boschetto B, Zuber C, et al: Pregnancy outcome following first-trimester exposure to fluoxetine (Prozac). JAMA 269:2246–2248, 1993

Pataki J, Zervas IM, Jandorf L: Catatonia in a university inpatient service (1985–1990). Convuls Ther 8:163–173, 1992

Paul SM, Extein I, Calil HM, et al: Use of ECT with treatment-resistant depressed patients at the National Institute of Mental Health. Am J Psychiatry 138:486–489, 1981

Pearlman CA: Electroconvulsive therapy for patient with cardiac pacemaker. JAMA 255:1501, 1986a

Pearlman CA: Neuroleptic malignant syndrome: a review of the literature. J Clin Psychopharmacol 6:257–273, 1986b

Pearlman C, Carson W, Metz A: Hemodialysis, chronic renal failure, and ECT. Convuls Ther 4:332–333, 1988

Pearlman CA, Richmond J: New data on the methohexital–thiopental–arrhythmia issue. Convuls Ther 6:221–223, 1990

Pearlman T, Loper M, Tillery L: Should psychiatrists administer anesthesia for ECT? Am J Psychiatry 147:1553–1556, 1990

Perris C: A study of cycloid psychoses. Acta Psychiatr Scand Suppl 253:1–77, 1974

Perris C, d'Elia G: A study of bipolar (manic-depressive) and unipolar recurrent depressive psychoses, IX: therapy and prognosis. Acta Psychiatr Scand Suppl 194:153–171, 1966

Peters M: Handedness and its relation to other indices of cerebral lateralization, in Brain Asymmetry. Edited by Davidson RJ, Hugdahl K. Cambridge, MA, MIT Press, 1995, pp 183–214

Peters SG, Wochos DN, Peterson GC: Status epilepticus as a complication of concurrent electroconvulsive and theophylline therapy. Mayo Clin Proc 59:568–570, 1984

Peterson GN: Training in ECT (letter). Am J Psychiatry 145:772, 1988

Petrides G: Continuation ECT: a review. Psychiatric Annals 28:517–523, 1998

Petrides G, Fink M: Atrial fibrillation, anticoagulation, and electroconvulsive therapy. Convuls Ther 12:91–98, 1996a

Petrides G, Fink M: The "half-age" stimulation strategy for ECT dosing. Convuls Ther 12:138–146, 1996b

Petrides G, Dhossche D, Fink M, et al: Continuation ECT: relapse prevention in affective disorders. Convuls Ther 10:189–194, 1994

Petrides G, Maneksha F, Zervas I, et al: Trimethaphan (Arfonad) control of hypertension and tachycardia during electroconvulsive therapy: a double-blind study. J Clin Anesth 8:104–109, 1996

Pettinati HM, Rosenberg J: Memory self-ratings before and after electroconvulsive therapy: depression- versus ECT-induced. Biol Psychiatry 19:539–548, 1984

Pettinati HM, Mathisen KS, Rosenberg J, et al: Meta-analytical approach to reconciling discrepancies in efficacy between bilateral and unilateral electroconvulsive therapy. Convuls Ther 2:7–17, 1986

Pettinati HM, Stephens SM, Willis KM, et al: Evidence for less improvement in depression in patients taking benzodiazepines during unilateral ECT. Am J Psychiatry 147:1029–1035, 1990

Pettinati HM, Tamburello TA, Ruetsch CR, et al: Patient attitudes toward electroconvulsive therapy. Psychopharmacol Bull 30:471–475, 1994

Pfaffenrath V, Rehm M: Migraine in pregnancy: what are the safest treatment options? Drug Safety 19:383–388, 1998

Philbrick KL, Rummans TA: Malignant catatonia. J Neuropsychiatry Clin Neurosci 6:1–13, 1994

Philibert RA, Richards L, Lynch CF, et al: Effect of ECT on mortality and clinical outcome in geriatric unipolar depression. J Clin Psychiatry 56:390–394, 1995

Pino RM, Ali HH, Denman WT, et al: A comparison of the intubation conditions between mivacurium and rocuronium during balanced anesthesia. Anesthesiology 88:673–678, 1998

Pippard J: Audit of electroconvulsive treatment in two national health service regions. Br J Psychiatry 160:621–637, 1992

Pippard J, Ellam L: Electroconvulsive Treatment in Great Britain. London, England, Gaskell, 1981

Pisvejc J, Hyrman V, Sikora J, et al: A comparison of brief and ultrabrief pulse stiumuli in unilateral ECT. J ECT 14:68–76, 1998

Pitts FJ: Medical physiology of ECT, in Electroconvulsive Therapy: Biological Foundations and Clinical Applications. Edited by Abrams R, Essman W. New York, Spectrum, 1982, pp 57–90

Pogue-Geile MF, Oltmanns TF: Sentence perception and distractability in schizophrenic, manic, and depressed patients. J Abnorm Psychol 89:115–124, 1980

Polster DS, Wisner KL: ECT-induced premature labor: a case report. J Clin Psychiatry 60:53–54, 1999

Pons G, Rey E, Matheson I: Excretion of psychoactive drugs into breast milk: pharmacokinetic principles and recommendations. Clin Pharmacokinet 27:270–289, 1994

Pope HG Jr, Lipinski JF: Diagnosis in schizophrenia and manic-depressive illness. Arch Gen Psychiatry 35:811–827, 1978

Pope HG Jr, Lipinski JF, Cohen BM, et al: "Schizoaffective disorder": an invalid diagnosis? A comparison of schizoaffective disorder, schizophrenia, and affective disorder. Am J Psychiatry 137:921–927, 1980

Pope HG Jr, Keck PE, McElroy SL: Frequency and presentation of neuroleptic malignant syndrome in a psychiatric hospital. Am J Psychiatry 143:1227–1233, 1986

Porac C, Coren S: Lateral Preferences and Human Behavior. New York, Springer Verlag, 1981

Pornnoppadol C, Isenberg K: ECT with implantable cardioverter defibrillator J ECT 14:124–126, 1998

Post F: The management and nature of depressive illness in late life: a follow-through study. Br J Psychiatry 121:393–404, 1972

Post RM, Putnam F, Uhde TW, et al: Electroconvulsive therapy as an anticonvulsant: implications for its mechanism of action in affective illness. Ann N Y Acad Sci 462:376–388, 1986

Poster E, Baxter LR Jr, Hammon CL: Nursing students' perception of electroconvulsive therapy: impact of instruction with an electroconvulsive therapy videotape. Convuls Ther 1:277–282, 1985

Pratt RT, Warrington EK, Halliday AM: Unilateral ECT as a test for cerebral dominance, with a strategy for treating left-handers. Br J Psychiatry 119:79–83, 1971

Price TR, McAllister TW: Response of depressed patients to sequential unilateral nondominant brief-pulse and bilateral sinusoidal ECT. J Clin Psychiatry 47:182–186, 1986

Price TR, McAllister TW: Safety and efficacy of ECT in depressed patients with dementia: a review of clinical experience. Convuls Ther 5:61–74, 1989

Price TR, McAllister TW, Peltier D, et al: Positive response to bilateral sinusoidal ECT in unilateral and bilateral brief-pulse "ECT-resistant" depressive illness. Convuls Ther 2:277–284, 1986

Pridmore S, Pollard C: Electroconvulsive therapy in Parkinson's disease: 30 month follow up. J Neurol Neurosurg Psychiatry 60:693, 1996

Prien R, Kupfer D: Continuation drug therapy for major depressive episodes; how long should it be maintained? Am J Psychiatry 143:18–23, 1986

Proakis AG, Harris GB: Comparative penetration of glycopyrrolate and atropine across the blood-brain and placental barriers in anesthetized dogs. Anesthesiology 48:339–344, 1978

Protheroe C: Puerperal psychoses: a long term study 1927–1961. Br J Psychiatry 115:9–30, 1969

Prudic J, Sackeim HA, Decina P, et al: Acute effects of ECT on cardiovascular functioning: relations to patient and treatment variables. Acta Psychiatr Scand 75:344–351, 1987

Prudic J, Devanand DP, Sackeim HA, et al: Relative response of endogenous and non-endogenous symptoms to electroconvulsive therapy. J Affect Disord 16:59–64, 1989

Prudic J, Sackeim HA, Devanand DP: Medication resistance and clinical response to electroconvulsive therapy. Psychiatry Res 31:287–296, 1990

Prudic J, Sackeim HA, Devanand DP, et al: The efficacy of ECT in double depression. Depression 1:38–44, 1993

Prudic J, Sackeim HA, Devanand DP, et al: Acute cognitive effects of subconvulsive electrical stimulation. Convuls Ther 10:4–24, 1994

Prudic J, Haskett RF, Mulsant B, et al: Resistance to antidepressant medications and short-term clinical response to ECT. Am J Psychiatry 153:985–992, 1996

Prudic J, Fitzsimons L, Nobler MS, et al: Naloxone in the prevention of the adverse cognitive effects of ECT: a within-subject, placebo-controlled study. Neuropsychopharmacology 21:285–293, 1999

Prudic J, Peyser S, Sackeim HA: Subjective memory complaints: a review of patient self-assessment of memory after electroconvulsive therapy. J ECT, in press

Pudenz RH, Bullara LA, Jacques S, et al: Electrical stimulation of the brain, III: neural damage model. Surg Neurol 4:389–400, 1975

Puri BK, Langa A, Coleman RM, et al: The clinical efficacy of maintenance electroconvulsive therapy in a patient with a mild mental handicap. Br J Psychiatr 161:707–709, 1992

Quitkin FM: The importance of dosage in prescribing antidepressants. Br J Psychiatry 147:593–597, 1985

Quitkin FM, Rabkin JG, Ross D, et al: Duration of antidepressant drug treatment: what is an adequate trial? Arch Gen Psychiatry 41:238–245, 1984

Quitkin FM, McGrath PJ, Stewart JW, et al: Can the effects of antidepressants be observed in the first two weeks of treatment? Neuropsychopharmacology 15:390–394, 1996

Rabbitt P: Development of methods to measure changes in activities of daily living in the elderly, in Alzheimer's Disease: A Report of Progress in Research. Edited by Corkin S, Davis KL, Growdon JH. New York, Raven, 1982, pp 127–131

Rabheru K, Persad E: A review of continuation and maintenance electroconvulsive therapy. Can J Psychiatry 42:476–484, 1997

Rachlin HL, Goldman GS, Gurvitz M, et al: Follow-up study of 317 patients discharged from Hillside Hospital in 1950. Journal of the Hillside Hospital 5:17–40, 1956

Rackowski D, Kalat JW, Nebes R: Reliability and validity of some handedness questionnaire items. Neuropsychologia 8:523–526, 1976

Rahman R: A review of treatment of 176 schizophrenic patients in the mental hospital Pabna. Br J Psychiatry 114:775–777, 1968

Rampton AJ, Griffin RM, Stuart CS, et al: Comparison of methohexital and propofol for electroconvulsive therapy: effects on hemodynamic responses and seizure duration. Anesthesiology 70:412–417, 1989

Randt CT, Brown ER: Randt Memory Test. Bayport, NY, Life Science, 1983

Randt CT, Brown ER, Osbourne DP: A memory test for longitudinal measurement of mild to moderate deficits. Clin Neuropsychol 2:184–194, 1980

Rao KM, Gangadhar RN, Janakiramaiah N: Nonconvulsive status epilepticus after the ninth electroconvulsive therapy. Convuls Ther 9:128–134, 1993

Räsänen J, Martin DJ, Downs JB, et al: Oxygen supplementation during electroconvulsive therapy. Br J Anaesth 61:593–597, 1988

Raskin DE: A survey of electroconvulsive therapy: use and training in university hospitals in 1984 (letter). Convuls Ther 2:293–296, 1986

Rasmussen KG, Abrams R: Treatment of Parkinson's disease with electroconvulsive therapy. Psychiatr Clin North Am 14:925–933, 1991

Rasmussen KG, Zorumski CF: Electroconvulsive therapy in patients taking theophylline. J Clin Psychiatry 54:427–431, 1993

Rasmussen KG, Zorumski CF, Jarvis MR: Possible impact of stimulus duration on seizure threshold in ECT. Convuls Ther 10:177–180, 1994

Rasmussen KG, Jarvis MR, Zorumski CF: Ketamine anesthesia in electroconvulsive therapy. Convuls Ther 12:217–223, 1996

Rasmussen T, Milner B: The role of early left-brain injury in determining lateralization of cerebral speech functions. Ann N Y Acad Sci 299:355–369, 1977

Ravn J: A comparison of past and present treatments of endogenous depression. Br J Psychiatry 112:501–504, 1966

Ray SD: Relative efficacy of ECT and CPZ in schizophrenia. J Indian Med Assoc 38:332–333, 1962

Rayburn BK: Electroconvulsive therapy in patients with heart failure or valvular heart disease. Convuls Ther 13:145–156, 1997

Reddy S, Nobler MS: Dangerous hyperglycemia associated with electroconvulsive therapy. Convuls Ther 12:99–103, 1996

Reid WH, Keller S, Leatherman M, et al: ECT in Texas: 19 months of mandatory reporting. J Clin Psychiatry 59:8–13, 1998

Reiter-Theil S: Autonomy and beneficence: ethical issues in electroconvulsive therapy. Convuls Ther 8:237–244, 1992

Remick RA, Maurice WL: ECT in pregnancy. Am J Psychiatry 135:761–762, 1978

Remick RA, Jewesson P, Ford RWJ: MAO inhibitors in general anesthesia: a reevaluation. Convuls Ther 3:196–203, 1987

Rey JM, Walter G: Half a century of ECT use in young people. Am J Psychiatry 154:595–602, 1997

Rice EH, Sombrotto LB, Markowitz JC, et al: Cardiovascular morbidity in high-risk patients during ECT. Am J Psychiatry 151:1637–1641, 1994

Rich CL, Woodruff RA, Cadoret R, et al: Electrotherapy: The effects of atropine on EKG. Diseases of the Nervous System 30:622–626, 1969

Rich CL, Spiker DG, Jewell SW, et al: The efficiency of ECT, I: response rate in depressive episodes. Psychiatry Res 11:167–176, 1984

Riddle WJ, Scott AI, Bennie J, et al: Current intensity and oxytocin release after electroconvulsive therapy. Biol Psychiatry 33:839–841, 1993

Ries RK, Bokan J: Electroconvulsive therapy following pituitary surgery. J Nerv Ment Dis 167:767–768, 1979

Ries RK, Wilson L, Bokan JA, et al: ECT in medication resistant schizoaffective disorder. Compr Psychiatry 22:167–173, 1981

Rifkin A: ECT versus tricyclic antidepressants in depression: a review of the evidence. J Clin Psychiatry 49:3–7, 1988

Roberts JM: Prognostic factors in the electroshock treatment of depressive states, I: clinical features from testing and examination. Journal of Mental Science 105:693–702, 1959a

Roberts JM: Prognostic factors in the electroshock treatment of depressive states, II: the application of specific tests. Journal of Mental Science 105:703–713, 1959b

Robertson AD, Inglis J: Memory deficits after electroconvulsive therapy: cerebral asymmetry and dual-encoding. Neuropsychologia 16:179–187, 1978

Robin A, de Tissera S: A double-blind controlled comparison of the therapeutic effects of low and high energy electroconvulsive therapies. Br J Psychiatry 141:357–366, 1982

Robin AA, Harris JA: A controlled comparison of imipramine and electroplexy. Journal of Mental Science 108:217–219, 1962

Robinson GE, Stewart DE: Postpartum psychiatric disorders. CMAJ 134:31–37, 1986

Roemer RA, Dubin WR, Jaffe R, et al: An efficacy study of single- versus double-seizure induction with ECT in major depression. J Clin Psychiatry 51:473–478, 1990

Rohde P, Sargant W: Treatment of schizophrenia in general hospitals. BMJ 2:67–70, 1961

Rohland BM, Carroll BT, Jacoby RG: ECT in the treatment of the catatonic syndrome. J Affect Disord 29:255–261, 1993

Roose SP, Glassman AH, Walsh BT, et al: Depression, delusions, and suicide. Am J Psychiatry 140:1159–1162, 1983

Roose SP, Glassman AH, Attia E, et al: Cardiovascular effects of fluoxetine in depressed patients with heart disease. Am J Psychiatry 155:660–665, 1998a

Roose SP, Laghrissi-Thode F, Kennedy JS, et al: Comparison of paroxetine and nortriptyline in depressed patients with ischemic heart disease. JAMA 279:287–291, 1998b

Rose JT: Reactive and endogenous depressions: response to ECT. Br J Psychiatry 109:213–217, 1963

Rosen AM, Mukherjee S, Shinbach K: The efficacy of ECT in phencyclidine-induced psychosis. J Clin Psychiatry 45:220–222, 1984

Rosenbach ML, Hermann RC, Dorwart RA: Use of electroconvulsive therapy in the Medicare population between 1987 and 1992. Psychiatr Serv 48:1537–1542, 1997

Ross AF, Tucker JH: Anesthesia risk, in Anesthesia, 3rd Edition. Edited by Miller RD. New York, Churchill Livingstone, 1990, pp 715–742

Ross JR, Malzberg B: A review of the results of the pharmacological shock therapy and the metrazol convulsive therapy in New York State. Am J Psychiatry 96:297–316, 1939

Rossi A, Stratta P, Nistico R, et al: Visuospatial impairment in depression: a controlled ECT study. Acta Psychiatr Scand 81:245–249, 1990

Roth LH: Data on informed consent for ECT. Psychopharmacol Bull 22:494–495, 1986

Roth LH, Meisel A, Lidz CW: Tests of competency to consent for treatment. Am J Psychiatry 134:279–284, 1977

Roth LH, Lidz CW, Meisel A, et al: Competency to decide about treatment and research: an overview of some empirical data. Int J Law Psychiatry 5:29–50, 1982

Roth SD, Mukherjee S, Sackeim HA: Electroconvulsive therapy in a patient with mania, parkinsonism, and tardive dyskinesia. Convuls Ther 4:92–97, 1988

Rothschild AJ, Samson JA, Bessette MP, et al: Efficacy of combination fluoxetine and perphenazine in the treatment of psychotic depression. J Clin Psychiatry 54:338–342, 1993

Rouse EC: Propofol for electroconvulsive therapy: a comparison with methohexitone. Preliminary report. Anaesthesia 43(suppl):61–64, 1988

Rowe TF: Acute gastric aspiration: prevention and treatment. Semin Perinatol 21:313–319, 1997

Royal Australian and New Zealand College of Psychiatrists: Electroconvulsive therapy (Clinical Memorandum #12). Melbourne, Australia, Royal Australian and New Zealand College of Psychiatrists, 1992

Royal College of Psychiatrists: The ECT Handbook: the second report of the Royal College of Psychiatrists' special committee on ECT. London, England, Royal College of Psychiatrists, 1995

Roy-Byrne PP, Gerner RH: Legal restrictions on the use of ECT in California: clinical impact on the incompetent patient. J Clin Psychiatry 42:300–303, 1981

Roy-Byrne PP, Weingartner H, Bierer LM, et al: Effortful and automatic cognitive processes in depression. Arch Gen Psychiatry 43:265–267, 1986

Rudorfer MV, Linnoila M, Potter WZ: Combined lithium and electroconvulsive therapy: pharmacokinetic and pharmacodynamic interactions. Convuls Ther 3:40–45, 1987

Rummans TA, Bassingthwaighte E: Severe medical and neurologic complications associated with near-lethal catatonia treated with electroconvulsive therapy. Convuls Ther 7:121–124, 1991

Rush AJ, Giles DE, Schlesser MA, et al: The inventory for depressive symptomatology (IDS): preliminary findings. Psychiatry Res 18:65–87, 1985

Rutala WA: APIC guideline for selection and use of disinfectants. Am J Infect Control 24: 313–342, 1996

Sachs GS: Treatment-resistant bipolar depression. Psychiatr Clin North Am 19:215–236, 1996

Sackeim HA: Acute cognitive side effects of ECT. Psychopharmacol Bull 22:482–484, 1986

Sackeim HA: The efficacy of electroconvulsive therapy in treatment of major depressive disorder, in The Limits of Biological Treatments for Psychological Distress: Comparisons with Psychotherapy and Placebo. Edited by Fisher S, Greenberg RP. Hillsdale, NJ, Erlbaum, 1989, pp 275–307

Sackeim HA: Are ECT devices underpowered? Convuls Ther 7:233–236, 1991

Sackeim HA: The cognitive effects of electroconvulsive therapy, in Cognitive Disorders: Pathophysiology and Treatment. Edited by Moos WH, Gamzu ER, Thal LJ. New York, Marcel Dekker, 1992, pp 183–228

Sackeim HA: The use of electroconvulsive therapy in late life depression, in Diagnosis and Treatment of Depression in Late Life. Edited by Schneider LS, Reynolds CF III, Liebowitz BD, et al. Washington, DC, American Psychiatric Press, 1993, pp 259–277

Sackeim HA: Continuation therapy following ECT: directions for future research. Psychopharmacol Bull 30:501–521, 1994

Sackeim HA: Comments on the "half-age" method of stimulus dosing. Convuls Ther 13:37–43, 1997a

Sackeim HA: What's new with ECT. American Society of Clinical Psychopharmacology Progress Notes 8:27–33, 1997b

Sackeim HA: The use of electroconvulsive therapy in late-life depression, in Geriatric Psychopharmacology, 3rd Edition. Edited by Salzman C. Baltimore, MD, Williams & Wilkins, 1998, pp 262–309

Sackeim HA: The anticonvulsant hypothesis of the mechanisms of action of ECT: current status. J ECT 15:5–26, 1999

Sackeim HA: Memory and ECT: from polarization to reconciliation. J ECT 16:87–96, 2000

Sackeim HA, Rush AJ: Melancholia and response to ECT. Am J Psychiatry 152:1242–1243, 1995

Sackeim HA, Steif BL: The neuropsychology of depression and mania, in Depression and Mania. Edited by Georgotas A, Cancro R. New York, Elsevier, 1988, pp 265–289

Sackeim HA, Stern Y: The neuropsychiatry of memory and amnesia, in The American Psychiatric Press Textbook of Neuropsychiatry, 3rd Edition. Edited by Yudofsky SC, Hales RE. Washington, DC, American Psychiatric Press, 1997, pp 501–518

Sackeim HA, Greenberg MS, Weiman AL, et al: Hemispheric asymmetry in the expression of positive and negative emotions: neurologic evidence. Arch Neurol 39:210–218, 1982

Sackeim HA, Decina P, Prohovnik I, et al: Anticonvulsant and antidepressant properties of electroconvulsive therapy: a proposed mechanism of action. Biol Psychiatry 18:1301–1310, 1983

Sackeim HA, Portnoy S, Neeley P, et al: Cognitive consequences of low-dosage electroconvulsive therapy. Ann N Y Acad Sci 462:326–340, 1986

Sackeim HA, Decina P, Kanzler M, et al: Effects of electrode placement on the efficacy of titrated, low-dose ECT. Am J Psychiatry 144:1449–1455, 1987a

Sackeim HA, Decina P, Portnoy S, et al: Studies of dosage, seizure threshold, and seizure duration in ECT. Biol Psychiatry 22:249–268, 1987b

Sackeim HA, Decina P, Prohovnik I, et al: Seizure threshold in electroconvulsive therapy: effects of sex, age, electrode placement, and number of treatments. Arch Gen Psychiatry 44:355–360, 1987c

Sackeim HA, Ross FR, Hopkins N, et al: Subjective side effects acutely following ECT: associations with treatment modality and clinical response. Convuls Ther 3:100–110, 1987d

Sackeim HA, Prudic J, Devanand DP, et al: The impact of medication resistance and continuation pharmacotherapy on relapse following response to electroconvulsive therapy in major depression. J Clin Psychopharmacol 10:96–104, 1990a

Sackeim HA, Prudic J, Devanand DP: Treatment of medication-resistant depression with electroconvulsive therapy, in Annual Review of Psychiatry, Volume 9. Edited by Tasman A, Goldfinger SM, Kaufmann CA. Washington, DC, American Psychiatric Press, 1990b, pp 91–115

Sackeim HA, Devanand DP, Prudic J: Stimulus intensity, seizure threshold, and seizure duration: impact on the efficacy and safety of electroconvulsive therapy. Psychiatr Clin North Am 14:803–843, 1991

Sackeim HA, Freeman J, McElhiney M, et al: Effects of major depression on estimates of intelligence. J Clin Exp Neuropsychol 14:268–288, 1992a

Sackeim HA, Nobler MS, Prudic J, et al: Acute effects of electroconvulsive therapy on hemispatial neglect. Neuropsychiatry Neuropsychol Behav Neurol 5:151–160, 1992b

Sackeim HA, Prudic J, Devanand DP, et al: Effects of stimulus intensity and electrode placement on the efficacy and cognitive effects of electroconvulsive therapy. N Engl J Med 328:839–846, 1993

Sackeim HA, Long J, Luber B, et al: Physical properties and quantification of the ECT stimulus, I: basic principles. Convuls Ther 10:93–123, 1994

Sackeim HA, Devanand DP, Nobler MS: Electroconvulsive therapy, in Psychopharmacology: The Fourth Generation of Progress. Edited by Bloom F, Kupfer D. New York, Raven, 1995, pp 1123–1142

Sackeim HA, Prudic J, Devanand DP, et al: A prospective, randomized, double-blind comparison of bilateral and right unilateral ECT at different stimulus intensities. Arch Gen Psychiatry 57:425–434, 2000

Saffer S, Berk M: Anesthetic induction for ECT with etomidate is associated with longer seizure duration than thiopentone. J ECT 14:89–93, 1998

Safferman AZ, Munne R: Combining clozapine with ECT. Convuls Ther 8:141–143, 1992

Saito S, Yoshikawa D, Nishihara, F, et al: The cerebral hemodynamic response to electrically induced seizures in man. Brain Res 673:93–100, 1995

Saito S, Miyoshi S, Yoshikawa D, et al: Regional cerebral oxygen saturation during electroconvulsive therapy: monitoring by near-infrared spectrophotometry. Anesth Analg 83:726–730, 1996

Sajatovic M, Meltzer HY: The effect of short-term electroconvulsive treatment plus neuroleptics in treatment-resistant schizophrenia and schizoaffective disorder. Convuls Ther 9:167–175, 1993

Salanave B, Bouvier-Colle MH, Varnoux N, et al: Classification differences and maternal mortality: a European study. MOMS Group. Mothers' mortality and severe morbidity. Int J Epidemiol 28:64–69, 1999

Salzman C: ECT and ethical psychiatry. Am J Psychiatry 134:1006–1009, 1977

Salzman C: The use of ECT in the treatment of schizophrenia. Am J Psychiatry 137:1032–1041, 1980

Salzman C, Schneider L, Alexopoulos G: Pharmacological treatment of depression in late life, in Psychopharmacology: Fourth Generation of Progress. Edited by Bloom F, Kupfer D. New York, Raven, 1995, pp 1471–1477

Sargant W: Drugs in the treatment of depression. BMJ 5221:225–227, 1961

Sargant W, Slater E: An Introduction to Physical Methods of Treatment in Psychiatry. Baltimore, MD, Williams & Wilkins, 1954

Savarese JJ: Some considerations on the new muscle relaxants. Anesth Analg l(suppl):119–127, 1998

Savarese JJ, Miller RD, Lien CA, et al: Pharmacology of muscle relaxants and their antagonists, in Anesthesia, 4th Edition. Edited by Miller RD. New York, Churchill Livingstone, 1994, pp 417–487

Sayer NA, Sackeim HA, Moeller JR, et al: The relations between observer-rating and self-report of depressive symptomatology. Psychological Assessment 5:350–360, 1993

Schaerf FW, Miller RR, Lipsey JR, et al: ECT for major depression in four patients infected with human immunodeficiency virus. Am J Psychiatry 146:782–784, 1989

Scheftner WA, Shulman RB: Treatment choice in neuroleptic malignant syndrome. Convuls Ther 8:267–279, 1992

Schneekloth TD, Rummans TA, Logan KM: Electroconvulsive therapy in adolescents. Convuls Ther 9:158–166, 1993

Schimmell MS, Katz EZ, Shaag Y, et al: Toxic neonatal effects following maternal clomipramine therapy. J Toxicol Clin Toxicol 29:479–484, 1991

Schnur DB, Mukherjee S, Silver J, et al: Electroconvulsive therapy in the treatment of episodic aggressive dyscontrol in psychotic patients. Convuls Ther 5:353–361, 1989

Schnur DB, Mukherjee S, Sackeim HA, et al: Symptomatic predictors of ECT response in medication-nonresponsive manic patients. J Clin Psychiatry 53:63–66, 1992

Schoenfeld A, Bar Y, Merlob P, et al: NSAIDs: maternal and fetal considerations. Am J Reprod Immunol 28:141–147, 1992

Schwarz T, Loewenstein J, Isenberg KE: Maintenance ECT: indications and outcome. Convuls Ther 11:14–23, 1995

Scott AI: Training and supervision, in Royal College of Psychiatrists: The ECT Handbook. The Second Report of the Royal College of Psychiatrists' Special Committee on ECT. London, England, Royal College of Psychiatrists, 1995, p 94

Scott AI, Riddle W: Status epilepticus after electroconvulsive therapy. Br J Psychiatry 155:119–121, 1989

Scott AI, Weeks DJ, McDonald CF: Continuation electroconvulsive therapy: preliminary guidelines and an illustrative case report. Br J Psychiatry 159:867–870, 1991

Scott AI, Rodger CR, Stocks RH, et al: Is old-fashioned electroconvulsive therapy more efficacious? A randomised comparative study of bilateral brief-pulse and bilateral sine-wave treatments. Br J Psychiatry 160:360–364, 1992

Seager CP, Bird RL: Imipramine with electrical treatment in depression: a controlled trial. Journal of Mental Science 108:704–707, 1962

Sedgwick JV, Lewis IH, Linter SP: Anesthesia and mental illness. Int J Psychiatry Med 20:209–225, 1990

Segman RH, Shapira B, Gorfine M, et al: Onset and time course of antidepressant action: psychopharmacological implications of a controlled trial of electroconvulsive therapy. Psychopharmacology (Berl) 119:440–448, 1995

Shapira B, Zohar J, Newman M, et al: Potentiation of seizure length and clinical response to electroconvulsive therapy by caffeine pretreatment: a case report. Convuls Ther 1:58–60, 1985

Shapira B, Lerer B, Gilboa D, et al: Facilitation of ECT by caffeine pretreatment. Am J Psychiatry 144:1199–1202, 1987

Shapira B, Kindler S, Lerer B: Medication outcome in ECT-resistant depression. Convuls Ther 4: 192–198, 1988

Shapira B, Gorfine M, Lerer B: A prospective study of lithium continuation therapy in depressed patients who have responded to electroconvulsive therapy. Convuls Ther 11:80–85, 1995

Shapira B, Lidsky D, Gorfine M, et al: Electroconvulsive therapy and resistant depression: clinical implications of seizure threshold. J Clin Psychiatry 57:32–38, 1996

Shapira B, Tubi N, Drexler H, et al: Cost and benefit in the choice of ECT schedule. Twice versus three times weekly ECT. Br J Psychiatry 172:44–48, 1998

Shaw IH, McKeith IG: Propofol and electroconvulsive therapy in a patient at risk from acute intermittent porphyria. Br J Anaesth 80:260–262, 1998

Shellenberger W, Miller MJ, Small IF, et al: Follow-up study of memory deficits after ECT. Can J Psychiatry 27:325–329, 1982

Sherer DM, D'Amico ML, Warshal DP, et al: Recurrent mild abruptio placentae occurring immediately after repeated electroconvulsive therapy in pregnancy. Am J Obstet Gynecol 165:652–653, 1991

Shettar SM, Grunhaus L, Pande AC, et al: Protective effects of intramuscular glycopyrrolate on cardiac conduction during ECT. Convuls Ther 5:349–352, 1989

Shnider SM, Levinson G: Anesthesia for Obstetrics, 3rd Edition. Baltimore, MD, Williams & Wilkins, 1993

Shoor M, Adams FH: The intensive electric shock therapy of chronic disturbed psychotic patients. Am J Psychiatry 107:279–282, 1950

Siesjö BK, Ingvar M, Wieloch T: Cellular and molecular events underlying epileptic brain damage. Ann N Y Acad Sci 462:207–223, 1986

Sikdar S, Kulhara P, Avasthi A, et al: Combined chlorpromazine and electroconvulsive therapy in mania. Br J Psychiatry 164:806–810, 1994

Simpson KH, Smith RJ, Davies LF: Comparison of the effects of atropine and glycopyrrolate on cognitive function following general anaesthesia. Br J Anaesth 59:966–969, 1987

Simpson KH, Halsall PJ, Carr CM, et al: Propofol reduces seizure duration in patients having anaesthesia for electroconvulsive therapy. Br J Anaesth 61:343–344, 1988

Sivan AB: Benton Visual Retention Test, 5th Edition. San Antonio, TX, Psychological Corporation, 1992

Small JG: Efficacy of electroconvulsive therapy in schizophrenia, mania, and other disorders, I: schizophrenia. Convuls Ther 1:263–270, 1985

Small JG, Milstein V: Lithium interactions: Lithium and electroconvulsive therapy. J Clin Psychopharm 10:346–350, 1990

Small JG, Kellams JJ, Milstein V, et al: Complications with electroconvulsive treatment combined with lithium. Biol Psychiatry 15:103–112, 1980

Small JG, Milstein V, Small IF, et al: Does ECT produce kindling? Biol Psychiatry 16:773–778, 1981

Small JG, Milstein V, Klapper M, et al: ECT combined with neuroleptics in the treatment of schizophrenia. Psychopharmacol Bull 18:34–35, 1982

Small JG, Klapper MH, Kellams JJ, et al: Electroconvulsive treatment compared with lithium in the management of manic states. Arch Gen Psychiatry 45:727–732, 1988

Small JG, Milstein V, Kellams JJ, et al: Hemispheric components of ECT response in mood disorders and shizophrenia, in The Clinical Science of Electroconvulsive Therapy. Edited by Coffey CE. Washington, DC, American Psychiatric Press, 1993, pp 111–123

Smetana GW: Preoperative pulmonary evaluation. N Engl J Med 340:937–944, 1999

Smith K, Surphlis WR, Gynther MD, et al: ECT-chlorpromazine and chlorpromazine compared in the treatment of schizophrenia. J Nerv Ment Dis 144:284–290, 1967

Smith LH, Hastings DW, Hughes J: Immediate and follow up results of electroshock therapy. Am J Psychiatry 99:351–354, 1943

Snaith RP: How much ECT does the depressed patient need?, in Electroconvulsive Therapy: An Appraisal. Edited by Palmer RL. New York, Oxford University Press, 1981, pp 61–64

Sobin C, Sackeim HA, Prudic J, et al: Predictors of retrograde amnesia following ECT. Am J Psychiatry 152:995–1001, 1995

Sobin C, Prudic J, Devanand DP, et al: Who responds to electroconvulsive therapy? A comparison of effective and ineffective forms of treatment. Br J Psychiatry 169:322–328, 1996

Solomons K, Holliday S, Illing M: Nonconvulsive status epilepticus complicating electroconvulsive therapy. Int J Geriatr Psychiatry 13:731–734, 1998

Sommer BR, Satlin A, Friedman L, et al: Glycopyrrolate versus atropine in post-ECT amnesia in the elderly. J Geriatr Psychiatry Neurol 2:18–21, 1989

Spencer MJ: Fluoxetine hydrochloride (Prozac) toxicity in a neonate. Pediatrics 92:721–722, 1993

Spielvogel A, Wile J: Treatment and outcomes of psychotic patients during pregnancy and childbirth. Birth 19:131–137, 1992

Spiker DG, Weiss JC, Dealy RS, et al: The pharmacological treatment of delusional depression. Am J Psychiatry 142:430–436, 1985

Squire LR: A stable impairment in remote memory following electroconvulsive therapy. Neuropsychologia 13:51–58, 1975

Squire LR: Memory functions as affected by electroconvulsive therapy. Ann N Y Acad Sci 462:307–314, 1986

Squire LR, Chace PM: Memory functions six to nine months after electroconvulsive therapy. Arch Gen Psychiatry 32:1557–1564, 1975

Squire LR, Miller PL: Diminution of anterograde amnesia following electroconvulsive therapy. Br J Psychiatry 125:490–495, 1974

Squire LR, Slater PC: Electroconvulsive therapy and complaints of memory dysfunction: a prospective three-year follow-up study. Br J Psychiatry 142:1–8, 1983

Squire LR, Zouzounis JA: Self-ratings of memory dysfunction: different findings in depression and amnesia. J Clin Exp Neuropsychol 10:727–738, 1988

Squire LR, Slater PC, Chace PM: Retrograde amnesia: temporal gradient in very long term memory following electroconvulsive therapy. Science 187:77–79, 1975

Squire LR, Chace PM, Slater PC: Retrograde amnesia following electroconvulsive therapy. Nature 260:775–777, 1976

Squire LR, Wetzel CD, Slater PC: Memory complaint after electroconvulsive therapy: assessment with a new self–rating instrument. Biol Psychiatry 14:791–801, 1979

Squire LR, Slater PC, Miller PL: Retrograde amnesia and bilateral electroconvulsive therapy. Long-term follow-up. Arch Gen Psychiatry 38:89–95, 1981

Squire L, Cohen N, Zouzounis J: Preserved memory in retrograde amnesia: sparing of a recently acquired skill. Neuropsychologia 22:145–152, 1984

Squire LR, Shimamura AP, Graf P: Independence of recognition memory and priming effects: a neuropsychological analysis. J Exp Psychol (Learn Mem Cogn) 11:37–44, 1985

Stack CG, Abernethy MH, Thacker M: Atracurium for ECT in plasma cholinesterase deficiency. Br J Anaesth 60:244–245, 1988

Standish-Barry HM, Deacon V, Snaith RP: The relationship of concurrent benzodiazepine administration to seizure duration in ECT. Acta Psychiatr Scand 71:269–271, 1985

Stanley WJ, Fleming H: A clinical comparison of phenelzine and electro-convulsive therapy in the treatment of depressive illness. Journal of Mental Science 108:708–710, 1962

Starkstein SE, Migliorelli R: ECT in a patient with a frontal craniotomy and residual meningioma. J Neuropsychiatry Clin Neurosci 5:428–430, 1993

Steffens DC, Krystal AD, Sibert TE, et al: Cost effectiveness of maintenance ECT (letter). Convuls Ther 11:283–284, 1995

Steif BL, Sackeim HA, Portnoy S, et al: Effects of depression and ECT on anterograde memory. Biol Psychiatry 21:921–930, 1986

Stephens SM, Pettinati HM, Greenberg RM, et al: Continuation and maintenance therapy with outpatient ECT, in The Clinical Science of Electroconvulsive Therapy. Edited by Coffey CE. Washington, DC, American Psychiatric Press, 1993, pp 143–164

Stern MB: Electroconvulsive therapy in untreated Parkinson's disease. Mov Disord 6:265, 1991

Stern RA, Nevels CT, Shelhorse ME, et al: Antidepressant and memory effects of combined thyroid hormone treatment and electroconvulsive therapy: preliminary findings. Biol Psychiatry 30:623–627, 1991

Sternberg DE, Jarvik ME: Memory function in depression: improvement with antidepressant medication. Arch Gen Psychiatry 33:219–224, 1976

Stiebel VG: Maintenance electroconvulsive therapy for chronic mentally ill patients: a case series. Psychiatr Serv 46:265–268, 1995

Stieper DR, Williams M, Duncan CP: Changes in impersonal and personal memory following electroconvulsive therapy. J Clin Psychol 7:361–366, 1951

Stoudemire A, Knos G, Gladson M, et al: Labetalol in the control of cardiovascular responses to electroconvulsive therapy in high-risk depressed medical patients. J Clin Psychiatry 51:508–512, 1990

Stoudemire A, Hill CD, Dalton ST, et al: Rehospitalization rates in older depressed adults after antidepressant and electroconvulsive therapy treatment. J Am Geriatr Soc 42:1282–1285, 1994

Strain JJ, Bidder TG: Transient cerebral complication associated with multiple monitored electroconvulsive therapy. Diseases of the Nervous System 32:95–100, 1971

Strain JJ, Brunschwig L, Duffy JP, et al: Comparison of therapeutic effects and memory changes with bilateral and unilateral ECT. Am J Psychiatry 125:50–60, 1968

Strober M, Rao U, DeAntonio M, et al: Effects of electroconvulsive therapy in adolescents with severe endogenous depression resistant to pharmacotherapy. Biol Psychiatry 43:335–338, 1998

Strömgren LS: Unilateral versus bilateral electroconvulsive therapy: investigations into the therapeutic effect in endogenous depression. Acta Psychiatr Scand Suppl 240:8–65, 1973

Strömgren LS: Therapeutic results in brief-interval unilateral ECT. Acta Psychiatr Scand 52:246–255, 1975

Strömgren LS: Is bilateral ECT ever indicated? Acta Psychiatr Scand 69:484–490, 1984

Strömgren LS: Electroconvulsive therapy in Aarhus, Denmark, in 1984: its application in nondepressive disorders. Convuls Ther 4:306–313, 1988

Strömgren LS: ECT in acute delirium and related clinical states. Convuls Ther 13:10–17, 1997

Strömgren LS, Juul-Jensen P: EEG in unilateral and bilateral electroconvulsive therapy. Acta Psychiatr Scand 51:340–360, 1975

Strömgren LS, Dahl J, Fjeldborg N, et al: Factors influencing seizure duration and number of seizures applied in unilateral electroconvulsive therapy: anaesthetics and benzodiazepines. Acta Psychiatr Scand 62:158–165, 1980

Summers WK, Robins E, Reich T: The natural history of acute organic mental syndrome after bilateral electroconvulsive therapy. Biol Psychiatry 14:905–912, 1979

Suppes T, Webb A, Carmody T, et al: Is postictal electrical silence a predictor of response to electroconvulsive therapy? J Affect Disord 41:55–58, 1996

Swan HD, Borshoff DC: Informed consent: recall of risk information following epidural analgesia in labour. Anaesth Intensive Care 22:139–141, 1994

Swartz CM: Electroconvulsive therapy emergence agitation and succinylcholine dose. J Nerv Ment Dis 178:455–457, 1990

Swartz CM: Propofol anesthesia in ECT. Convuls Ther 8:262–266, 1992

Swartz CM: ECT emergence agitation and methohexital-succinylcholine interaction: case report. Gen Hosp Psychiatry 15:339–341, 1993

Swartz CM: Asymmetric bilateral right frontotemporal left frontal stimulus electrode placement for electroconvulsive therapy. Neuropsychobiology 29:174–178, 1994

Swartz CM, Larson G: ECT stimulus duration and its efficacy. Ann Clin Psychiatry 1:147–152, 1989

Swartz CM, Lewis RK: Theophylline reversal of electroconvulsive therapy (ECT) seizure inhibition. Psychosomatics 32:47–51, 1991

Swartz CM, Saheba NC: Comparison of atropine with glycopyrrolate for use in ECT. Convuls Ther 5:56–60, 1989

Swindells SR, Simpson KH: Oxygen saturation during electroconvulsive therapy. Br J Psychiatry 150:695–697, 1987

Szenohradszky J, Caldwell JE, Wright PM, et al: Influence of renal failure on the pharmacokinetics and neuromuscular effects of a single dose of rapacuronium bromide. Anesthesiology 90:24–35, 1999

Szuba MP, Guze BH, Liston EH, et al: Psychiatry resident and medical student perspectives on ECT: influence of exposure and education. Convuls Ther 8:110–117, 1992

Tassorelli C, Joseph SA, Buzzi MG, et al: The effects on the central nervous system of nitroglycerin: putative mechanisms and mediators. Prog Neurobiol 57:607–624, 1999

Taub S: Electroconvulsive therapy, malpractice, and informed consent. Journal of Psychiatry and Law 15:7–54, 1987

Taylor MA, Abrams R: Catatonia: prevalence and importance in the manic phase of manic-depressive illness. Arch Gen Psychiatry 34:1223–1225, 1977

Taylor MA, Abrams R: Short-term cognitive effects of unilateral and bilateral ECT. Br J Psychiatry 146:308–311, 1985

Taylor P, Fleminger JJ: ECT for schizophrenia. Lancet 1:1380–1382, 1980

Tenenbaum J: ECT regulation reconsidered. Medical Disability Law Reporter 7:148–159, 211, 1983

Tew JD Jr, Mulsant BH, Haskett RF, et al: Acute efficacy of ECT in the treatment of major depression in the old-old. Am J Psychiatry 156:1865–1870, 1999

Thase ME, Rush AJ: Treatment-resistant depression, in Psychopharmacology: The Fourth Generation of Progress. Edited by Bloom F, Kupfer D. New York, Raven, 1995, pp 1081–1098

Thienhaus OJ, Margletta S, Bennett JA: A study of the clinical efficacy of maintenance ECT. J Clin Psychiatr 51:141–144, 1990

Thomas J, Reddy B: The treatment of mania: a retrospective evaluation of the effects of ECT, chlorpromazine, and lithium. J Affect Disord 4:85–92, 1982

Thompson D, Hylan TR, McMullen W, et al: Predictors of a medical-offset effect among patients receiving antidepressant therapy. Am J Psychiatry 155:824–827, 1998

Thompson JW, Blaine JD: Use of ECT in the United States in 1975 and 1980. Am J Psychiatry 144:557–562, 1987

Thompson JW, Weiner RD, Myers CP: Use of ECT in the United States in 1975, 1980, and 1986. Am J Psychiatry 151:1657–1661, 1994

Thornton JE, Mulsant BH, Dealy R, et al: A retrospective study of maintenance electroconvulsive therapy in a university-based psychiatric practice. Convuls Ther 6:121–129, 1990

Thorogood M, Cowen P, Mann J, et al: Fatal myocardial infarction and use of psychotropic drugs in young women. Lancet 340:1067–1068, 1992

Tomac TA, Rummans TA, Pileggi TS, et al: Safety and efficacy of electroconvulsive therapy in patients over age 85. Am J Geriatr Psychiatry 5:126–130, 1997

Treiman DM, Meyers PD, Walton NY, et al: A comparison of four treatments for generalized convulsive status epilepticus. Veterans Affairs Status Epilepticus Cooperative Study Group. N Engl J Med 339:792–798, 1998

Trollor JN, Sachdev PS: Electroconvulsive treatment of neuroleptic malignant syndrome: a review and report of cases. Aust N Z J Psychiatry 33:650–659, 1999

Trzepacz PT, Weniger FC, Greenhouse J: Etomidate anesthesia increases seizure duration during ECT. A retrospective study. Gen Hosp Psychiatry 15:115–120, 1993

Tsuang MT, Dempsey GM, Fleming JA: Can ECT prevent premature death and suicide in "schizoaffective" patients? J Affect Disord 1:167–171, 1979

Tsui BC, Reid S, Gupta S, et al: A rapid precurarization technique using rocuronium. Can J Anaesth 45:397–401, 1998

Tubi N, Calev A, Higal D, et al: Subjective symptoms in depression and during the course of electroconvulsive therapy. Neuropsychiatry Neuropsychol Behav Neurol 6:187–192, 1993

Üçok A, Üçok G: Maintenance ECT in a patient with catatonic schizophrenia and tardive dyskinesia. Convuls Ther 12:108–112, 1996

Ulett GA, Gleser GC, Caldwell BM, et al: The use of matched groups in the evaluation of convulsive and subconvulsive photoshock. Bull Menninger Clin 18:138–146, 1954

Ulett GA, Smith K, Gleser G: Evaluation of convulsive and subconvulsive shock therapies utilizing a control group. Am J Psychiatry 112:795–802, 1956

Ungvári G, Pethö B: High-dose haloperidol therapy: its effectiveness and a comparison with electroconvulsive therapy. Journal of Psychiatric Treatment and Evaluation 4:279–283, 1982

Unsworth J, d'Assis-Fonseca A, Beswick DT, et al: Serum salicylate levels in a breast fed infant. Ann Rheum Dis 46:638–639, 1987

Valentine M, Keddie KM, Dunne D: A comparison of techniques in electroconvulsive therapy. Br J Psychiatry 114:989–996, 1968

Valentine SJ, Marjot R, Monk CR: Preoxygenation in the elderly: a comparison of the four-maximal-breath and three-minute techniques. Anesth Analg 71L:516–519, 1990

Van Den Berg AA, Honjol NM: Electroconvulsive therapy and intraocular pressure. Middle East J Anesthesiol 14:249–258, 1998

Vanelle JM, Loo H, Galinowski A, et al: Maintenance ECT in intractable manic-depressive disorders. Convuls Ther 10:195–205, 1994

Viby-Mogensen J, Hanel H: Prolonged apnea after suxamethonium. Acta Anaesth Scand 22:371–380, 1978

Viguera A, Rordorf G, Schouten R, et al: Intracranial haemodynamics during attenuated responses to electroconvulsive therapy in the presence of an intracerebral aneurysm. J Neurol Neurosurg Psychiatry 64:802–805, 1998

Villalonga A, Bernardo M, Gomar C, et al: Cardiovascular response and anesthetic recovery in electroconvulsive therapy with propofol or thiopental. Convuls Ther 9:108–111, 1993

Wainwright AP, Broderick PM: Suxamethonium in myasthenia gravis. Anaesthesia 42:950–957, 1987

Walker MC: The epidemiology and management of status epilepticus. Curr Opin Neurol 11:149–54, 1998

Walker R, Swartz CM: Electroconvulsive therapy during high-risk pregnancy. Gen Hosp Psychiatry 16:348–353, 1994

Walter G, Rey JM: An epidemiological study of the use of ECT in adolescents. J Am Acad Child Adolesc Psychiatry 36:809–815, 1997

Walter G, Rey JM, Starling J: Experience, knowledge, and attitudes of child psychiatrists regarding electroconvulsive therapy in the young. Aust N Z J Psychiatry 31:676–681, 1997

Walter G, Koster K, Rey JM: Electroconvulsive therapy in adolescents: experience, knowledge, and attitudes of recipients. J Am Acad child Adolesc Psychiatry 38:594–599, 1999a

Walter G, Rey JM, Mitchell PB: Practitioner review: electroconvulsive therapy in adolescents. J Child Psychol Psychiatry 40:325–334, 1999b

Walter-Ryan WG: ECT regulation and the two-tiered care system. Am J Psychiatry 142:661–662, 1985

Warmflash VL, Stricks L, Sackeim HA, et al: Reliability and validity of measures of seizure duration. Convuls Ther 3:18–25, 1987

Warner MA, Shields SE, Chute CG: Major morbidity and mortality within 1 month of ambulatory surgery and anesthesia. JAMA 270:1437–1441, 1993

Watt DC, Katz K, Shepherd M: The natural history of schizophrenia: a 5 year prospective follow-up of a representative sample of schizophrenics by means of a standardized clinical and social assessment. Psychol Med 13:663–670, 1983

Watterson D: The effect of age, head resistance and other physical factors of the stimulus threshold of electrically induced convulsions. J Neurol Neurosurg Psychiatry 8:121–125, 1945

Webb MC, Coffey CE, Saunders WR, et al: Cardiovascular response to unilateral electroconvulsive therapy. Biol Psychiatry 28:758–766, 1990

Wechsler D: Wechsler Memory Scale, 3rd Edition. San Antonio, TX, Psychological Corporation, 1997

Weeks D, Freeman CP, Kendell RE: ECT, III: enduring cognitive deficits? Br J Psychiatry 137:26–37, 1980

Weiner RD: The psychiatric use of electrically induced seizures. Am J Psychiatry 136:1507–1517, 1979

Weiner RD: ECT and seizure threshold: effects of stimulus wave form and electrode placement. Biol Psychiatry 15:225–241, 1980

Weiner RD: Does ECT cause brain damage? Behav Brain Sci 7:1–53, 1984

Weiner RD, Coffey CE: Use of electroconvulsive therapy in patients with severe medical illness, in Treatment of Psychiatric Disorders in Medical-Surgical Patients. Edited by Stoudemire A, Fogel B. New York, Grune & Stratton, 1987, pp 113–134

Weiner RD, Coffey CE: Indications for use of electroconvulsive therapy, in Review of Psychiatry, Volume 7. Edited by Frances A, Hales R. Washington, DC, American Psychiatric Press, 1988, pp 458–481

Weiner RD, McCall WV: Dental examination for ECT. Convuls Ther 8:146–147, 1992

Weiner RD, Krystal AD: EEG monitoring of ECT seizures, in The Clinical Science of Electroconvulsive Therapy. Edited by Coffey CE. Washington, DC, American Psychiatric Press, 1993, pp 93–109

Weiner RD, Sibert TD: Use of ECT in treatment of depression in patients with diabetes mellitus. J Clin Psychiatry 57:3, 1996

Weiner RD, Volow MR, Gianturco DT, et al: Seizures terminable and interminable with ECT. Am J Psychiatry 137:1416–1418, 1980a

Weiner RD, Whanger AD, Erwin CW, et al: Prolonged confusional state and EEG seizure activity following concurrent ECT and lithium use. Am J Psychiatry 137:1452–1453, 1980b

Weiner RD, Rogers HJ, Davidson JR, et al: Effects of electroconvulsive therapy upon brain electrical activity. Ann N Y Acad Sci 462:270–281, 1986a

Weiner RD, Rogers HJ, Davidson JR, et al: Effects of stimulus parameters on cognitive side effects. Ann N Y Acad Sci 462:315–325, 1986b

Weiner RD, Weaver LA, Sackeim HA: Reporting of technical parameters in ECT publications: recommendations for authors. Convuls Ther 4:88–91, 1987

Weiner RD, Coffey CE, Krystal AD: The monitoring and management of electrically induced seizures. Psychiatr Clin North Am 14:845–869, 1991

Weiner RD, Coffey CE, Krystal AD: Electroconvulsive therapy in the medical and neurologic patient, in Psychiatric Care of the Medical Patient, 2nd Edition. Edited by Stoudemire A, Fogel BS, Grenberg D. New York, Oxford University Press, 2000, pp 419–428

Weiner SJ, Ward TN, Ravaris CL: Headache and electroconvulsive therapy. Headache 34:155–159, 1994

Weingartner H, Silberman E: Cognitive changes in depression, in Neurobiology of Mood Disorders. Edited by Post RM, Ballenger JC. Baltimore, MD, Williams & Wilkins, 1984, pp 121–135

Weinger MB, Partridge BL, Hauger R, et al: Prevention of the cardiovascular and neuroendocrine response to electroconvulsive therapy, I: effectiveness of pretreatment regimens on hemodynamics. Anesth Analg 73:556–562, 1991

Weinstein R: Migraine occurring as sequela of electroconvulsive therapy. Headache 33:45, 1993

Weisberg LA, Elliott D, Mielke D: Intracerebral hemorrhage following electroconvulsive therapy. Neurology 41:1849, 1991

Welch CA: ECT in medically ill patients, in The Clinical Science of Electroconvulsive Therapy. Edited by Coffey CE. Washington, DC, American Psychiatric Press, 1993, pp 167–182

Welch C, Drop L: Cardiovascular effects of ECT. Convuls Ther 5:35–43, 1989

Weller M, Kornhuber J: Electroconvulsive therapy in a geriatric patient with multiple bone fractures and generalized plasmocytoma. Pharmacopsychiatry 25:278–280, 1992

Wells DA: Electroconvulsive treatment for schizophrenia: a ten-year survey in a university hospital psychiatric department. Compr Psychiatry 14:291–298, 1973

Wells DG, Bjorkstein AR: Monoamine oxidase inhibitors revisited. Can J Anaesth 36:64–74, 1989

Wells DG, Davies GG, Rosewarne F: Attenuation of electroconvulsive therapy induced hypertension with sublingual nifedipine. Anaesth Intensive Care 17:31–33, 1989

Wengel SP, Burke WJ, Pfeiffer RF, et al: Maintenance electroconvulsive therapy for intractable Parkinson's disease. Am J Geriatr Psychiatr 6:263–269, 1998

Wesner RB, Winokur G: The influence of age on the natural history of unipolar depression when treated with electroconvulsive therapy. European Archives of Psychiatry and Neurological Sciences 238:149–154, 1989

Wessels WH: A comparative study of the efficacy of bilateral and unilateral electroconvulsive therapy with thioridazine in acute schizophrenia. S Afr Med J 46:890–892, 1972

West ED: Electric convulsion therapy in depression: a double-blind controlled trial. BMJ 282:355–357, 1981

Westreich L, Levine S, Ginsburg P, et al: Patient knowledge about electroconvulsive therapy: effect of an informational video. Convuls Ther 11:32–37, 1995

Wettstein RM, Roth LH: The psychiatrist as legal guardian. Am J Psychiatry 145:600–604, 1988

Wijeratne C, Shome S: Electroconvulsive therapy and subdural hemorrhage. J ECT 15:275–279, 1999

Williams K, Smith J, Glue P, et al: The effects of electroconvulsive therapy on plasma insulin and glucose in depression. Br J Psychiatry 161:94–98, 1992

Willoughby CL, Hradek EA, Richards NR: Use of electroconvulsive therapy with children: an overview and case report. J Child Adolesc Psychiatr Nurs 10:11–17, 1997

Wilson IC, Vernon JT, Guin T, et al: A controlled study of treatments of depression. Journal of Neuropsychiatry 4:331–337, 1963

Wilson WC, Benumof JL: Pathophysiology, evaluation, and treatment of the difficult airway. Anesthesiol Clin North Am 16: 29–75, 1998

Wingard LB, Cook DR: Clinical pharmacokinetics of muscle relaxants. Clin Pharmacokinet 2:330–343, 1977

Wingate BJ, Hansen-Flaschen J: Anxiety and depression in advanced lung disease. Clin Chest Med 18:495–505, 1997

Winslade WJ: Electroconvulsive therapy: legal regulations, ethical concerns, in Review of Psychiatry, Vol 7. Edited by Frances AJ, Hales RE. Washington, DC, American Psychiatric Press, 1988, pp 513–525

Winslade WJ, Liston EH, Ross JW, et al: Medical, judicial, and statutory regulation of ECT in the United States. Am J Psychiatry 141:1349–1355, 1984

Wise MG, Ward SC, Townsend-Parchman W, et al: Case report of ECT during high-risk pregnancy. Am J Psychiatry 141:99–101, 1984

Wisner KL, Perel JM: Psychopharmacologic agents and electroconvulsive therapy during pregnancy and the puerperium, in Psychiatric Consultation in Childbirth Settings: Parent and Child-Oriented Approaches. Edited by Cohn REL. New York, Plenum, 1988, pp 165–206

Wittman P: A scale for measuring prognosis in schizophrenic patients. Elgin Papers 4:20–33, 1941

Wolfersdorf M, Barg T, Konig F, et al: Paroxetine as antidepressant in combined antidepressant-neuroleptic therapy in delusional depression: observation of clinical use. Pharmacopsychiatry 28:56–60, 1995

Wolff GE: Electric shock treatment. Am J Psychiatry 111:748–750, 1955

Woodbury LA, Davenport VD: Design and use of a new electroshock seizure apparatus, and analysis of factors altering seizure threshold and pattern. Archives Internationales de Pharmacodynamie et de Therapie 92:97–107, 1952

Working Group on Status Epilepticus: Treatment of convulsive status epilepticus: recommendations of the Epilepsy Foundation of America's Working Group on Status Epilepticus. JAMA 270:854–859, 1993

World Health Organization: Schizophrenia: An International Follow-up Study. New York, Wiley, 1979

Wrede G, Mednick SA, Huttunen MO, et al: Pregnancy and delivery complications in the births of an unselected series of Finnish children with schizophrenic mothers. Acta Psychiatr Scand 62:369–381, 1980

Wyant GM, MacDonald WB: The role of atropine in electroconvulsive therapy. Anaesth Intensive Care 8:445–450, 1980

Wyatt RJ: Neuroleptics and the natural course of schizophrenia. Schizophr Bull 17:325–351, 1991

Wyatt RJ: Early intervention for schizophrenia: can the course of the illness be altered? Biol Psychiatry 38:1–3, 1995

Yager J, Borus JF, Robinowitz CB, et al: Developing minimal national standards for clinical experience in psychiatric training. Am J Psychiatry 145:1409–1413, 1988

Yassa R, Hoffman H, Canakis M: The effect of electroconvulsive therapy on tardive dyskinesia: a prospective study. Convuls Ther 6:194–198, 1990

Yesavage JA, Brink TL, Rose TL, et al: Development and validation of a geriatric depression screening scale: a preliminary report. J Psychiatr Res 17:37–49, 1982–1983

Yoshida K, Smith B, Kumar R: Psychotropic drugs in mothers' milk. J Psychopharmacol 13:64–80, 1999

Young RC, Biggs JT, Ziegler VE, et al: A rating scale for mania: reliability, validity and sensitivity. Br J Psychiatry 133:429–435, 1978

Zakzanis KK, Leach L, Kaplan E: On the nature and pattern of neurocognitive function in major depressive disorder. Neuropsychiatry Neuropsychol Behav Neurol 11:111–119, 1998

Zeifert M: Results obtained from the administration of 12,000 doses of metrazol to mental patients. Psychiatr Q 15:772–778, 1941

Zervas IM, Fink M: ECT for refractory Parkinson's disease (letter). Convuls Ther 7:222–223, 1991

Zervas IM, Fink M: ECT and delirium in Parkinson's disease. Am J Psychiatry 149:1758, 1992

Zervas IM, Jandorf L: The Randt Memory Test in electroconvulsive therapy: relation to illness and treatment parameters. Convuls Ther 9:28–38, 1993

Zervas IM, Calev A, Jandorf L, et al: Age-dependent effects of electroconvulsive therapy on memory. Convuls Ther 9:39–42, 1993

Zielinski RJ, Roose SP, Devanand DP, et al: Cardiovascular complications of ECT in depressed patients with cardiac disease. Am J Psychiatry 150:904–909, 1993

Zimmerman M, Coryell W, Pfohl B: The treatment validity of DSM-III melancholic subtyping. Psychiatry Res 16:37–43, 1985

Zimmerman M, Coryell W, Pfohl B, et al: ECT response in depressed patients with and without a DSM-III personality disorder. Am J Psychiatry 143:1030–1032, 1986a

Zimmerman M, Coryell W, Stangl D, et al: An American validation study of the Newcastle scale, III: course during index hospitalization and six-month prospective follow-up. Acta Psychiatr Scand 73:412–415, 1986b

Zimmerman M, Coryell W, Pfohl B, et al: What happens when ECT does not work? A prospective follow-up study of ECT failures. Ann Clin Psychiatry 2:47–51, 1990

Zis AP: Acute administration of fluoxetine and the duration of electrically induced seizures. Convuls Ther 8:38–53, 1992

Zis AP, McGarvey KA, Clark CM, et al: Effect of stimulus energy on electroconvulsive therapy-induced prolactin release. Convuls Ther 9:23–27, 1993

Zorumski CF, Rutherford JL, Burke WJ, et al: ECT in primary and secondary depression. J Clin Psychiatry 47:298–300, 1986

Zwil AS, Pelchat RJ: ECT in the treatment of patients with neurological and somatic disease. Int J Psychiatry Med 24:1–29, 1994

Zwil AS, Bowring MA, Price TRP, et al: Prospective electroconvulsive therapy in the presence of intracranial tumor. Convuls Ther 6:299–307, 1990

Zwil AS, McAllister TW, Price TR: Safety and efficacy of ECT in depressed patients with organic brain disease: review of a clinical experience. Convuls Ther 8:103–109, 1992

APPENDIX A

Individuals and Groups Providing Input to the Document Revision Process

To ensure that these practice recommendations were as accurate and comprehensive as possible, the American Psychiatric Association (APA) Committee on Electroconvulsive Therapy solicited and encouraged input from relevant groups both inside and outside the APA. The initial draft of the revision was distributed to approximately 500 individuals and groups. Among these were academic experts and practitioners in relevant areas of psychiatry, anesthesiology, cardiology, nursing, and psychology. Device manufacturers were given the opportunity to comment, as were regulatory organizations such as the Joint Commission on Accreditation of Health Care Organizations, the U.S. Food and Drug Administration, and governmental agencies such as the National Institute of Mental Health and the Veterans Administration. In addition, professional and scientific societies with an interest in ECT were asked to provide formal comments. Finally, major lay organizations representing consumers and their families were also provided with the opportunity to review and comment on the guidelines.

Within the APA component structure, the initial draft was shared with representatives focusing on problems of children, aging, law, governmental relations, public affairs, and education. In addition, it was made available to members of the Assembly of District Branches, and all drafts were reviewed in total by members of the Committee on Research on Psychiatric Treatments, the Council on Research, the Joint Reference Committee, and finally by members of the Board of Trustees.

Below is a listing of organizations followed by a listing of individuals who actually provided input into this document. Other individuals and groups were provided with the opportunity to comment but did not do so.

Representatives of the following organizations provided input into these guidelines:

• American Association of Directors of Psychiatric Residency Training
• American College of Neuropsychopharmacology
• American Geriatrics Society
• American Society of Anesthesiologists
• Association for Academic Psychiatry
• Association for Convulsive Therapy
• Black Psychiatrists of America
• Department of Veterans Affairs
• MECTA Corporation
• National Institute of Mental Health
• Somatics, Inc.

Specific reviewers providing comments:

Richard Abrams, M.D.
Hagop S. Akiskal, M.D.
Robert J. Applegate, M.D.
James F. Arens, M.D.
Samuel H. Bailine, M.D.
Richard Balon, M.D.
Mark Beale, M.D.
Carl C. Bell, M.D.
Jules R. Bemporad, M.D.
Henry Bibr, M.D., F.R.C.P.
Donald Black, M.D.
Dan G. Blazer, M.D.
Luc Bourgon, M.D.
Walter A. Brown, M.D.
Michael Burke, M.D.
Carol M. Burns, M.S.N., R.N., C.S.
Avi Calev, Ph.D.
Marc Cantillon, M.D.
Worrawat Chanpattana, M.D.
Eric Christopher, M.D.
Bruce Cohen, M.D.
Raymond Crowe, M.D.
Ramona Davis, M.D.
Karon Dawkins, M.D.

Himasin De Silva, M.D.
D.P. Devanand, M.D.
Roberto A. Dominguez, M.D.
Anne Donahue
Steven Lew Dubovsky, M.D.
David L. Dunner, M.D.
Norman S. Endler, Ph.D.
Randall Espinoza, M.D.
Raymond Faber, M.D.
Max Fink, M.D.
Herbert Fox, M.D.
Fred Frankel, M.B.Ch.B., D.P.M.
B. N. Ganadhar, M.D.
Enrique S. Garza-Trevino, M.D.
John C. Gillin, M.D.
Frank Guerra, M.D., F.A.P.A.,
    F.A.C.A.
Grace Gunderson-Falcone,
    R.N., M.S.N., A./G.N.P., F.N.P.
Roger F. Haskett, M.D.
Donald P. Hay, M.D.
Mustafa Husain, M.D.
Vaclav Hyrman, M.D.
Richard L. Jaffe, M.D.

James W. Jefferson, M.D.
Russell T. Joffe, M.D., F.R.C.P.(C).
Gordon F. Johnson, M.D.
Barry Kramer, M.D.
Stephen Kramer, M.D.
Ranga Krishnan, M.D.
Andrew D. Krystal, M.D., M.S.
Laurent Lehmann, M.D.
Stuart Levy, D.O.
Steven Lippmann, M.D.
Bill Lyndon, M.D.
Leslie F. Major, M.D.
Barry Maletzky, M.D.
Sidney Malitz, M.D.
Laurel Malson
Barry A. Martin, M.D.
John McAllister, M.D.
Frances McCafferty, M.D.
W. Vaughn McCall, M.D.
William McDonald, M.D.
Herbert Y. Meltzer, M.D.
Jeffrey Metzner, M.D.
Laura J. Miller, M.D.
Thomas M. Milroy, M.D.
Philip Mitchell, M.D.
Timothy S. Mitzel, M.D.
Jose C. Montes, M.D.
Scott Moore, M.D., Ph.D.
Benoit H. Mulsant, M.D.
John I. Nurnberger Jr., M.D., Ph.D.
Herbert Pardes, M.D.
Chester Pearlman, M.D.

Marquerite Poreda, M.D.
Fred Quitkin, M.D.
Lewis Ray, M.D.
David Reiss, M.D.
Michelle Riba, M.D.
Richard Ries, M.D.
Steven Roose, M.D.
Raymond Roy, M.D.
Matt Rudorfer, M.D.
Teresa Rummans, M.D.
Carl Salzman, M.D.
Diane Schetky, M.D.
David B. Schnur, M.D.
Steven S. Sharfstein, M.D.
Iver F. Small, M.D.
Joyce G. Small, M.D.
David Solomon, M.D.
Deborah Spitz, M.D.
Jagannathan Srinivasaraghavan, M.D.
David Steffens, M.D.
Nada Stotland, M.D.
Stephen Strakowski, M.D.
Lizzie Sand Stromgren, M.D.
Mark Teitelbaum, M.D., PhD
James Thompson, M.D.
Paula Trzepacz, M.D.
Gary J. Tucker, M.D.
Leon Wanerman, M.D.
Tim Webb, M.D., Ph.D.
Thomas N. Wise, M.D.
Sidney Zisook, M.D.
Charles F. Zorumski, M.D.

APPENDIX B

Sample ECT Consent and Patient Information Documents

1. Consent Form: Acute Phase

2. Consent Form: Continuation/Maintenance ECT

3. Patient Information Sheet

Note: These are sample documents and, if used in a particular clinical setting, should be modified to be consistent with local policies, procedures, and requirements.

Electroconvulsive Therapy (ECT) Consent Form: Acute Phase

Name of Patient: _____

My doctor, _____, has recommended that I receive treatment with electroconvulsive therapy (ECT). This treatment, including the risks and benefits that I may experience, has been fully described to me. I give my consent to be treated with ECT.

Whether ECT or an alternative treatment, like medication or psychotherapy, is most appropriate for me depends on my prior experience with these treatments, the features of my illness, and other considerations. Why ECT has been recommended for me has been explained.

ECT involves a series of treatments that may be given on an inpatient or outpatient basis. To receive each treatment I will come to a specially equipped area in this facility. The treatments are usually given in the morning. Because the treatments involve general anesthesia, I will have had nothing to eat or drink for several hours before each treatment. Before the treatment, a small needle will be placed in my vein so that I can be given medications. An anesthetic medication will be injected that will quickly put me to sleep. I will then be given another medication that will relax my muscles. Because I will be asleep, I will not experience pain or discomfort or remember the procedure. Other medications may also be given depending on my needs.

To prepare for the treatment, monitoring sensors will be placed on my head and body. Blood pressure cuffs will be placed on an arm and leg. This monitoring involves no pain or discomfort. After I am asleep, a carefully controlled amount of electricity will be passed between two electrodes that have been placed on my head.

I may receive bilateral ECT or unilateral ECT. In bilateral ECT, one electrode is placed on the left side of the head, the other on the right side. In unilateral ECT, both electrodes are placed on the same side of the head, usually the right side. Right unilateral ECT (electrodes on the right side) is likely to produce less memory difficulty than bilateral ECT. However, for some patients bilateral ECT may be a more effective treatment. My doctor will carefully consider the choice of unilateral or bilateral ECT.

The electrical current produces a seizure in the brain. The amount of electricity used to produce the seizure will be adjusted to my individual needs, based on the judgment of the ECT physician. The medication used to relax my muscles will greatly soften the contractions in my body that would ordinarily accompany the seizure. I will be given oxygen to breathe. The seizure will last for approximately 1 minute. During the procedure, my heart, blood pressure, and brain waves will be monitored. Within a few minutes, the anesthetic medications will wear off and I will awaken. I will then be observed until it is time to leave the ECT area.

The number of treatments that I will receive cannot be known ahead of time. A typical course of ECT is 6 to 12 treatments, but some patients may need fewer and some may need more. Treatments are usually given three times a week, but the frequency of treatment may also vary depending on my needs. If I need more than _____ treatments, my written consent will be reobtained.

ECT is expected to improve my illness. However, I understand that I may recover completely, partially, or not at all. After ECT, my symptoms may return. How long I will remain well cannot be known ahead of time. To make the return of symptoms less likely after ECT, I will need additional treatment with medication, psychotherapy, and/or ECT. The treatment I will receive to prevent the return of symptoms will be discussed with me.

Like other medical treatments, ECT has risks and side effects. To reduce the risk of complications, I will receive a medical evaluation before starting ECT. The medications I have been taking may be adjusted. However, in spite of precautions, it is possible that I will experience a medical complication. As with any procedure using general anesthesia, there is a remote possibility of death from ECT. The risk of death from ECT is very low, about 1 in 10,000 patients. This rate may be higher in patients with severe medical conditions.

ECT very rarely results in serious medical complications, such as heart attack, stroke, respiratory difficulty, or continuous seizure. More often, ECT results in irregularities in heart rate and rhythm. These irregularities are usually mild and short lasting but in rare instances can be life threatening. With modern ECT technique, dental complications are infrequent and bone fractures or dislocations are very rare.

If serious side effects occur, I understand that medical care and treatment will be instituted immediately and that facilities to handle emergencies are available. I understand, however, that neither the institution nor the treating physicians are required to provide long-term medical treatment. I shall be responsible for the cost of such treatment whether personally or through medical insurance or other medical coverage. I understand that no compensation will be paid for lost wages or other consequential damages.

The minor side effects that are frequent include headache, muscle soreness, and nausea. These side effects usually respond to simple treatment.

When I awaken after each treatment, I may be confused. This confusion usually goes away within 1 hour. During the treatment course I may have new difficulties in attention and concentration and other aspects of thinking. These problems rapidly go away after completion of ECT.

I understand that memory loss is a common side effect of ECT. The memory loss with ECT has a characteristic pattern, including problems remembering past events and new information. The degree of memory problems is often related to the number and type of treatments given. A smaller number of treatments is likely to produce less memory difficulty than a larger number. Shortly following a treatment, the problems with memory are greatest. As time from treatment increases, memory improves.

I may experience difficulties remembering events that happened before and while I received ECT. The spottiness in my memory for past events may extend back to several months before I received ECT, and, less commonly, for longer periods of time, sometimes several years or more. Although many of these memories should return during the first few months following my ECT course, I may be left with some permanent gaps in memory.

For a short period following ECT, I may also experience difficulty in remembering new information. This difficulty in forming new memories should be temporary and typically disappears within several weeks following the ECT course.

The majority of patients state that the benefits of ECT outweigh the problems with memory. Furthermore, most patients report that their memory is actually improved after ECT. Nonetheless, a minority of patients report problems in memory that remain for months or even years. The reasons for these reported long-lasting impairments are not fully understood. As with any medical treatment, people who receive ECT differ considerably in the extent to which they experience side effects.

Because of the possible problems with confusion and memory, I should not make any important personal or business decisions during or immediately after the ECT course. During and shortly after the ECT course, and until discussed with my doctor, I should refrain from driving, transacting business, or other activities for which memory difficulties may be troublesome.

The conduct of ECT at this facility is under the direction of Dr. _____. I may contact him/her at _____ if I have further questions.

I am free to ask my doctor or members of the ECT treatment team questions about ECT at this time or at any time during or following the ECT course. My decision to agree to ECT is being made voluntarily, and I may withdraw my consent for further treatment at any time.

I have been given a copy of this consent form to keep.

_____   _____
Signature   Date

Person Obtaining Consent:

_____   _____
Name   Signature

Electroconvulsive Therapy (ECT) Consent Form: Continuation/Maintenance Treatment

Name of Patient: _____

My doctor, _____, has recommended that I receive continuation or maintenance treatment with electroconvulsive therapy (ECT). This treatment, including the risks and benefits that I may experience, has been fully described to me. I give my consent to be treated with this type of ECT.

I will receive ECT to prevent return of my illness. Whether ECT or an alternative treatment, like medication or psychotherapy, is most appropriate for me at this time depends on my prior experience with these treatments in preventing the return of symptoms, the features of my illness, and other considerations. Why continuation/maintenance ECT has been recommended for me has been explained.

Continuation/maintenance ECT involves a series of treatments with each usually separated in time by 1 or more weeks. Continuation/ maintenance ECT is usually given for a period of several months or longer. These treatments may be given on an inpatient or outpatient basis.

To receive each continuation/maintenance treatment I will come to a specially equipped area in this facility. The treatments are usually given in the morning. Because the treatments involve general anesthesia, I will have had nothing to eat or drink for several hours before each treatment. Before the treatment, a small needle will be placed in my vein so that I can be given medications. An anesthetic medication will be injected that will quickly put me to sleep. I will then be given another medication that will relax my muscles. Because I will be asleep, I will not experience pain or discomfort or remember the procedure. Other medications may also be given depending on my needs.

To prepare for the treatment, monitoring sensors will be placed on my head and body. Blood pressure cuffs will be placed on an arm and leg. This monitoring involves no pain or discomfort. After I am asleep, a carefully controlled amount of electricity will be passed between two electrodes that have been placed on my head.

I may receive bilateral ECT or unilateral ECT. In bilateral ECT, one electrode is placed on the left side of the head, the other on the right side. In unilateral ECT, both electrodes are placed on the same side of the head, usually the right side. Right unilateral ECT (electrodes on the right side) is likely to produce less memory difficulty than bilateral ECT. However, for some patients bilateral ECT may be a more effective treatment. My doctor will carefully consider the choice of unilateral or bilateral ECT.

The electrical current produces a seizure in the brain. The amount of electricity used to produce the seizure will be adjusted to my individual needs, based on the judgment of the ECT physician. The medication used to relax my muscles will greatly soften the contractions in my body that would ordinarily accompany the seizure. I will be given oxygen to breathe. The seizure will last for approximately 1 minute. During the procedure, my heart, blood pressure, and brain waves will be monitored. Within a few minutes, the anesthetic medications will wear off and I will awaken. I will then be observed until it is time to leave the ECT area.

The number of continuation/maintenance treatments that I will receive will depend on my clinical course. Continuation ECT is usually given for at least 6 months. If it is felt that continuation ECT is helpful and should be used for a longer period (maintenance ECT), I will be asked to consent to the procedure again.

ECT is expected to prevent the return of my psychiatric condition. Although for most patients ECT is effective in this way, I understand that this cannot be guaranteed. With continuation/maintenance ECT I may remain considerably improved or I may have a partial or complete return of psychiatric symptoms.

Like other medical treatments, ECT has risks and side effects. To reduce the risk of complications, I will receive a medical evaluation before starting ECT. The medications I have been taking may be adjusted. However, in spite of precautions, it is possible that I will experience a medical complication. As with any procedure using general anesthesia, there is a remote possibility of death from ECT. The risk of death from ECT is very low, about one in 10,000 patients. This rate may be higher in patients with severe medical conditions.

ECT very rarely results in serious medical complications, such as heart attack, stroke, respiratory difficulty, or continuous seizure. More often, ECT results in irregularities in heart rate and rhythm. These irregularities are usually mild and short lasting, but in rare instances can be life threatening. With modern ECT technique, dental complications are infrequent and bone fractures or dislocations are very rare.

If serious side effects occur, I understand that medical care and treatment will be instituted immediately and that facilities to handle emergencies are available. I understand, however, that neither the institution nor the treating physicians are required to provide long-term medical treatment. I shall be responsible for the cost of such treatment whether personally or through medical insurance or other medical coverage. I understand that no compensation will be paid for lost wages or other consequential damages.

The minor side effects that are frequent include headache, muscle soreness, and nausea. These side effects usually respond to simple treatment.

When I awaken after each treatment, I may be confused. This confusion usually goes away within 1 hour.

I understand that memory loss is a common side effect of ECT. The memory loss with ECT has a characteristic pattern, including problems remembering past events and new information. The degree of memory problems is often related to the number and type of treatments given. A smaller number of treatments is likely to produce less memory difficulty than a larger number. Shortly following a treatment, the problems with memory are greatest. As time from treatment increases, memory improves.

I may experience difficulties remembering events that happened before and while I received ECT. The spottiness in my memory for past events may extend back to several months before I received ECT, and, less commonly, for longer periods of time, sometimes several years or more. Although many of these memories should return during the first few months following continuation/maintenance ECT, I may be left with some permanent gaps in memory.

For a short period following each treatment, I may also experience difficulty in remembering new information. This difficulty in forming new memories should be temporary and will most likely disappear following completion of continuation/maintenance ECT.

The effects of continuation/maintenance ECT on memory are likely to be less pronounced than those during an acute ECT course. By spreading treatments out in time, with an interval of a week or more between treatments, there should be substantial recovery of memory between each treatment.

Because of the possible problems with confusion and memory, it is important that I not drive or make any important personal or business decisions the day that I receive a continuation/maintenance treatment. Limitations on my activities may be longer depending on the side effects I experience following each treatment and will be discussed with my doctor.

The conduct of ECT at this facility is under the direction of Dr. _____. I may contact him/her at _____ if I have further questions.

I am free to ask my doctor or members of the ECT treatment team questions about ECT at this time or at any time during or following the ECT course. My decision to agree to continuation/maintenance ECT is being made voluntarily, and I may withdraw my consent for future treatment at any time.

I have been given a copy of this consent form to keep.

_____   _____
Signature   Date

Person Obtaining Consent:

_____   _____
Name   Signature

Sample Patient Information Booklet

Electroconvulsive Therapy

What is Electroconvulsive Therapy?

Electroconvulsive therapy (ECT; called "shock treatment" by some) is an extremely safe and effective medical treatment for certain psychiatric disorders. With this treatment, a small amount of electricity is applied to the scalp and this produces a seizure in the brain. The procedure is painless because the patient is asleep under general anesthesia.

Who is Treated with ECT?

ECT has been used for over 60 years. In the United States, about 100,000 individuals are estimated to receive ECT each year. ECT is most commonly given when patients have severe depressive illness, mania, or some forms of schizophrenia. Frequently, ECT is given when patients have not responded to other treatments, when other treatments appear to be less safe or difficult to tolerate, when patients have responded well to ECT in the past, or when psychiatric or medical considerations make it particularly important that patients recover quickly and fully.

Not all patients improve when treated with medications or psychotherapy (talk therapy). Indeed, when illnesses such as depression become particularly severe, it is doubtful that psychotherapy alone will be sufficient. For some patients, the medical risks of medications may be greater than the medical risks of ECT. Typically, these are people with serious medical problems, such as certain types of heart disease. When patients have life-threatening psychiatric problems, such as suicidal tendencies, ECT is also often recommended because it usually provides faster relief than medications. Overall, the great majority of depressed patients treated with ECT show substantial improvement. Even the majority of those who have not been helped by medications respond to ECT. This makes ECT the most effective of the antidepressant treatments.

Who Administers ECT?

A treatment team administers ECT. The team consists of a psychiatrist, an anesthesiologist, and nurses. The physicians responsible for administering ECT are experienced specialists. ECT is administered in a dedicated suite at the ___(name of facility)___. The suite contains a waiting area, a treatment room, and a recovery room.

How is ECT Given?

Before ECT is administered, the patient's medical condition is carefully assessed. This includes a medical history, physical examination, and medical tests as needed. The treatments are usually given three times per week in the morning on Monday, Wednesday, and Friday. Before each treatment, the patient should not eat or drink anything for several hours. Patients should also try to refrain from smoking during the morning prior to the treatment.

When the patient comes to the ECT treatment room, an intravenous line is started. Sensors for recording EEG (electroencephalogram, a measure of brain activity) are placed on the head. Other sensors are placed on the chest for monitoring ECG (electrocardiogram). A cuff is wrapped around an arm for monitoring blood pressure. When everything is connected and in order, an anesthetic medication (methohexital) is injected through the intravenous line that will cause the patient to sleep for 5 to 10 minutes. Once the patient falls asleep, a muscle relaxing medication (succinylcholine) is injected. This prevents movement, and during the seizure there are only minimal contractions of the muscles.

When the patient is completely asleep and the muscles are well relaxed, the treatment is given. A brief electrical charge is applied to electrodes on the scalp. This stimulates the brain and produces the seizure, which lasts for about 1 minute. Throughout the procedure, the patient receives oxygen through a mask. This continues until the patient resumes breathing on his or her own. When the treatment is completed, the patient is taken to a recovery area for monitoring by trained staff. Usually within 30 to 60 minutes, the patient can leave the recovery area.

How Many Treatments are Needed?

ECT is given as a course of treatments. The total number needed to successfully treat psychiatric disturbance varies from patient to patient. For depression, the typical range is from 6 to 12 treatments, but some patients may require fewer and some patients may require more treatments.

Is ECT Curative?

ECT is extremely effective in providing relief from psychiatric symptoms. However, permanent cures for psychiatric illness are rare, regardless of the treatment given. To prevent relapse after ECT, most patients require further treatment with medications or with ECT. If ECT is used to protect against relapse, it is usually administered to outpatients on a weekly to monthly basis.

How Safe is ECT?

It is estimated that death associated with ECT occurs in 1 of 10,000 patients. This rate may be higher in patients with severe medical conditions. ECT appears to have less risk of death or serious medical complications than a number of the medications used to treat psychiatric conditions. Because of this strong safety record, ECT is often recommended to treat mental disorders in patients with serious medical conditions. With modern anesthesia, fractures and dental complications are very rare.

What Are the Common Side Effects of ECT?

The patient will experience some confusion on awakening following the treatment. This is partly due to the anesthesia and partly due to the treatment. The confusion typically clears within 1 hour. Some patients have headaches following the treatment. This usually improves with pain relievers, such as Tylenol (acetaminophen) or aspirin. Other side effects, such as nausea, last for a few hours at most and are relatively uncommon. In patients with heart disease, the risk of cardiac complications is increased. Cardiac monitoring and other precautions, including the use of additional medications if required, help to ensure a safe treatment.

The side effect of ECT that has received the most attention is memory loss. ECT results in two types of memory loss. The first involves rapid forgetting of new information. For example, shortly after the treatment, patients may have difficulty remembering conversations or things they have recently read. This type of memory loss is short-lived and has not been shown to last for more than a few weeks after the completion of ECT. The second type of memory loss concerns events from the past. Some patients will have gaps in their memory for events that occurred in the weeks to months and, less commonly, years before the treatment course. This memory problem also improves after the completion of ECT. However, permanent gaps in memory may exist for some events, particularly those that occurred close in time to the treatment. As with any treatment, patients differ in the extent to which they experience side effects, and more extensive memory loss has been reported. It is known that the effects on memory are not necessary to obtain the benefits of ECT.

Many psychiatric illnesses result in impairments of attention and concentration. Consequently, when the psychiatric disturbance improves after ECT, improvement in these aspects of thinking often occurs. Shortly after ECT, most patients show improved scores on tests of intelligence, attention, and learning.

Does ECT Cause Brain Damage?

The scientific evidence strongly speaks against this possibility. Careful studies in animals have shown no evidence of brain damage from brief seizures such as those given with ECT. In the adult, seizures must continue for hours before brain damage can occur, yet the ECT seizure lasts only about 1 minute. Brain scans after ECT have shown no injury to the brain. During ECT, the amount of electricity that reaches the brain is too small to cause electrical injury.

How Does ECT Work?

Like many other treatments in medicine, the exact process that underlies the effectiveness of ECT is uncertain. It is known that the benefits of ECT depend on producing a seizure in the brain and on technical factors in how the seizure is produced. Biologic changes that result from the seizure are critical to effectiveness. Most investigators believe that specific changes in brain chemistry produced by ECT are the key to restoring normal function. Considerable research is being conducted to isolate the critical biochemical processes.

Is ECT Frightening?

ECT has often been portrayed in the movies and on television as a painful procedure used to control or punish patients. These portrayals have no resemblance to modern ECT. One survey found that after ECT most patients reported that it was no worse than going to the dentist, and many found ECT less stressful. Other research has shown that that the vast majority of patients report that, if needed, they would receive ECT again.

Where Can I Find First-Person Accounts of ECT?

ECT is an extremely effective form of treatment. It is often safer and more effective than medications or no treatment at all. If you have any questions about ECT, please discuss them with your physician. You may also wish to read *Holiday of Darkness* by Norman S. Endler (Revised Edition, Toronto, Canada, Wall & Thompson, 1990) and/or *Undercurrents: A Therapist's Reckoning With Depression* by Martha Manning (San Francisco, CA, Harper, 1995). Both books were written by psychologists who were against people having ECT until they experienced severe depression themselves and needed ECT treatment. Drs. Endler and Manning describe their illness, their experience in treatment with medication and psychotherapy, and their experience with ECT.

Index

*Page numbers printed in **boldface** type refer to tables or figures.*